Back to Balance

Back to Balance

A Holistic Self-Help Guide to Eastern Remedies

By Dylana Accolla with Peter Yates, L. Ac.

KODANSHA INTERNATIONAL
Tokyo • New York • London

Distributed in the United States by Kodansha America, Inc., 114 Fifth Avenue, New York, N.Y. 10011, and in the United Kingdom and continental Europe by Kodansha Europe Ltd., 95 Aldwych, London WC2B 4JF. Published by Kodansha International Ltd., 17-14 Otowa 1-chome, Bunkyo-ku, Tokyo 112, and Kodansha America, Inc.

First edition, 1996.
96 97 98 10 9 8 7 6 5 4 3 2 1

ISBN 4-7700-1923-8

Library of Congress Cataloging-in-Publication Data

Accolla, Dylana, 1963–
        Back to balance: a holistic self-help guide to Eastern remedies /
    Dylana Accolla, with Peter Yates: illustrations by Lisa Miller.
            p. cm.
        Includes bibliographical references and index.
        ISBN 4-7700-1923-8
        1. Self-care, Health. 2. Medicine, Oriental. I. Yates, Peter,
    1951– . II. Title.
    RA776. 95. A25 1996
    613'. 095—dc20
95-40330
CIP

In memory of:
Donald Michael Lembitz
1933-1976
D.A.

To My Mother and Father
P.Y.

CONTENTS

Part II: Self-Care

11

Acknowledgments

To everyone who helped and supported my efforts along the way:

Diane Lembitz, my mother, and Heather Moden Jones, for her clarity and lessons on style and tone, and David Jones for the writer's garret. To all the editors who made up the editing "dream team:" Meagan Calogeras, our editor at Kodansha, who has supported my work through many life changes; Meg Seaker, our copy editor, whose caring hand chiseled this project into a bona fide book; Oriental medical practitioners and our medical editors, Jacqueline Young and Anne Harper Kubota; to Lisa Dale Miller, for her inspired illustrations and unshakable belief in our ability to graphically depict Qi. To Nigel Dawes, for his invaluable contributions and suggestions. I would also like to thank our editors, Ethne Ashizawa, formerly of the *Mainichi Daily News*, and Fukushima Kazuhiko and the *Asahi Evening News* staff, for their support of our health columns. Thanks also to photographer and friend Richard White; and to Solid Grounds Cafe in Buffalo, New York, for prolonged use of their wall socket. To Hatanaka Nobusuke, for his *joie de vivre* and for bravely taste-testing my Japanese cooking and many of the recipes in this book; to Hua Guo Luo; Dearbhaile Bradley; Takeuchi Nobuyuki and Wakabayashi Akihiko of the Akahigedo clinic in Yoyogi, Tokyo; to Tokyo yoginis: Rajay Mahtani, whose fax made this international project possible and whose yoga instruction changed my life; Liane Grunberg, for her writing support; Michal Mugrage for her magic; and Barbara Seymour, my kung fu sister. To soul brothers: Andy Boerger, David Brickler (our valued go-between), and Yukio Fujimi. To Paolino Accolla, for holding my hand through the hardest times. To Scott, Amy, and Laurie Lembitz, for loving me and accepting me back home. And finally, to Roland Legiardi-Laura.

D.A.

To my teachers, students, patients past and present, Nigel Dawes, Jackie Young, and all at Kodansha International—a big thanks.

P.Y.

FOREWORD

To translate the Oriental concept of balance into the context of Western civilisation and appeal to the Western mind is a tremendous challenge. It involves resisting the temptation of over simplifying key Oriental concepts and keeping faith with the essence of the Oriental approach stressing health maintenance and disease prevention. This differs sharply from the Western medical model in which germ theory dictates that the presence of pathological microorganisms identifies the disease process. The World Health Organisation has defined health as "the absence of disease" while illness is associated with the activity of invasive pathogenic agents. The role of the medicine is to relieve suffering by removing the influence of such agents, by aggressive means if necessary. The role of the physician is to actively provide such relief and that of the patient to tolerate both illness and treatment.

Oriental medicine, like any medical tradition, is also aimed at relieving suffering. Yet health is perceived in a complex and subtle manner, not based on the notion of the elimination of disease but rather emphasising health maintenance. It requires more than the skills of the physician and tolerance of the patient to effect a cure. It is a system based on re-activating the body's own, innate powers of self-healing, something which demands active and committed collaboration between practitioner and client. The one making skilled technical decisions about treatment strategies and offering support and guidance, the other being willing and open to change both lifestyle and psychological, emotional and physical patterns of behaviour. This process involves getting to know the patient deeply, not just discovering the pathogenic agent.

The opening line of this book is "You heal yourself," and Dylana Accolla is careful to emphasise the importance of both the "body's innate intelligence" and the patient/ practitioner collaborative relationship in this process of self-healing. In doing so, the book clearly identifies itself in the self-help genre but with a notable difference. It is a bold attempt to convey the essence of the healing process; how to learn what it takes to influence one's own healing potential and when to trust the professional skills of another. It is careful to avoid giving prescriptive "to do" lists while concentrating on conveying a very real sense of what it takes in "action, practice and consistency" to activate self-healing as well as when to listen to our bodies and seek professional help. This book offers no quick fixes and instead highlights the effort and commitment that true healing demands and defines the responsibilities of both client and practitioner in their collaborative relationship.

The text mixes the vitality of a personal story with well-informed facts, observations and advice. This in part comes from the unique relationship of the author with Peter Yates, the principal medical advisor who became her healer and teacher. Though the book is not only a personal testimonial, the author's own experience lends appeal and a powerful sense of authenticity to the subject matter. The reader is constantly invited to share, not only in the practical results and effects of various treatments but also in the entire healing experience. Added to this very personal tone, there is the constant sense that the range and power of the Oriental healing tradition is being fully explored through Peter Yates' profound skills and knowledge. The information in the book is a clear reflection of the depth and understanding he has acquired from both his own training and from varied clinical experience. The book is divided so that more than half is devoted to a comprehensive self-care section including healing approaches with both standard, folk and personally concocted internal and external applications. But there is also an intelligent and fascinating first section offering a mixture of classical knowledge and practical explanations of topics such as the Oriental concept of balance (a key to appreciating the book), the role of diet and exercise in healthcare and the different Oriental treatment modalities. Peter displays his deep appreciation of the philosophical origins of the medicine by including chapters on seasonal balance, pain and vitality and even on choosing a practitioner, all significant elements in the Taoist principle of harmonising Yin and Yang.

The ultimate message of the book asserts that balance is a natural state and like the seasons cannot be rushed or contrived; that health and disease, vitality and pain are both two sides of the same coin and that finding "your way" and "your doctor" is perhaps the most significant factor in the healing process. This is a book you can use both to gain quick, practical, safe and effective advice for treating many common complaints and also one to be read and re-read in depth to absorb and appreciate the full potential of the Oriental healing tradition as experienced and practiced by one of its more gifted, Western exponents. Peter and I are long time friends and colleagues, having begun our acupuncture studies together in Tokyo in the early 1980s. His continued commitment to the study of Oriental healing and martial arts both in China and Japan, where he still lives, leads me to believe that he is one of the very few Westerners to have really mastered these complex disciplines. I respect him and his work immensely and believe this book conveys the depth and originality as well as the purity of his knowledge and understanding both of the Oriental mind and of its healing tradition.

NIGEL DAWES
Director, Department of Herbology, New Center for Holistic Health, Education and Research
August 1995 New York

Introduction

You heal yourself. This is the basic premise of this book. You and nature heal you. Whatever illness you come down with, whatever medicine you take for it, whatever modality of medicine you choose, and whichever doctor you see, the bottom line is that your body does the work. Your mind can join in with the effort, play a passive role in the process, take a victim stance, or sabotage healing.

Back to Balance has been written to provide lay readers with tools to help them return to their individual states of balance: the state at which the body is capable of adapting appropriately to challenges, instead of buckling under or losing stability. Illness is a challenge your body issues to prompt changes in your life that will get you back to a state of relative balance from where your body can function at its best. It is an opportunity to shift gears, figure out a way to become more comfortable, change perspectives, reflect on your values, and uncover negative systems of belief that increase stress and discomfort.

Redirecting those belief systems promotes health, as obstacles that block the flow of energy during metabolism are removed. Sitting quietly and reevaluating and questioning our lives puts us in contact with the body's innate intelligence. That intelligence not only regulates our body's internal workings but holds inner knowledge of our disorders and of the ways in which we can nurse ourselves back to health. Schools of traditional and folk medicine in China, Japan, India, and Western Europe have always depended on (and still do) this intelligence to bring about healing.

Back to Balance has been written with the intent to guide readers to becoming in tune with that intelligence through Traditional Chinese Medicine concepts, herbs, massage, and folk wisdom that has existed for thousands of years in the Far East. It is also a guide to becoming your practitioner's partner in a team bent on improving your condition and the quality of your life. With your support, your doctor is bound to do a better job. With a capable and trustworthy practitioner, you are likely to feel good about the treatment you are receiving. We believe this partnership is going to become a recognized aspect of medical care and that people will come to expect medical treatment that is a collaborative effort between doctors and themselves.

In China, the patient/doctor relationship is venerated in the Confucian scheme of the universe as one of the most important types of relationships in society. As such, it represents a type of spiritual connection—*yuan* (pronounced "yoon") in Chinese or *en* in Japanese. The patient/doctor *yuan* that Peter and I have has had a profound effect on our lives. Peter, the doctor in this relationship, has guided me toward self-reliance in my healing process and schooled me in preventative maintenance. I, in turn, became so excited about these lessons in healing that I felt the impetus to share his knowledge and experience with others. Thus began our writing collaborations, which have carried on for several years, culminating with *Back to Balance*.

Peter, a native of Lancashire, England, has 15 years of experience in Oriental medicine. He is a graduate of the East-West Center of Oriental Medicine in Australia, the International Institute of Oriental Medicine in Japan, and the Guangzhou College of Traditional Chinese Medicine in China. He has also studied with several important teacher-practitioners in Japan, including Todō Yuki. Peter is a dedicated martial artist, holding a second-degree black belt in Goju Ryu karate and a first-degree black belt in Kempo karate, and has studied a number of body/mind practices in addition to karate, including Oki yoga, qigong, tai'chi, and Chen, Hsing Yi, and Hun-gar styles of kung fu. Master Share Lew and Master Luo Hua Guo are two martial arts teachers who have influenced Peter's practice and work. Currently he teaches acupuncture and qigong in Tokyo, where he also runs a thriving medical practice and regularly gives lectures and workshops on healing, relaxation, and martial arts.

I first went to see Peter for acupuncture seven years ago, while I was a student of Japanese and a beginning journalist in Tokyo, for a nine-year case of chronic amenorrhea, compounded by an eating disorder and addictions to cigarettes, coffee, and alcohol. My initial course of treatment with him lasted about half a year, during which time he taught me many of the basic healing and stress management techniques we include in the book: meditation, visualization, and simple deep-breathing exercises. He brought the issue of diet into focus in a gentle, non-threatening way, and under his tutelage, with the support of a Twelve-Step program, a therapist, and my soon-to-be husband, I began to learn how to eat again.

After six months of weekly treatments my menstrual cycle appeared in fits and starts, but Peter felt there was nothing more he could do for me; we agreed to stop the treatments. At that point I took responsibility for my own healing and began an exploration of various modalities of healing and mind-body unification: qigong, yoga, and meditation. I worked with herbs, chakras, shamans, Qi healers, and Buddhist priests, and explored tai'chi, art, journaling, magic, and myths. I visited half-a-dozen clinics and hospitals in the Tokyo area for acupuncture, shiatsu, and herbal medicine for varying periods of time and became familiar with the different styles and techniques of medicine practiced in those places. The eating disorder and addictions disappeared, but the menstrual problems continued, remaining the proverbial thorn in the side that kept me seeking other therapies and philosophies.

The menstrual problem eventually turned into a healing crisis when a particularly long and painful case of PMS brought me back to Peter for help. We used meditation and acupuncture to work with the pain, and the treatment shifted the energy in my body dramatically, causing a release of my blood-engorged uterus.

Hemorrhage and surgery resulted, and the doctors also found two large ovarian cysts that they said would require surgical removal. I felt as if my entire reproductive system were slowly but surely breaking down. In despair, I turned to Western allopathy for hormonal treatment and set a future date for the surgical removal of the cysts.

Before the second surgery took place, two synchronistic events came into play whose results rendered surgery unnecessary: Peter introduced me and three of his other women qigong students to his kung fu master, Dr. Luo Hua Guo, in China; and an Irish counselor, Dearbhaile Bradley, called me after hearing of my story the day she arrived in Tokyo. Dearbhaile practices what she calls "metaphor work," which she describes as a combination of Neurolinguistic Programming ideas with psychosynthesis and Gestalt approaches. She takes the metaphors people use to describe their illness or imbalance, expands, and develops that through the "information-rich way they store their feelings." Dearbhaile taught me how to dialogue with the energy of illness in my body and put me in touch with the deep pain I felt about being a woman. We worked with the Sumerian myth of Erishkigal and Inanna as part of our "descent" into my illness.

A few weeks later, I traveled with three other Western women to China to study kung fu with Sifu (Master) Luo. He spoke little English, but we communicated about my illness by writing in Chinese and Japanese. He assured me that Chinese medicine could heal my cysts, advised me to go off the hormones, and gave me a series of qigong exercises and meditation to practice. I trusted his judgment completely. My fellow students and I were drilled daily in qigong, tai'chi, and kung fu, and walked and bicycled often. Our diet consisted of fresh vegetables, soup, meat, large quantities of organ meat, eggs, occasional herbs, rice, and Chinese tea. He never restricted our diets in any way, and indulged in an evening beer and peanuts with us, but I went off caffeine and sugar on my own.

My health immediately improved, the color returned to my complexion, and within ten days the anemia was clearly arrested, leaving me feeling full of energy and vitality. I had a strange, painful experience with meditation about a week after starting the regimen that forced me to acknowledge the suffering Erishkigal inside me. This vision ended in a physical sensation of burning energy shooting upward from my lower abdomen. Several days later, Sifu Luo brought me to a Chinese hospital to have the cysts checked, and they had disappeared. I went on to have a healthy menstrual cycle, which continues except during times of intense stress. My cycle has become an effective "stress barometer," telling me when I am overextended by not appearing.

The experience of being sick was terrifying and the struggle to become healthy long and arduous. There were many times when I doubted I could ever stop starving myself or binging and purging, that emotions would ever stabilize to allow me to work and earn a living again, that I would ever menstruate regularly without pain, breast distention, and worry and depression. Breast and uterine cancer runs in my family, but my experiences in Asia, and with Oriental medicine in particular, have given me tools to confront the deeply ingrained belief that I, too, would die of it. Instead, I am building a new, more positive set of beliefs about my health.

In the years since going to China that first time, besides working full-time as a journalist for the daily *Asahi Evening News*, I have gone on to teach qigong, meditation, and to practice body work and massage in Tokyo. I also work in an informal way as a support for women with eating disorders, and am beginning training in Oriental medicine.

This book is meant to provide beginners on the search for health with a system of support, to help them carry out healing and transformation in their own lives. Rather than glibly pronouncing "If I can do it, you can, too," Peter and I want to communicate our shared experience of healing and being healed and provide the tools and methods we have used effectively in the process. Please do not feel intimidated by the amount of seeking and experimenting I did to heal myself; much of that fit into my journalism work. Moderate reading and close work with a practitioner are likely to be just as helpful.

Peter is the main font of medical knowledge in the text. The first eight chapters are based on the material he uses to teach his acupuncture courses and on our discussions over the years of issues basic to self-healing. The Self-Care sections are composed of Peter's suggestions based on his clinical experience and traditional Japanese folk remedies, some recommended by Japanese acupuncturists, others compiled from printed collections of folk remedies, which I have personally translated—mainly from Gakken's *Kanpō Jitsuyō Jiten*, *Shizen Ryōhō* by Tojō Yuriko, *Yoku Kiku Kampō to Minkan Ryōhō* by Yamanouchi Shinichi, *Oishiku Naosō* by Marumoto Yoshio, *Yasōcha de Utsukushiku Kenko ni Naru Hō* by Morishita Keiichi and Satō Narusei, and *Yakutō* by Ōumi Jun. Nigel Dawes, a British-born Oriental medicine practitioner who trained in Japan and China and is now the director of the New Center for Holistic Health's Herbology Department in Long Island, New York, generously lent his expertise with invaluable contributions to the "Adapting and Building the Immune System" and "Fatigue" sections in Part II. For the energetic properties of food, I have relied principally on Bob Flaws and Honora Wolfe's *Prince Wen Hui's Cook*, supported by Henry Lu's *Chinese System of Food Cures*, while information on tonic herbs comes from Bensky and Gamble's *Chinese Herbal Medicine Materia Medica*, Ron Teegarden's *Chinese Tonic Herbs*, and Michael Tierra's *Planetary Herbology*.

We could have made an encyclopedic presentation of syndromes and remedies, for example, listing all of the energetic and nutritional properties of the foods that are included in the self-care sections. While this information is useful, it can also become a trap: our intellects get stuck in too much information. Self-healing requires action, practice, and consistency—actually preparing and applying a remedy provides a lot more healing impetus than almost any amount of reading.

Oriental medicine can be used to cure or aid the healing of almost every imbalance and illness. According to Dr. Felix Mann, an early practitioner and researcher in the efficacy of Oriental medicine, diseases and conditions that may be treated with acupuncture include headache, the early stages of cerebral arteriosclerosis, and neuralgia; problems with the limbs and muscles, such as sciatica and rheumatoid arthritis or osteoarthritis; almost any digestive disorder, and many others. A more complete list has been included in the Appendix.[1]

Acupuncture works in conjunction with diet, exercise, rest, herbs, and physical manipulation to stimulate energy deeply and bring about the conditions that allow the body to rebalance itself, but it is not 100 percent effective for all illnesses in all people. Certainly it is useful for more than its analgesic abilities, and particularly in these days of increased interest in preventative medicine, it warrants much more research.

Although we are firm proponents of the Oriental view of health, we respect Western allopathic medicine's ability to deal with emergencies faster and more effectively than organic medicine, which does not rely on sophisticated machines and the intervention of chemical drugs. The two do not have to contradict one another; they can be used together in a meaningful way. A broken leg can be reset and placed in a cast at the hospital, but an Oriental practitioner would say that this treatment does not restore the full flow of Qi running through a broken bone, torn muscle, and ligaments. In this case acupuncture and acupressure can augment incomplete allopathic therapy to result in a more thorough healing.

This type of complementary action can be applied to many types of illness, particularly chronic illness, and immune, endocrine, and nervous system disorders. Lay people and members of the medical establishment are beginning to gradually accept the term "complementary medicine" in acknowledgement of the fact that the two forms of medicine can exist side by side.[2]

A plurality of complementary therapies is rapidly becoming available, and we applaud this opening in Western cultures. The more choice a patient has, the higher the chance that she or he will find a therapy that works. It is also important that practitioners remain open to recommending another type of therapy if it seems appropriate for the client. Not all therapies are right for all people. Fasting, for example, could severely weaken someone with a dysfunctional digestive system, while this person could reap real benefit from a therapy that strengthened the entire body. *Back to Balance* is meant to help readers determine their body types and appropriate treatment for imbalance, according to the principles of Oriental medicine. Serious and long-term chronic illness should be brought to the attention of a professional.

Finally, Peter and I are as much explorers on this road to healing as you, the reader, are. As we follow our paths, discovering and observing the function and movement of Qi (vital energy) through martial arts, medicine, and meditation, we have seen this energy interact with the body's intelligence in countless ways. It has brought me healing and has allowed Peter to facilitate spectacular recoveries. We hardly propose to know the ins and outs of the Tao's mysteries, but we would like to share some of what we have learned in the hope that we can serve as helpful signs along the road in your search for health and balance.

Life, at best, is a rich compendium of experience, full of growth. Adopting this point of view moves you far beyond simplistic expectations of a happy, beautiful life. A life that is satisfying and "perfect" is so with all its blemishes intact.

The ancient Taoists sought longevity with an attitude of practicality toward the body and purpose toward the soul. The longer they lived, they reasoned, the closer they could come to finding wisdom and reaching the highest state of being.

May you live long and discover your wisdom.

Endnotes

[1] Although the World Health Organization has assembled a list of over a hundred conditions that experts agree are treatable by acupuncture/herbs, the authors feel WHO's list is limited in scope, since it places emphasis on Oriental medicine's analgesic effects.

[2] Americans are turning to alternative therapies *en masse*, as statistics from the January 28, 1993, *New England Journal of Health* demonstrate. In 1990, one out of three Americans was using alternative therapies and spending $10.3 billion for it (compare this to $12.8 billion spent out of pocket for conventional hospital treatment the same year). *Science* magazine reported in May, 1994, that an estimated 90 million acupuncture treatments are given annually in the United States, a figure that is rising "exponentially," according to Joseph Helms, president of the American Academy of Medical Acupuncture. Alternative medicine is becoming recognized by academia—witness the creation of Columbia University's *Journal of Alternative and Complementary Medicine*. On a national level, the Department of Education recognizes acupuncture education and has formed the National Accreditation Commission for Schools and Colleges of Acupuncture and Oriental Medicine (NACSCAOM), which recognizes schools in several states, making them eligible for federal tuition aid. Regulatory standards have been established by the National Commission for Certification of Acupuncturists (NCCA), and 23 states and the District of Columbia have legislated laws requiring that students pass a competency exam before certifying them as acupuncturists. In addition to the legal and academic recognition of Oriental medicine, health insurance—Mutual of Omaha, Blue Cross and Blue Shield of Washington and Alaska, and Medicaid programs—is beginning to cover acupuncture under certain conditions.

How to Use this Book

Back to Balance is meant to be a guide for the layperson seeking to under-stand illness and health in terms of the energetics of Oriental medicine. It is a prac-tical handbook to be used to bring a body suffering from slight disorders, chronic conditions, or acute, non-life-threatening illnesses back into balance. The book can be used by itself or, for deeper, more serious chronic conditions, as an adjunct to professional help.

The individual remedies in *Back to Balance* are by no means cure-alls. They can, and should, be used in combination with one another; when appropriate, con-traindications are listed. Not every remedy will work for every person. Some will attract you, others may repel you. Choose what sounds appealing; the efficacy of self-help remedies depends on your intuition, on your willingness to follow the nat-ural intelligence of your body. Sometimes choosing a remedy is a question of prac-ticality. Often people opt for the simplest healing method; readers who are genuinely curious about traditional healing in the Far East, and committed to get-ting well using natural means, will find the more complicated formulas, recipes, and other recommendations calling for less familiar ingredients from both the folk and the Chinese medicinal traditions, extremely beneficial.

One important point to remember is that the remedies will take longer to work than an over-the-counter allopathic drug. Natural methods harmonize with the rhythms of the body and allow it to heal in its own time. If you are sick, it's proba-bly because you have allowed yourself to be run-down, and, more than a palliative or something to squelch the symptoms, what you really need is rest and nourish-ment. A person living a fast-paced life tends to find a rest-and-nourishment approach impossibly exasperating. We understand. Of this person we ask an extra measure of patience and respect for the body, which is not a machine. If you find yourself thinking of illness as a cog out of line that hinders your productivity, be aware of that pattern of thinking. It is probably the most health-undermining atti-tude pervading Western society.

If you have a serious health condition or a systemic disorder—diabetes, AIDS, any kind of lump or tumorous growth, arthritis—we assume you are already under the care of a qualified practitioner. You may want to discuss self-help mea-sures with him or her, using this book's nutrition and immune chapters as a springboard for the development of your own health program. Oriental medicine is truly an art form, and the remedies included here are far more effective if used in conjunction with the guidance of a professional.

Read the beginning sections of *Back to Balance* all the way through to famil-iarize yourself with the theory of the meridians and organs, the energetics of food and tonic herbs, and the diagnostic terms used in Oriental medicine. We considered eliminating the specialized terminology completely, discussing illness only in Western terms readers would readily recognize, but ultimately we felt this would not contribute to a true understanding of the principles of Oriental medicine on any level. The modality is still rather new to this country, and unfortunately, it does not translate literally into Western thought and patterns of logic. Just as a good literary translation demands interpretation from the translator, so have we tried to interpret to heighten understanding. The fact is that Oriental medicine is stubborn; if you want to understand it, be prepared to make room for it on its own terms.

You may feel a degree of frustration at first. You may want more correspondences with Western medicine. You may feel that there *has* to be an acceptable Western way of expressing a certain idea. Sometimes there is. Often there is not. If it helps, think of the energetic descriptions as metaphors for your condition. In this way you can visualize and work with an imbalance on the mental level. The mind is a powerful ally in healing, and Oriental medicine facilitates the mind's cooperation.

Once you have become familiar with the concept of energetics, you can refer to the Self-Care sections in Part II whenever you need to. They include common patterns that cause each imbalance as it is diagnosed according to Oriental medicine and then go on to define treatment goals. Please remember that these patterns are general and reflect only part of the imbalance in your own body. In actuality, other influences and symptoms complicate the situation, sometimes to the point that the description seems to have nothing in common with your pattern of symptoms. If that is the case, don't dismiss Oriental medicine as a possibility for healing. See a practitioner for individual diagnosis and treatment. Techniques for proper Oriental medicine diagnosis, such as tongue and phlegm diagnoses and pulse reading, have not been included. These tools and medicines are best left in the physician's black bag, practiced by a trained practitioner with the expertise to administer them wisely.

A Note on Capitalization and Terminology:

Words that represent Oriental medicine energetics appear capitalized in the text to differentiate them from their Western meanings. Thus organ names appear beginning with a capital letter, e.g., Liver, Lung, Kidney, etc., when referring to the organs in an Oriental medical context. This can get a bit confusing, particularly in the case of b/Blood. But we felt that a complete lack of differentiation would have been more, not less, obfuscating.

Chinese words appear in the pinyin transliteration, with some exceptions, such as Tao, with which Western readers are more familiar, as opposed to Dao. Chinese names of herbs and acupuncture points appear in the margins of the text, in the Glossary, and on the BodyMap, with their written characters where appropriate. Japanese pronunciations have also been provided.

The usage of herb names is mixed; it is based more on familiarity and common usage than on a consistent rule. Westerners are slowly becoming familiar with Chinese herbs through the herbs' widespread availability in natural food and health stores. We decided to use Chinese names if we noticed their Chinese names on products currently on the market. Dang gui (*Angelica sinensis*), ma huang (*Ephedra*), and di huang (*Rehmannia*) are three examples of herbs being sold by their Chinese names. Codonopsis, on the other hand, is a frequently used Chinese herb that is never sold by its Asian name. Therefore, it is referred to only by its English name in the text. Additionally, the herbs appear in the Glossary with Chinese and Japanese pronunciations and Chinese characters.

Elements of
Balance

C H A P T E R 1

The Oriental View of Health and Illness

The sages lived peacefully under heaven on earth, following the rhythms of the planet and the universe. They adapted to society without being swayed by cultural trends. They were free from emotional extremes and lived a balanced, contented existence. Their outward appearance, behavior, and thinking did not reflect the conflicting norms of society. The sages appeared busy but abided in calmness, recognizing the empty nature of phenomenological existence. The sages lived over one hundred years because they did not scatter and disperse their energies.[1]

The Yellow Emperor's Classic of Medicine

Balance as an Ideal for Health

Balance is the great regulator of life. It is what we invoke whenever we rest after working, whenever we eat less for breakfast after feasting the night before. Balance is an invigorating leap out into the spring sunshine on the first warm day after the long winter. It's a weekend of golf after a week of business travel. It's a meal of greens after a breakfast of bagels and cream cheese. Balance is taking a walk when you are feeling anxious and reaching out when you are lonely. It is laughter after an argument.

Balance is the art of simplicity that helps us adapt to the complexities of our modern world. It is awareness of the pull of opposites and steering the center course. Balance is letting your fishing nets out, and pulling them back in, exploring the waters near shore then turning back into the deeper stream where the flow is steady and strong, where you won't get stuck.

Balance encompasses order and harmony, which can be seen preeminently in our bodies as the many systems—circulatory, endocrine, immune, respiratory,

The Yellow Emperor's
Classic of Medicine
(25–220 A.D.)

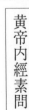

黄
帝
内
經
素
問

HUANG
DI
NEI
JING SU
WEN

digestive, and elimination—that keep us alive. These systems work together wondrously efficiently, maintaining your health without your having to think about it or control the process.

How does the body know how to do this? Deepak Chopra, M.D., director of the Institute for Mind/Body Medicine and Human Potential and author of the best-selling *Quantum Healing*, talks about the "intelligence" of the body that keeps track of us, our concepts of self, and keeps the mind and body inseparably interwoven as a functioning, self-regulating whole. Chopra mentions Oriental medicine in several of his books, pointing out that the Chinese and Japanese have long understood the interaction of mind and body. The "intelligence" of the human mind, body, and spirit, the Chinese wrote over 2,000 years ago, is Qi, the life force.

Before discussing the hazards of imbalance, it is important that we clarify what health means to us within the context of this book. The American Medical Association defines health as the absence of physical or mental disease, but the definition needs to be articulated in the positive.

"When the body and the mind are attuned," wrote the Zen master Hakuin (1686–1769), "they say that even if one is a hundred years old, the hair does not turn white, the teeth remain firm, the eyesight is clearer than ever before, and the skin acquires a luster."[2]

Whatever health is, it would seem to necessitate cooperation between the mind and the body, according to Hakuin.

Lao-tzu says that a healthy man is one "having deep roots and a firm foundation," which help him discover "the Tao of long life and eternal vision." Deep roots and a firm foundation imply some sort of thinking and action that is grounding, balanced, and that supports life and the life principle. The clearest place one sees the life principle at work is in nature, and the ancient Taoists spent long hours contemplating the movement of nature.

> *Movement overcomes cold.*
> *Stillness overcomes heat.*
> *Stillness and tranquility set things in order in the universe.*[3]

Much of the thought in the *Tao Te Ching* has to do with contemplation of the nature of the opposite pulls of energy in the universe, which the Chinese call Yin and yang. Yin refers to that which is cold, slow, inactive, dark, sticky and viscous, deep, damp, and earthy. Yang is that which is hot, high, heavenly, light, dry, and active. These two forces interact dynamically, ceaselessly, and to borrow from the Indian tradition, they are like Shiva and Shakti locked in an eternal embrace.

> *The 10,000 things carry Yin and embrace Yang.*
> *They achieve harmony by combining these forces.*[4]

By constantly moving through and around each other, these two forces under-lie the constant change that characterizes life. I remember being struck with the recognition of the meaning and nature of change for the first time. I was ill and desperate to get well, and a woman I'd just met in a Twelve-Step program sat in a coffee shop telling me to stay hopeful, "because this too shall pass. The only thing you can really count on is change." Her wisdom has never failed me.

One can gain health by becoming aware of the movement of these opposing forces and how they affect body, mind, and spirit. In this sense, the road to health is the road of knowledge. Ancient wisdom holds, "Knowing ignorance is strength; ignoring knowledge is sickness."

The Taoists cultivated their energy and practiced healthy eating, hygiene, and sexuality in order to increase their longevity and spend more time developing their spiritual natures. Living long was not an end in itself, but was the means by which they could develop and cultivate the spirit within. Without sound mind and body, successful cultivation of the spiritual nature could not be done, they acknowledged. The sages used nature as their guide on the journey toward long life and spiritual fulfillment. They watched animals: what and how they ate, how they slept, how they moved. They paid close attention to babies and to young growth. They watched the movements of land, rocks, sea, fire, rivers, clouds, stars, and sky. They learned to read the winds and developed the ability to interpret natural phenomena and eventually to discern the rules of the changes.

The sages postulated that the rules of the changes are contained within some-thing called the Tao, the unknowable and the unnameable. The patterns of the changes that occur within the Tao were observable in nature; watching and living by the dynamics of nature best nurtures the human being, they thought.

Early Chinese philosophers taught that man's purpose on earth is to become one with the Tao; to do that requires long years of self-study and practice, "avoid-ing extremes, excesses, and complacency."[3] Through diligent practice of the Middle Way, as the Buddhists call it, the body and mind begin to work better than ever. Eating wholesome food, getting plenty of exercise, working, playing, relaxing in balance, taking in clean air, being in nature, and spending moments alone fills us with Qi, with energy, the life force.

Following this prescription for health gives us the tools we need to steer our rudders clear of life's snags and obstacles—or at least through them without tip-ping over. You can have more energy than you ever dreamed possible. You can eat with gusto and relish your food, sleep well and deeply, and enjoy emotional stabil-ity while riding above an underlying river of joy. This is our vision of health for you.

Imbalance as the Cause of Illness

Tai'chi is a form of movement that was born out of the martial arts in China thousands of years ago. To practice tai'chi, the practitioner begins by centering the body, connecting with heaven and earth—as the Taoists called subtle and material forms of energy—connecting the tongue to the roof of the mouth, and breathing deeply. Ideally, as he moves through his form, he attunes his mind to the movement to become one with his body and its motions. The outside world, worries, and extraneous thoughts are shut out as mind becomes arm— shoulder, elbow, wrist, hand, fingers—and arm becomes the fluid arc that cuts through the air. The mind focuses on the lower abdomen (the *hara* in Japanese, *dan tian* in Chinese), keeping the body grounded. From this position, the practitioner is poised for anything. When his mind is open and aware, he can spot things coming from any direction as he keeps moving, from side to side, turning, turning. He is in balance.

The reality of the tai'chi practitioner is that there are days when he has a great practice, when the energy is flowing and he really feels connected to the practice, to the natural environment he is practicing in, to the world around him. And there are days when nothing goes right, when he forgets part of the form, and when he has to begin again because he loses concentration halfway through. Perhaps he doesn't feel well, has a headache or an upset stomach. Whatever the cause, the world is not in order. He falls during his one-legged Standing Crane. He is off balance.

Balance is the ideal. It's where we imagine ourselves to be when the world is in order. Life doesn't make finding that equilibrium easy, however, and balance is elusive. Some days, no matter how hard you try, life rains on your parade—trains are missed, communication breaks down, computers make mistakes, and tempers fly. Part of being balanced is recognizing that those challenging days come. And they pass. But if life is a constant flurry of activity that moves by so quickly you can't even remember the last time you felt something like balance, it may be helpful to sit down quietly, perhaps with a notebook, and write out a scenario of balance for yourself.

Quickly jotting down priorities is an effective way to identify the component parts of life as you lead it. Typically, these could include family, friends, work, your art, ways to unwind, recovery, emotional growth, community service or activism, and spiritual development. Some or all of these may be important to you; that's fine. You may have your own categories. The longer the list is, the more juggling you will do, however—an important acknowledgement. Number priorities according to how important they really are to you, not according to the expectations or demands of others. Now, imagine a day in your life as you would *like* to live it. Describe your activities from the moment you wake up until you go to bed. Use your imagination to create balance among your component parts on a daily and/or weekly basis.

Each day, do you leave ample time to attend to your personal details? Is the morning packed with chores that keep you so busy that you don't even have time to go to the bathroom before leaving the house? Can you prepare for the morning in some ways the evening before? Have you created space to meditate, take a walk, do morning tai-chi, to read? Have you left more alone time than the time in the car commuting to and from work? Is there space in your balanced life to communicate with loved ones? Can you consistently dedicate part of your day to some health-related activity? Once you finish this daily list, review it. Does it leave you feeling good about what you are doing with your life? Are you satisfied that your priorities are being met? Does joy bubble under the surface because you are allowing yourself to do what you really want to do?

If your life is complicated by many duties and activities, in addition to a balanced-day scenario, try writing out a weekly agenda and see if everything that needs to be there can fit in comfortably without making you feel overwhelmed or overloaded. Once it is written down, review it, take several deep breaths and imagine yourself going through the motions of this "balanced" week, day by day. Is it comfortable; can you breathe into this way of life with ease? Or does your breath become constricted during any part of the review? If so, reconsider that component's place in your ideal of balance. You may feel trapped by it, but imagine your life without that component. What would you be doing instead? How would you do things differently? If you come up with blanks at first, breathe deeply, relax, and ask yourself the questions again. Give yourself permission to come up with other options. The key to this exercise is freeing your mind up to allow the imagination to create new possibilities for yourself. Once you hit upon a scenario that makes you excited, enthusiastic, or light and easy, and you decide this is really how you would like life to feel, commit to concentrating on this image daily. Ten to fifteen minutes a day is enough. Eventually you may find yourself taking steps to actualize your ideal. Imagining and writing out this scenario is an important first step to actualizing it.

Man is a microcosm of the universe, according to the Taoists. Our bodies replicate the same laws that activate the universe as a whole. We are powerful beings in that we have the free will and choice to follow the law of nature or not, to take care of the body, our vehicle, or not. Everything we do to follow what is right and natural for us will bring us closer to center. When we move out of balance and moderation, we move away from center. The longer we stay out on the extreme ends of this scale the further we move away from balance, and movement from balance can easily become movement toward illness.

In Oriental medicine terms, illness is imbalance manifesting in the body. Healthy organs, science now says, exhibit the same behavior as their component cells: they function efficiently and effectively and have the immune ability to fight off disease. Unhealthy organs, on the other hand, are characterized by the disorder of their component cells that have split from the harmony and balance of the rest of the body to create a whirlpool of chaos on their own.

This bodily imbalance is caused, as the reader is no doubt aware, by a combination of stress, overwork, or not eating and sleeping regularly or enough. Overindulgence in partying, excessive sex, and a wild lifestyle contribute to or cause imbalance; so do unreasonable rigidity or living by too many rules that come out of your head, rather than allowing your body to tell you what you need. Imbalance can stem from experiencing an excess of a single emotion for too long. Any excess that continues for a prolonged period—and how long is too long depends on one's own body—will block the body's harmonious flow, that intelligence that keeps things in order, to become the eventual root of disease.

A Closer Look at Lifestyle

"Lifestyle" is a vague term that means different things to different people. It may be helpful to stop for a minute and break down the elements that make up a balanced body and lifestyle to discover the areas in your life, if any, that require more balancing attention than others, which might be fairly well balanced already. On a physical level, we want to be neither too hot nor too cold. We don't want to be too active and overextend, nor do we want to remain sedate all day every day. We want to get enough sleep, but again, not too much. Work is fine and necessary, but overwork takes away from play and rest, two other essentials to equilibrium. We all need to connect with people, yet time alone is important too. In terms of diet, eating natural, unrefined foods is good for us. A steady flow of deep-fried fast food and coffee is a guaranteed way of losing constitutional and/or emotional balance. Eating too much strains your system and overtaxes the liver and the other internal organs. Eating too little does not supply the minimum nourishment needed to maintain basic metabolic functions. You'll find yourself working at half-power.

Your environment is important. Are you doing what you can to make yourself comfortable? Do you have the opportunity to get outside, breathe clean air deeply, frolic in the grass, walk by some running water? Growing a garden is an exquisite lesson in balance. When is the last time you sank your hands in some real soil, seeded, weeded, plucked, and harvested?

What about your home? Do you have a clean, comfortable place to live and work? Can you properly maintain it? Is it spacious enough to allow you to let down your inner guards and walls and completely permeate the space when you need to? What about other basic material goods for survival—do you have what you need to survive? Chances are you're bogged down in stuff. Having too much can be complicated and burdensome. Taking care of two or three houses, two or three cars, and whatever else becomes a part of your personal holdings requires a great amount of time and energy, often to the detriment of other areas in your life. This leads you away from center.

Is work enjoyable? Are you getting what you want out of it? Do you put into it what you want to? Do you feel like a valuable contributor to your work environment? Answering yes to these questions points toward balance. Long hours may leave you feeling drained at times, but if you derive satisfaction from your work you are probably not that far from maintaining the balance that is right for you.

Sometimes work leaves us frazzled. We wake up to a sensational sunrise, run through our morning practice or prayers, ablutions, workout, and then just as we get into the car or board the train, we start feeling nervous. Our stomachs knot up, and by the time we get there we may have run through any number of possible confrontations and difficulties in our minds. In response to this stress, the chest, abdomen, and diaphragm begin to tense up and constrict. You want to do a good job, you want to be alert, so you have a cup or two of coffee.

A couple of years of this can have a devastating effect on your system. Twenty years of it spells angina, high blood pressure, stomach or duodenal ulcer, and a host of other stress-related disorders.

> *Better stop short than fill to the brim.*
> *Oversharpen the blade and the edge will soon blunt...*
> *This is the way of heaven.*[5]

Regaining Balance

We have to work to regain our balance; it's not usually something that you just pick up, like the hula hoop. It requires effort because you are taking on the downward-spiralling forces of entropy, the natural tendency things (objects, plants, bodies) have to decay. This is why it is so important to try to stem imbalance in the bud. If you wander a little off the path, as humans are wont to do, steering yourself back to the main road is not so difficult. But the further astray you go, the more time and effort are required to find your way back.

• Effort

Putting yourself back on course is really challenging if you are facing serious health difficulties. One reason for this is, simply, that it took a lot of time for your body to develop a serious illness and in that time your less than health-promoting actions have become thoroughly ingrained habits that are probably quite dear to you. Getting well could mean having to recognize that those habits have contributed to your illness, giving some of them up, and developing new ones to replace them. It takes effort, but that effort doesn't have to be unpleasant. Learn to see this as an interesting process, a process of getting to know yourself.

Some people have trouble with this concept of changing to become well. They don't want to feel deprived of their cherished after-dinner drink, chocolate splurges, Sunday afternoon ice creams, cigarettes, or Porterhouse steaks. Some people argue that life is only lived once and is meant to be enjoyed, so why give up bad habits. Others are afraid to give up habits that they perceive as lifeboats on the rough sea of life. Frankly, if these thoughts stand in your way of changing to become well again, perhaps it is time to take a hard look at your life, your personal priorities, and ask yourself how much longer you really want to live. Balance may be a dance, but it can be a deadly dance if taken up cavalierly. It's fine to feel that you don't want to live that much longer, too. There is no judgment here. It is better to be clear about these things, however, and take responsibility for the path of your life. You do have a choice, to some extent, in the matter.

- Nature

Getting back to nature is one of the most important and profound steps a person whose life is out of balance can take to move toward balance again. All of us have experienced serenity while being in nature, and this experience can be tapped to bring about life-transforming change. It doesn't require a splendid natural scene; a park with trees and birds will do. Being in nature reminds us of life's natural rhythms. Spending ample amounts of time there can lead to the realization that you are not a separate entity from nature. Experiencing a oneness with that energy is your ticket to the burrowing of roots and building of foundations that were mentioned previously.

The most balanced people tend to lead natural lives irrespective of the location of their homes. Europeans, especially Italians, have this down to an art. Business is based on the rhythms of the body. People wake up early, start work by 7 or 8 A.M., stop around 12:30 for lunch—they often go home to eat—take a long break while their food is digested, then work again from around 2:30 till sundown.

The Chinese live a similar way, very simply. They allow the day to follow the course of sunlight and temperature. Our kung fu master, a doctor in Canton, lives an extraordinarily simple life with no telephone and no hot running water. He wastes nothing, protects his privacy, and lives a very earthy, quiet life despite the dirt and noise of the outside world. In that sanctum of asceticism both Peter and I have experienced healing and clearings of emotions and turmoil that had been contributing to imbalances.

- Prayer and Inner Practice

It is important to acknowledge that just living keeps us pretty well occupied. We all feel the pushes and strains of daily existence, no matter how simplified a form we have life pared down to. "Trying to stay alive keeps me pretty busy," admits Hui-yuan, a woman hermit living on Nanwutai mountain in China. And then, addressing the problem of stress, she adds, "I get up every day before dawn and chant the Lotus Sutra and the Tisang Sutra. At night, I meditate and chant the name of the Buddha. Practice depends on the individual. This is my practice."[6]

This form of ritualized quietude is crucial to the process of aligning yourself with your inner intelligence. So important, in fact, that we would venture to say that you probably can't locate that balance without it. Only in the silencing of extraneous thought can you perceive the inner working of the Tao, the motions of the energy inside you. Only in the silence can you discern the way you're being guided to shift, to maintain balance. This is the space where you create mental images of health and nurture them into reality. This is your center.

> *The space between Heaven and Earth is like a bellows.*
> *The shape changes but not the form;*
> *The more it moves, the more it yields.*
> *More words count less.*
> *Hold fast to the center.*[7]

• Love and Compassion

Lao-tzu's *Tao Te Ching* doesn't make much mention of it, the rest of the Taoists didn't write much about it, and one hardly hears of it in classes, treatment sessions, and workshops on Oriental medicine. Martial arts practitioners often seem more bent on detaching from it and cultivating their warrior spirits than on meditating on its power. Current books on Oriental medicine discuss theory, practice, even the philosophical beauty of Oriental medicine.... All in all, love gets short shrift in terms of its recognition as a healing tool. Which is interesting because the great healers, therapists, and martial artists I know are all brimming over with love.

Love is the greatest transformer of energy, more so than any practice, meditation, or remedy we have included in this book. Love alone can reverse entropy if channeled properly. The flows of love and Qi are inseparable, and when you have opened a flow to both, healing ensues. There is no question about it. Learning to love yourself will bring healing to you in some form. Having compassion for others will extend that healing out into the world. Love provides us with insight into the meaning and reasons for our struggle to survive at all.

Love can manifest itself as friendship and reaching out, it is expressed through positiveness, smiles, laughter, and good cheer. It is a touch at the appropriate moment, a hug when needed. It can be a song to yourself or a barrage of uplifting music every morning. It can be sharing a meal, offering a massage, giving the right book or a letter to someone in need. It can be the glow of being together with someone, or it can be the glow of connecting with the power of love inside yourself. This is the lubrication of healing.

Having the love and support of other people makes healing that much more possible. A good practitioner—from the medical modality of your choice—is essential. Working with a competent counselor or therapist, who can help plough through old thought patterns, can help tremendously. Having other people around you who have fought for their health and won is a great boost to healing. These people live with zest and vitality and their presence is an inspiration to your own struggle. Good therapists and people who have healed themselves can frequently act as energy conductors, or as mirrors who reflect images of our healthy selves back to us while we work toward claiming that image for ourselves. They are important lights and guideposts down the road to health.

Endnotes

*1 *The Yellow Emperor's Classic of Medicine*, Chapter 1, trans. Maoshing Ni (Boston: Shambhala Publications, 1995), p.4.

*2 *Zen Master Hakuin, Selected Writings*, ed. Philip B. Yampolsky, (New York: Columbia University Press, 1971), p. 42.

*3 *Tao Te Ching*, trans. Stephen Mitchell (New York: HarperCollins, 1989), No.45.

*4 *Tao Te Ching*, No.42.

*5 *Tao Te Ching*, No.9.

*6 Bill Porter, *Road to Heaven, Encounters with Chinese Hermits* (San Francisco: Mercury House, 1993) p. 170.

*7 *Tao Te Ching*, No.5.

C H A P T E R 2

Building Blocks of the Energetics of Imbalance

In approaching an understanding of the energetics of Oriental medicine, its diagnoses and remedies described in this book, the reader will be required to let go of the Western concept of pathology. This may be confusing at first, but it is possible to achieve two different ways of understanding the body, resulting in a completely new set of options in approaching personal wellness. Apparently unrelated problems may suddenly come together in a pattern that lends itself to treatment that consists of the best of Western and Oriental medical practices.

Organs are Energy Zones

The organs as understood in Oriental medicine are never as material as in Western medicine. Doctors in ancient China explored the body through outward symptoms and signs, assessing the clarity of the eyes and skin and the modulation of the voice, observing pulse and tongue, palpating, and questioning the patient. Healers followed a strict code of "least intervention"—believing that nature heals, and that anything that disturbs the flow of energy in the body inhibits the healing process. When a doctor in ancient China actually performed surgery so he could explore the internal organs, he was caustically criticized by the medical profession for what were described as his barbaric methods.

Rather than emphasizing the substance and anatomical location of an organ, Oriental medicine sees organs as zones of concentrated energy. This energy is responsible for carrying out certain functions within the body. Harmony results when the interdependent zones are in balance and functioning correctly. Imbalance in any one zone affects the whole body and is manifested in any number of disorders.

The Viscera and
Bowels

ZANG FU

As an example, an imbalance in the energetic function of the organ, the Liver, and its corresponding meridian system could be manifested as red, sore eyes, irritability, pain in or under the ribs, digestive upsets, and a tendency to shout. To the Western practitioner, there would often be no apparent connection between liver function and such symptoms.

There are 14 paths or meridians and 365 points identified in Traditional Chinese Medicine (TCM), which is actually Oriental medicine as it has been codified in China since the Cultural Revolution. Prior to present codification, Chinese practitioners of traditional medicine identified as many as 70 pathways and up to 2,000 points, depending on the particular "school" of medicine.[1] The TCM version used here is the form that is becoming accepted in the United States, and is adequate for carrying out the self-help remedies contained in this book.

Of these meridians, ten correspond with organs whose names are familiar to us. These are grouped in Yin/Yang pairs as the Lung (Yin)/ Large Intestine (Yang), Spleen (Yin)/ Stomach (Yang), Heart (Yin)/ Small Intestine (Yang), Kidney (Yin)/ Bladder (Yang), Liver (Yin)/ Gallbladder (Yang).

The four other meridians are called the Triple Heater (consisting of the Upper Burner, Middle Burner, and Lower Burner), the Pericardium, the Conception Vessel, and the Governor channel.

Lung / Large Intestine

The Lung

—controls Qi

—controls respiration, the process of inhaling clean Qi (oxygen) and exhaling impure Qi (toxins and CO_2)

—controls the refinement of nutrients it receives from the Spleen and air. It combines these two to produce Chest Qi.

—is responsible—together with the Heart—for the correct circulation of Qi

—is in charge of the functions of descending and dispersing. As the uppermost organ in the body, the energy of the Lungs flows downward; the Lung is responsible for the descending action of fluids, sending them to the Kidney and Bladder for reabsorption and excretion. This function works in coordination with the Spleen and Kidney. If impaired, Lung Qi stagnates in the chest, producing asthma, fullness and pain in the chest, and edema in the face and arms.

—controls the Protective Qi (Wei Qi) or immune function, sending Protective Qi circulating beneath the skin throughout the body. The body becomes easily susceptible to colds and flu when this function is impaired.

—controls the opening and closing of the pores, sweating, and the evaporation of body fluids, which are distributed over the skin as a fine mist

—regulates fluid metabolism. Receives fluids from the Spleen and distributes them throughout the body, to the skin, and the Kidneys. When fluids descend to the Kidneys to be eliminated, part is retained by the Kidney, warmed by its heating function, called the Kidney Yang energy, and is then sent back up to the Lung to keep it moist.

—controls moisture and life of skin and hair. Rough, dry, flaccid or lifeless hair, and rough and dry skin may result from imbalance.

—opens into the nose and controls the sense of smell.

The Large Intestine

—receives wastes from the Small Intestine, separates them, and then either excretes or reabsorbs the usable fluid. Imbalance sometimes causes the Large Intestine to absorb too much fluid, resulting in constipation. Failure to absorb results in diarrhea.

Spleen / Stomach

The Spleen

—is the main organ of digestion

—controls the transformation and transportation of food and the distribution of nutrients and energy to the various organs

—controls muscles and limbs and keeps them well nourished

—controls healthy appetite, absorption of food, and normal bowel movements. If this function is impaired, anorexia, abdominal distention, loose stool, undigested food in the stool, and lassitude can result.

—controls, together with the Stomach, transportation of food energy to muscles. If this function is impaired, weak limbs and a desire to lie down all the time result.

—transforms, transports, and distributes fluids. If this function is impaired, fluid accumulation, internal Damp, edema, and heaviness in the mid- and lower body and legs can result.

—keeps the Blood in the vessels. This holding action works in combination with the circulating function of the Heart and the regulating action of the Liver. Disharmony in this function can appear as blood in the stool or urine, tendency to bruise easily, and excessive menstruation.

—opens into the mouth and manifests in the lips. The Spleen is believed to produce saliva, which begins the process of digestion. A healthy Spleen will allow clear differentiation of tastes and keeps the lips moist, full, and reddish. A disharmony of Spleen energy may result in a "sticky" taste or feeling in the mouth and an inability to taste food. Heat in the Spleen may give the mouth a sweetish taste and dry lips. A weak Spleen results in pale lips and there may be dribbling of saliva during sleep.

—controls the energy that keeps the organs up and in place. Weakness of this function results in organ prolapse or the sensation that the organ is heavy or

Lung

FÈI
HAI

Large Intestine

DÀ CHÁNG
DAI CHŌ

Spleen

PÍ
HI

dropping, most often affecting the stomach, bladder, uterus, and anus.

Stomach

WÈI
I

The Stomach
—is in charge of digestion, breaks down food, and sends nutrients to the Spleen and wastes to the Small Intestine
—controls the descending energy of food into the alimentary canal. Dysfunction results in belching, nausea, and vomiting.

Heart / Small Intestine

Heart

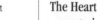

XIN
SHIN

The Heart
—controls the Blood, blood circulation, amount of blood
—maintains the condition of the blood vessels
—keeps the complexion healthy
—houses the Shen, the spiritual energy of the body, which regulates mental activity, emotional stability, and consciousness
—determines the color, form, and appearance of the tongue, which controls the faculty of speech. Speech abnormalities and stuttering are often related to and treated through the Heart channel.

Small Intestine

XIǍO CHAŃG
SHO CHŌ

The Small Intestine
—separates and assimilates food and liquid, continues the process of decomposition, and separates nutrients and wastes, sending the nutrients to the Spleen and the wastes to the Large Intestine and Bladder
—is connected energetically to the Bladder. Urinary problems can sometimes be treated through the Small Intestine channel.

Kidney / Bladder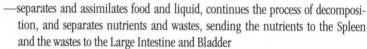

Kidney

SHÈN
JIN

The Kidney
—stores primary Yin and Yang energy at birth. These are the energies that make up the foundations of life, controlling growth, sexual development and maturity, reproduction, and the aging process. Both energies begin dissipating from birth and must be continually fortified from energy acquired from food and air.
—stores Jing (the Generative Qi that produces bone marrow), nourishes the brain and spinal cord, creates clear thinking, good memory, the ability to reason, and nourishes the bones. Deficiency results in poor memory, unclear thinking, poor bone formation, deterioration of bones, and a weak lumbar spine and knee joint.
—controls water—the amount and function of urination, sends fluids for excretion to the Bladder, and receives and warms fluid from the Lungs and sends it back to warm the Lungs
—interacts with the Spleen to regulate fluid separation

—holds Qi from the Lung. Failure to do so could congest the Lung, resulting in asthma.

—opens into the ear, controls the sense of hearing. As people get older and the energy of the Kidney decreases, so does hearing ability. Fleshy, long earlobes are considered to be a sign of longevity.

—stores the strongest Fire, the source of body heat, in the Gate of Life (located between the Kidneys). If this fire declines, a deficiency of Yang energy can result leading to impotence, menstrual problems, infertility, leukorrhea, digestion problems, poor absorption, and diarrhea.

—is closely connected to the uterus, which is also intimately connected to the Blood. Kidneys aid menstruation, pregnancy, and fetal development. Abnormality in Jing energy or the lack of Yang fire in the Gate of Life can result in painful menstruation, a lack of menses, or infertility. The uterus is also closely connected to the Heart, which moves the Blood; the Liver, which stores the blood; and the Spleen, which keeps the Blood in the vessels.

The Bladder
—receives and excretes urine. Imbalance can result in incontinence, cystitis, painful urination, or lack of urination.

Urinary Bladder

膀
胱

GUĀNG PÁNG
BŌKŌ

Liver / Gallbladder

The Liver
—stores the Blood. It is believed that when the body is at rest blood circulation decreases and some of the blood returns to the Liver where it is stored. When the body resumes activity the Liver releases the Blood, affecting the amount circulating in the body at any one time.

Liver

肝

GĀN
KAN

—influences menstruation; a lack of Blood stored in the Liver can result in amenorrhea or infertility. Heat in the Liver can result in excessive menstruation.

—is in charge of moistening the eyes and tendons with stored Blood. Deficiency could result in blurred vision and tightness or contracture of the tendons. Heat in the Liver manifests as red eyes.

—promotes the free flow of Qi throughout the body, making sure there are no obstacles in its path

—is in charge of the smooth flow of emotions. When the Liver Qi flows smoothly and the Liver function is normal, the emotions are in balance. When the Liver Qi is blocked, depression, anger, emotional instability, hypochondriacal distress, tightness in the chest and headache, PMS accompanied by swelling in the breasts, abdominal distention, irritability, and depression may result.

—promotes healthy digestion through the smooth flow of Liver Qi. Stagnant Liver Qi can invade the Stomach and Spleen, resulting in vomiting, nausea, belching, pain in the abdomen, abdominal distention, and a loose stool. Also, the secretion of bile relies upon the free flow of Qi; disturbance may result in a bitter taste, belching, abdominal distention, and jaundice.

—nourishes the fingernails and toenails. Dry, brittle nails indicate Liver problems.

—controls tendons, ensuring their correct contraction and relaxation, makes movement of the joints possible. If Blood is deficient and cannot nourish the tendons, contractions, spasms, impaired flexion and extension, numbness of limbs, and loss of power in the limbs may result.

—opens into the eyes and controls sight, the ability to distinguish colors. Many other meridians pass through the eyes and affect them. Fire from the Heart can make the eyes painfully bloodshot, while a deficiency of Kidney Yin energy will dull the vision.

Gallbladder

DĂN
TAN

The Gallbladder

—stores and secretes bile manufactured by the Liver. Disharmony may result in the vomiting of bitter fluid, constipation, jaundice, an inability to make decisions or the tendency to make rash decisions.

Fluids, Qi, and Blood

These are three frequently used terms in the Self-care sections of the book. Their meanings differ slightly from Western medical terms. They are liquid substances (in the cases of fluid and blood), but practitioners of Oriental medicine also think of them as the body's environmental matrix, the routes by which nutrient, waste, and energy are distributed, and the function of that distribution.

Liquids

JÌN
SHIN

Body Fluids

Body fluids are divided into the clear/Yang type and the thick/Yin type. The clear/Yang type moisturizes the skin and warms and nourishes the muscles. Perspiration is an example of this type of fluid.

Thick/Yin type fluid circulates to nourish and lubricate the joint cavities (synovial fluid), brain and spinal cord (cerebrospinal fluid), bone marrow, and sense organ orifices. It appears as a greasy secretion of the sweat glands on the skin.

Humors

YÈ
EKI

Each organ is associated with a specific type of fluid: the Lungs with mucus, the Kidneys with sexual secretions and cerebrospinal fluid, the Liver with bile and tears, the Heart with blood and sweat, and the Spleen with lymph, saliva, and chyme. Fluid imbalance appears as asthma; dry eyes, skin, and lips; or edema.

Qi

Qi is the force that animates all life. It is formless, tasteless, and invisible. Nevertheless, paradoxically, it permeates all matter. The Taoist scholar Chuang-tzu said, "The Tao can be divided but remains one." So, too, Qi may assume various roles but remains a single entity. Oriental medicine says that when Qi flows smoothly through the body, disease can find no place to reside. Our heredity, the quality and quantity of food and drink ingested, and the air breathed all affect Qi.

Qi coexists with the body's organs in a dynamic relationship: the proper functioning of the organs is necessary to obtain Qi, and Qi influences the correct functioning of the organs.

Prenatal Qi and Congenital Qi are derived from one's parents. They are essential for the proper development of the fetus, growth of the organism, regeneration, and aging. Acquired Qi, or Nutritive Qi, as it is also called, is energy derived from the air, sunlight, and food and drink. Air Qi is one example—nutritive energy gained from the air we breathe. Chest Qi nourishes the Heart and Lungs and promotes circulation and respiration. Yuan Qi, or True Qi, is energy in the body in its most refined and readily usable state. Wei Qi, or Protective Qi, circulates below the skin and protects the body from attack by external invaders. Ying Qi is another form of Protective Qi that flows through the channels and organs, protecting the body's internal cavities from pathogens.

Blood

Blood is best thought of in a functional sense as the fluid that nourishes the organs, which in turn produce and regulate Qi. For this reason, Blood is called the "Mother of Qi." The relationship between Blood and Qi is interactive, since the Qi is the force that moves Blood and keeps it in the vessels. Blood is derived from two sources: the combined "essence" of food and air and the Kidney Jing, which produces Marrow, an energetic matrix from which the brain, the spinal column, and bone marrow are formed. The bone marrow, in turn, produces Blood. The Blood nourishes the body, promotes the correct operation of the organs, and moistens the tissues, tendons, and eyes.

Blood is moved by the power of the Heart Qi and the Chest Qi. If the Qi fails to move Blood, stagnation will occur. If Qi fails to hold Blood in the vessels, hemorrhaging will result.

Blood

XUÈ
KETSU

The Five Elements

The interrelationship of what Oriental medical practitioners call the Five Elements is key to understanding the patterns of imbalance.

The ancient Taoists formulated the interaction of the elemental energies in the universe according to the model called the Five Elements. The Five Element Theory represents the movement of energy on the macrocosmic and the microcosmic level, which is to say, the theory supports the idea that changes in small systems replicate the patterns of change that take place in large systems.

The Five Elements are Wood, Fire, Earth, Metal, and Water. Each element relates to a time of day, a taste or flavor, an organ of the body, a color, a sound, a smell, an emotion, a season, and a direction. These elements, or groups of characteristics and energies, interact with one another in predetermined patterns toward and away from each other, in what are called the Creative and Controlling Cycles.

The Five Elements

WŪ XIEŃG
GO GYŌ

As you see in the diagram below, there is a circle drawn through the five pairs of organ systems. Arrows are drawn on the circle to demonstrate that energy moves from one organ to the next, nourishing the element/organ that follows it. Find the Liver/Gallbladder on the diagram and notice the arrow that follows the circle toward the Heart/Small Intestine. This means that the Liver derives energy from the Wood Element, which it then passes to the Fire Element—the Heart organ and meridian system.

The Creative Cycle

XIÀNG SHĒNG GŪAN
XĪ
SO SEI KAN KEI

The Five Element Cycle

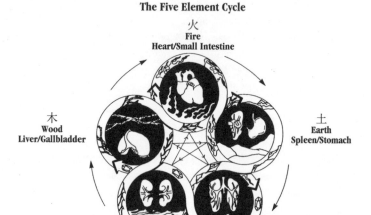

火
Fire
Heart/Small Intestine

木
Wood
Liver/Gallbladder

土
Earth
Spleen/Stomach

水
Water
Kidney/Bladder

金
Metal
Lung/Large Intestine

The ramifications of the Creative Cycle are enormous, suggesting that when an imbalance exaggerates the energy of one organ within the system, another organ will be Deficient because it cannot receive the nourishment it must have. For example, a Deficiency in the Heart could mean that: 1) the Heart is not getting the proper nourishment it needs from the Liver; 2) it might benefit the Heart to tonify the Liver; 3) the Stomach and Spleen systems (next in the series following the Heart), or the digestive system, are also affected.

The second part of the Five Elements' cycle, the Controlling Cycle, helps prevent the organs and their energy from working on overdrive, either to ultimately burn themselves out, drain energy from the nourishing organ preceding, or overwhelm the organ following. In this cycle

Wood controls the Earth (like a tree holding soil in place);
Earth controls Water (keeping its water contained);
Water controls Fire (putting out its flames);
Fire controls Metal (like fire melting ore);
Metal controls Wood (like an axe chopping wood).

This translates into:
Liver/Gallbladder limit the energy of the Stomach/Spleen;
Stomach/Spleen limit the energy of the Kidney/Bladder;
Kidney/Bladder limit the energy of the Heart/Small Intestine;
Heart/Small Intestine limit the energy of the Lung/Large Intestine;
Lung/Large Intestine limit the energy of the Liver/Gallbladder.

The Control Cycle

XIÀNG KÈ GŪAN XÌ
SO KOKU KAN KEI

The actions of the Controlling Cycle suggest: 1) we can treat an Excess condition by stimulating the organ that controls it on the Controlling Cycle; 2) ailing or Deficient organs and systems can be helped by toning down the activity of the organ that controls it on the Controlling Cycle; and 3) going back to our Deficient Heart/Small Intestine example, the condition could very well be treated by balancing and tonifying the Kidney/Bladder system.

In addition, each organ system is nourished and controlled by five different types of tastes or food energies, colors, times, seasons, and sounds.

When we listen to our bodies and become aware of the basic qualities that make up our constitutions, of how much energy we have and put out, whether we feel warm or cool most of the time, how fast we metabolize food, what kind, color, and amount of phlegm, urine, and feces we secrete and excrete, and so forth, we can relate this information to the Five Elements and work to establish balance among the organs involved.

The Four Phases

The Four Phases

SÌ XÍŊG
SHI GYŌ

An Oriental medical practitioner diagnoses patients according to which phase of life the patient is in. Traditionally the Chinese divided the life cycle into four phases: infancy/childhood, adolescence, adulthood, and old age. Bodies have different dietary, exercise, and rest requirements depending on what stage of the cycle they are in.

Infants and young children, for example, are somewhat delicate creatures. Their digestive tracts are still forming and they can't stomach red meat and grains without special preparation. They need space and freedom to play, roam around, and develop, but their stamina is limited. They need more sleep than older children and adults. Adolescents are entering their growth spurt into physical maturity. They need a lot of physical exercise, sleep, and food, and they change in unfamiliar ways. Adults have stabilized in terms of growth, and generally the aging process is said to begin at about age 30. Adults are in their prime and should enjoy it, but they should also remember to nurture their strength and energy in preparation for old age. Seniors are winding down, though older people today enjoy an increased life expectancy that can be enhanced if they choose foods that do not strain the digestive tract but promote strength, vigor, and healthy elimination. Regular exercise that keeps muscles and tendons stretched and used to moving also contributes to a healthy old age. Practicing yoga, tai'chi, or a similar discipline actually increases energy levels and builds immunity. Rest needs may change as well.

Types of Bodies

Knowing your body type is a good starting point in determining how to treat any imbalance. Certain body types tend to have certain types of imbalances, and imbalances will run a different course depending on the body's constitutional type.

The Chinese divide the world into two distinct yet ever-interpenetrating spheres of energy, Yin and Yang. You have probably heard of these even if you're not sure exactly what they mean. For purposes of conveying information clearly in this chapter, we are going to simplify the concepts for now and identify Yin with cold/cool energies and Yang with hot/warm. All bodies fall somewhere on the continuum between cold and hot.

Yang bodies are hot, red, strong, full of energy, and easily excitable. People with a predominance of Hot, Yang energy tend to have stiff bodies, and strong, loud voices; their manner is often aggressive, they breathe heavily, and they tend to have cracked lips and reddish skin—dark-skinned people will exhibit a reddish tinge. The mucus of a Hot constitution will be yellow or even red, as will the urine; the feces tend to be hard, and bowel movements are difficult due to constipation.

As Hot moves toward balance the Heat starts cooling, the red becomes pinkish and takes on a healthy glow, and the energy level evolves from less excitable and restless to active and participatory. Warm people tend to respond openly, with an enthusiasm that can easily take control, but they are less overbearing than Hot people. They tend to breathe heavily, but less noisily and gratingly than one with a Hot constitution. The lips and skin are still dryish, but not cracking and peeling. Mucus in the Warm person is green or yellow and thick. The urine is dark yellow, the stool hard and somewhat dark, and the body odor is fairly strong.

Balanced people are of a "normal" weight and condition. They are not too thin nor are they overweight. They have some muscle tone but are not overladen with muscle. They move with fluidity and seem comfortable and relaxed in their bodies. They know when to move and when to rest. The voice is melodic and its pleasant modulation is easy to listen to. The breath is unnoticeable, the lips and skin smooth and moist. Their body secretions are white mucus, and golden urine, and the body is gently scented and fragrant.

Cool people seem somewhat emotionally muted in comparison with Warm and Hot types; they are quieter and self-effacing, seeming to lack confidence or the ability to assert themselves. Their movements are reserved and smaller, and their breath is light or shallow, often taken only from the upper cavities of the lungs.

Their voices are soft. Light-skinned people appear pale or very light in color, while dark-skinned people exhibit a grayish tinge. The lips are moist but pale, veering toward gray, the mucus is thin, clear, or white, and the urine is a pale yellow while the stool is light and loose.

Yin bodies may be either overweight or emaciated. The posture is slack or droopy. Cold people may seem unhappy or depressed. They move very little, preferring to sit huddled up or curled around themselves like cats. The voice is quiet, even whispery, the breath very shallow and faint, the skin is pale and clammy, the lips are pale and very moist. Mucus is clear and wet, the body gives off almost no odor, the urine is clear and the stool is loose, and there may be chronic diarrhea.

These body types are generalizations, of course. You probably fall in between, as most of us do. As you read through the characteristics, check off the ones you find most frequently in yourself. The section you've made the most checks in is your primary type. Pay attention to the other checks as well, since you're probably a little Warm or Cool with some movement toward another part of the continuum.

Also remember that as you begin to modify your diet and lifestyle, you may find yourself shifting on the continuum. In a few months you may want to refer once more to the chart to see if anything has changed and adjust your diet and lifestyle accordingly.

Types of Imbalances

Oriental medicine practitioners diagnose illness according to the signs and symptoms manifested in a pattern of disharmony rather than concerning themselves with identifying a specific germ as the cause of pathology. The symptoms analyzed are predominantly of a Heat or of a Cold nature, which can arise from internally generated imblance or through the invasion of external influences. Excessive and Deficient are terms used to describe the degree of Heat or Cold the imbalance represents.

Hot people, or those lacking in Yin energy—Yin Deficient types—tend to exhibit symptoms of Excess Heat: thirst, fever, constipation, green and thick sticky mucus. They refuse to be covered with blankets and prefer cooling compresses; the appetite is hardy, the digestion is strong or a burning sensation may even be experienced. There may be red in the face and eyes. Inflammation and infections are common Heat symptoms.

Cold people, those lacking Yang energy—Yang Deficient types—tend to feel cold when they get sick. They become pale, bluish, and will exhibit very low energy. The urine becomes very light, the mucus is clear and abundant, and they may have diarrhea. Craving warmth, people with Cold imbalance will want to bundle themselves under mounds of blankets. The appetite may disappear, the digestion may stagnate, and the body may ache, particularly in the joints and muscles.

Heat

RÈ
NETSU

Cold

HÁN
KAN

The tendency for Hot people to exhibit Hot illnesses and Cold people to have Cold imbalances is not a hard and fast one. A Hot/Warm person can acquire a Cold illness. The best thing to do in confusing cases is to make a quick survey of characteristics (in Types of Bodies, above) to find your normal constitution (Hot and Cold conditions when you are not sick), then compare your symptoms to the following Heat and Cold Symptoms charts. This will help you decide which of the self-help remedies in Part II to employ.

Excessive Heat Symptoms

Hot body	Constipation
Intense dislike of heat	Extreme sweating
A craving for cold drinks	Normal appetite
Continuous thirst	Strong or burning digestion
Fever	Inflammation
Red face and eyes	Infection
Dark, concentrated urine	

Fire is used to describe conditions of extreme Heat generated by the body as a result of invasion by external pathogenic factors such as Wind, Summer Heat, and Dryness (see below). All of these can turn into Fire if left untreated and the signs of Heat in these instances will be severe, potentially damaging the body's cooling moisture element, its Yin. The Yin of the Liver is especially vulnerable to Fire. When Fire combines with internal Wind, stiff neck and shoulders, convulsions, upwardly staring eyes, delirium, and convulsions could result.

Excessive Cold Symptoms

Chills in part of or entire body	Diarrhea
Desire for warmth	Low blood pressure
Aching and numbness relieved by heat	Pale and cold appearance
Frequent urination	Poor or no appetite
No desire to move	Poor digestion
Slow movement	
A craving for warm or hot drinks	
Difficulty in keeping warm	
Excretion of large volumes of clear urine	
Desire to sleep	

The lower portion of the list includes symptoms of Yang Deficiency usually related to a problem with the Kidney organ and energy system, which is said to produce Heat in the body. Prolonged exposure to Cold or a congenital Yang Deficiency can result in this pattern of Cold.

External Influences

Wind, Summer Heat, Damp, and Dryness

In addition to Cold and Heat, Wind, Summer Heat, Damp, and Dryness, are referred to throughout this book. In Oriental terms, they describe external factors that invade the body and cause imbalance or illness. In Western terms we think of these invaders as pathogens, more specifically, as germs, bacteria, and viruses. We do not use Western science's terms in Oriental medicine, but for the Western reader it might be helpful at first to think of them interchangeably.

Wind can refer to wind in the normal sense. It can also mean the sudden changes in the weather that are often seen in spring and fall. In nature, wind is fast and changes quickly. It is capricious. Just so in the body, where in Oriental medicine it is considered to be an invasion of a force of movement. Try picturing it as something leaping around the inside of the body, outside of your control, usually manifesting as aches and pains. Wind can combine with Cold, Heat, Damp, or Dryness to strengthen their effects and drive them deeper into the body. For instance, Cold may enter the body through the Kidneys in the winter, chilling the body and producing low-grade cold and flu symptoms, but if it combines with Wind, the flu can travel around the body, manifesting as aching joints and muscles and/or chills in various parts of the body. Or it can enter the Stomach and cause digestive disorders or a "stomach flu."

Wind is light and Yang in quality; it attacks from the top—it tends to attack the upper parts (again the top, or Yang) of the body first: the face, head, neck and shoulders, and Lungs. Wind enters easily after the body sweats and starts to cool. The Chinese say that an invasion of Wind at this time affects the opening and closing of the pores and can lead to respiratory problems.

Internal Wind is usually associated with disharmony in the Liver organ and its corresponding meridian system. The Oriental practitioner would diagnose sudden outbursts of anger, tremors, spasms, shaking, convulsions, and strokes as complications of Internal Wind.

Summer Heat is excess Heat that is very Yang in nature and leads to a Deficiency of Yin; the condition is common in China where people spend long hours working the fields and overexposing themselves to the sun. Summer Heat problems can also surface in people who work in abnormally warm environments such as a foundry or a bakery. Summer Heat can manifest as dizziness, thirst, nausea, concentrated

Six Environmental Excesses

六淫

LÌN YÍN
MUTSU IN

Wind

風

FĒNG
FU

Summer Heat

暑

SHǓ
SHO

urine, lassitude, constipation, and in severe cases, palpitations, delirium, and coma, or disturbed Shen energy (see Chapter 6, Pain and Vitality).

Yin Summer Heat is a condition of Coldness that arises from overingesting quantities of cold or frozen food and iced beverages in summer. In this case, the excess Yin (ice) is said to combine with excess Yang (Heat), resulting in chills, a dull headache, abdominal pain with diarrhea, and profuse sweating—the summer cold.

Dampness

SHĪ
SHITSU

Damp symptoms include a feeling of heaviness that usually occurs in the lower limbs, sluggishness, a tight feeling in the head as if it were wrapped in an elastic bandage, edema, dizziness, a sticky mouth with a sweet taste, a thick, greasy coating on the tongue. Damp is a feeling of heaviness and congestion. It tends to sink in the solar plexus and lower abdominal areas (two centers of energy in Oriental medicine that are part of the Triple Heater meridian system—the Middle Burner is in the area of the stomach and the Lower Burner is a couple of inches below the bellybutton) to cause indigestion, nausea, diarrhea, and fullness in the abdomen. Damp also manifests as skin eruptions, discharges like leukorrhea, and turbid urine.

Damp diseases often appear in late summer in humid climates or during the rainy season (where there is one). Such diseases also result from working or living in a wet or damp environment, wearing wet clothes, or eating too many foods that aggravate Damp—deep-fried foods, cold and raw foods, and dairy products. If Damp combines with Heat, any discharge or inflammation already in the body will become more severe. Damp is one of the most difficult invaders to clear and diseases involving Damp often require long-term treatment.

Dryness

ZÀO
SŌ

Dryness and Dry conditions most frequently occur when the air is driest. In China and Japan, the driest time of year runs from late autumn to the end of winter, which is why autumn and dryness are associated with one another under the Five Element Theory. Dryness is Yang and can lead to a Deficiency of Yin. The Lungs are most vulnerable in autumn. Dry symptoms may include dry, rough, or chapped skin; a dry nose, mouth, and lips; dry, sore throat; dry cough with little phlegm; and dry stools.

External Influence	Nature	Symptoms/Manifestations
Wind	Light, Yang, movement, changes quickly	Aches, pain, outbursts, trembling, spasms, stroke
Summer Heat	Yang, drains Yin	Thirst, dizziness, nausea, concentrated urine, weakness, fatigue, constipation, palpitations, delirium, disturbed Shen

External Influence	Nature	Symptoms/Manifestations
Damp	Heavy, sluggish, tightness, congestion	Edema, dizziness, sweet sticky mouth, indigestion, nausea, diarrhea, fullness in abdomen, skin eruptions, leukorrhea
Dry	Drying	Dry skin, nose, throat, stool

Emotions and Imbalance

For thousands of years the Chinese have classified seven categories of emotions and discussed their effects on the internal organs and energy systems. Rather than focusing on the emotional condition of the client, however, in making a diagnosis the Oriental practitioner considers the main emotion exhibited by the patient to be another symptom in his or her pattern of imbalance.

In China and Japan, both of which existed long before the West evolved the idea of the primacy of the individual, emotional factors were taken into consideration, along with internal and external factors, when a practitioner determined the progression of a patient's illness. But traditionally, the role of the emotions was not particularly emphasized nor overemphasized in this determination. Most holistic practitioners today also agree that disease has an emotional component to a greater or lesser degree and that serious diseases include a significant emotional component.

It is hard to say just how great or small this component actually is—surely that depends on the individual. However, emotional imbalance and illness do interact in a dynamic way. The person experiencing great anger may experience an imbalance in the Liver. Conversely, a person abusing the Liver by ingesting too much alcohol, caffeine, and food additives and preservatives in refined and processed foods may begin to exhibit anger and emotional instability more frequently. Emotional factors can cause disease; they can also be the symptoms of a disease.

Joy, Excitement, Fright

The Heart and the energy it houses, the Shen, are affected most by the emotions of joy, excitement, and fright. Insomnia, bursts of laughter or fits of tears, an inability to think clearly, delirium, or hysteria may result. The exhaustion of Blood and/ or Yin Deficiency from overwork, childbirth, and hemorrhaging affect the Heart and may bring about emotional disturbances such as anxiety, insomnia, and phobias.

The Seven Emotions

QĪ QÍNG
NANA JŌ

Grief, Sadness

Grief and sadness affect the Lungs, weakening the body, causing lassitude, creating a desire to be alone, and paling the complexion. The body may weaken; it may slump: shoulders hunch forward, the chest is compressed, the breath is shallow, and energy does not circulate. Left untreated, this condition can lead to Lung problems.

Worry, Obsessive Thought

Worry and obsessive thoughts affect the Spleen. Worry also damages the Lungs. Constant worry and obsession can lead to digestive problems—from minor discomfort, such as feelings of fullness and distention after eating only small amounts, and diarrhea—to problems as severe as anorexia. Imbalance in the Spleen can also cause worrying and obsession.

Fear, Fright

Fear weakens the Kidneys. It also drives the body's Qi downward to the intestines, bladder, urethra, and anus. Sudden fright can impair the Kidneys and lead to fluid imbalance. Persons with weak Kidneys may seem fearful by nature, fear commitment, or suffer from phobias or paranoia. Physically they may suffer from edema, swollen face, and bags under the eyes. Long-term fearful feelings can lead to serious Kidney imbalance, while a Kidney imbalance can lead to experiencing feelings of fear.

Anger, Frustration, and Depression

Anger affects the Liver, which is probably the organ most sensitive to emotional influence. Anger causes Qi and Blood to rise to the head, neck, and shoulders resulting in stiffness, pain, headache, ringing in the ears, redness in the eyes, and sinus problems. Prolonged anger can cause Liver Fire (convulsions, coma, delirium) and may cause the Liver Qi to invade the Stomach/Spleen organs and energy systems, leading to indigestion, pain in the ribs and abdomen, abdominal distention, belching, nausea, acid reflux, and hypertension. Anger can also affect the Liver's function of storing and regulating Blood, leading to irregular or difficult menstrual periods. Liver Qi imbalance also leads to irritability, anger, frustration, and depression.

Shock

Shock affects the respiration and circulation of Qi by injuring the Heart and "Chest Qi," which nourishes the chest and the Lungs. Traditionally shock was said to evict the Shen from the Heart, leaving the body's spiritual center displaced. Severe shock can lead to a loss of consciousness. Long-term shock affects emotional stability.

Endnote

*1 Some people are able to intuit or "see" the connections between points along the body's meridians and have counted up to 350 points in the body. This brings up the interesting topic of the plurality of schools that, looking in from the outside, appear to make up one uniform school of Traditional Oriental Medicine. Proponents of schools of Oriental medicine have long held differing opinions concerning the number of points and meridians.

C H A P T E R 3

Eating Alive

O ne should be mindful of what one consumes to ensure proper growth, reproduction, and development of bones, tendons, ligaments, channels, and collaterals: This will help generate the smooth flow of Qi and Blood, enabling one to live to a ripe age.[1]

The Yellow Emperor's Classic of Medicine

Oriental Folk Wisdom of Food

The Japanese story *The Tale of the Making of the Jewel*, contained in the early Heian Period book, *Six Major Poets (Rokkasen)*,[2] is about the life and times of "the most beautiful woman in the world, Ono No Komachi." The story documents the daily life and eating habits of Ono no Komachi, a woman of modest means who became a lady of great privilege. What did the lady eat? All kinds of fish, game—duck, bear, rabbit, and deer—and her grain of choice was an unrefined brown rice cooked down to easily digestible gruel. Her favorite food, however, was barley mixed with *yamaimo* (literally, mountain potato), known to doctors of herbal medicine as dioscorea.

In those days the yamaimo was considered a delicacy that could only be found growing in the wild. It was listed in Shen Nung's *Chronicles of Trees and Grasses (Shinnō Honzōkyō)* as having a salutary effect on the internal organs, supplementing a weak constitution, and if eaten for a prolonged period of time, stretching the earlobe—a metaphor for increasing longevity.

Today, in dried root form, dioscorea is used in Chinese medicinal cooking as a secondary tonic—meaning that it supports and rounds out primary tonics. It is also an important Yin tonic, promoting the intellect, the spirit, and a long life. It

ONO NO KOMACHI

Chronicles of Trees and Grasses or *The Divine Husbandman's Classic of the Materia Medica.* (Later Han Dynasty)

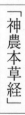

SHÉN NÓNG BĚN CAŎ JĪNG
SHINNŌ HONZŌKYŌ

strengthens and tonifies the Stomach/Spleen system, nourishes the Lungs, and supplements Kidney Qi. It has also been found to have steroid precursors.

Ono no Komachi ate yamaimo grated over barley (a mixture called *mugi-toro*). When the root is grated, it becomes sticky. High in mannan and amino acids, it expands when it enters the stomach. When barley and yamaimo are eaten together, they make the diner feel full and prevent overeating. In the intestines, the water-soluble dietary fiber of the yamaimo meets with the non-water-soluble fiber in barley to clear the stool and cleanse the intestines. Clear intestines result in healthy and clear skin and Lungs, while the body stays slender and attractive.

In other words, the yamaimo is a perfect beauty-enhancing food. Yamaimo is traditionally grated and mixed with raw tuna; the combination of the white of the ground root and the vivid fleshy pink or red of the tuna aesthetically pleases the eye and stimulates the palate and the digestive juices. It also combines harmoniously with many other foods to facilitate digestion—characteristics of this root that wise Japanese cooks have always appreciated.

Ono no Komachi's food preferences, based on a knowledge of food's effects on the body, became common wisdom in Japan in later centuries. A mother feeding her brood, who was constantly aware of the physical condition of everyone in her house, chose foods that would contribute to her family's general well-being and at the same time correct imbalances suffered by a particular family member.

The knowledge of food's effects on the body was also commonly held folk wisdom in China, and Chinese cooks rely on this wisdom even today. In both China and Japan, martial artists, Oriental medical practitioners, priests, monks, and nuns have traditionally cooked this way for themselves as well. Whenever Peter and I go to study with our kung fu master in Canton we are fed foods specifically chosen to strengthen or stimulate a particular organ channel that the forms we are learning are also stimulating.

On my first trip to China to study kung fu, I went with three other women—I had had a uterine hemorrhage only a few weeks before. After explaining this to my teacher, my kung fu partners and I found ourselves eating heart several times a week—it builds the Blood. After a couple of weeks of eating this way, our bodies were terribly confused by the whole thing, and we all became constipated. After complaining to our teacher, we found a particular type of green vegetable on the table for a week straight. "Good for this," the master would say, pointing to his large intestine. Food is enormously important in China, and was obviously the subject of much of the discussion that went on between our teacher and the cook at dinner time. Even though we could understand little of their conversation, it was clear that our teacher and Ma Yi, or Auntie Yi, the cook, spent countless evenings talking about the effects of food on the body, proper preparation, and how much of what foods we should eat.

We were never urged to cut coffee, black tea, sugar, or alcohol out of our diets, probably because we were basically healthy and were practicing kung fu for six hours a day. On such a schedule the normal body can handle practically any toxin in limited amounts. But I was there to heal cysts and anemia, and cut out sugar and caffeine of my own volition. My teacher understood and approved. He never encouraged extreme ways of eating, however. Eating regularly and healthily, getting plenty of exercise, and building Qi are the foundations of health—extreme acts do not cultivate a firm foundation, especially for a relatively young person.

One of the most important differences between the way foods are prepared in China and the way we cook here is that the Chinese food-shop daily. This is probably a main factor in the effectiveness of dietary therapy. Once in a while I would go shopping with Auntie Yi, a round, bashful woman with a ready smile. The market, teeming with shoppers at 9:30 in the morning, is like no other for its chaos and crowds. Chickens squawk, children squeal, hawkers hawk. Stalls—piled high with greens plucked fresh from the fields that morning—line several blocks of side streets. Butchers hang slabs of freshly slaughtered beef, pork, dog, and fowl. The blood runs into the street and mixes with fish innards, feathers, dung, and spit. Tofu, ginger, garlic, red peppers, and various strange balls of fish and meat pastes—all of it so fresh that it still smells like the tofu factory, the chicken coop, or the ground it came from—give the market its distinctive Asian mark. The strong smells emanating from mountains of dried mushrooms, thousand-year-old preserved duck eggs, and fresh coriander satiate the senses. A kind of rough lusciousness is built into the concept of eating from the moment food is sold.

In China, food is usually the first course of treatment employed to correct an imbalance. Practitioners are taught to try food and qigong to get the energy flowing and shifting before they dispense herbs. The foods contain Cooling or Warming energies, and have dispersing, consolidating, ascending, and descending properties (see Food Energetics, pages 62 to 64). To determine which foods are best to use in your case, first read Types of Imbalances (pages 47–52). Consider whether you have a Hot, Cold, Excess, or Deficient condition. Sometimes you will manifest a combination of imbalances. This is usually the case. Eat to balance the condition that is most acute. If constipation is the problem, you will want to eat quantities of fresh vegetables with high water and fiber contents, and whole grains. If you are down with the flu and chills, easy-to-digest thin rice porridge with warming ginger and scallions would be the way for you to nourish and warm your body without spending too much of the body's energy, which is needed for healing, on digestion.

In Japan, until the current generation (which counts calories and reads recipe books just like Western cooks do), mothers and others in charge of food combinations followed a traditional list of foods to combine, called the *Tabeawase Hyo*. It was part of the common wisdom, said to be derived from the *Yōjokun* by Kaibara Masuken, the first recorded list of food combinations in Japan. Historians are fairly certain that Kaibara's work, in turn, was derived from various similar Chinese works on proper diet, hygiene, and food combining.

Although the traditional food combination lists have gone the way of the kimono and jinrikisha, on them one finds combinations classic to the cuisine: tofu with bonito flakes, miso soup with *abura age* (a type of deep-fried tofu), grilled fish with grated daikon root and soy sauce, and so forth. Close scientific examination of these traditional food combinations has shown that in many instances they do indeed have numerous beneficial effects on the body. The ancients knew why they were eating various foods.

Basic Eating Guidelines

> *The superior man is careful of his words and temperate in eating and drinking.*[3]
>
> I-Ching

To avoid building complication into your life, keep general guidelines in your head concerning food, meal planning, cooking, and eating. The following list of guidelines expresses the attitude of the Middle Way; it is meant to be followed flexibly, in a style that suits your needs.

1) Eat meals at the same time daily. But don't force yourself to eat if you do not feel hungry.
2) Eat enough to satisfy but never until you are full.
3) Vary the type of foods at each meal and from day to day.
4) Don't mix too many types of food at any one time.
5) Chew your food well.
6) Refrain from eating too much of any one type of food.
7) Make sure your food is well washed and properly cooked. Do not reheat food more than once, but reheat thoroughly.
8) When possible eat natural and organically grown food.
9) Eat food that is as fresh as possible.
10) Avoid eating a meal before bed.

In Lancashire, where Peter comes from, it is said that one should "Eat breakfast like a king, lunch like a prince, and dinner like a pauper." The Stomach's most active time of day is from 7–9 A.M., the optimum time to break-the-fast. Food is digested more efficiently in the morning, and most people have more energy during the day if they eat an adequate breakfast. At night the body is winding down, the body's energy is more slow, and one is less apt to be active. Food takes more time to digest, and eating late does not allow the Stomach to take a much-needed break. A healthier option is to eat the last meal of the day about 12 hours before you wake to begin the next day.

Oriental medical practitioners agree that there is no single method of food-choosing suitable for everyone. Oriental medical practitioners studiously avoid rules such as "Eat raw food, or cooked as little as possible," "Drink eight glasses of water a day," or "Eat 2 ounces or less of meat a day." Instead, they counsel that each of us needs to determine what types of food are most appropriate to our needs. Meat may benefit the health of a Cold, weakened constitution by building up strength, while it could actually be detrimental to a person with a Hot constitution on the verge of manifesting a serious heart or liver problem. Likewise, raw foods are beneficial for a healthy person or one with a Normal or Warm constitution, but they can aggravate someone with a weak Spleen, causing nausea, belching, abdominal pain, and distention, and showing up undigested in the stool.

The Four Phases and Eating

The Four Phases described in Chapter 2 also affect our eating patterns. Each phase of growth and development presents special dietary needs and limitations.

Babies and young children, for example, have weak digestive systems that the Chinese feel cannot handle large amounts of meat, whole grains, deep-fried, and cold foods. Straining the developing digestive system can produce an excess of phlegm.

Teenagers need to eat larger quantities of food to provide their growing bodies with adequate nourishment, but budding sexual maturity can create an excess of Heat in the body, appearing later as acne and also as rambunctiousness, irritability, instability, and a proneness to temper tantrums. Adolescents should avoid excessively spicy, rich, deep-fried, and fatty foods.

As a rule, adults can eat freely but should do so in moderation. Eat when hungry, not out of habit or by the clock. Eat sitting down, in a serene environment where you can concentrate on eating. Take extra care when eating out and try to choose the restaurant if you can. Stay away from heavy, fatty, deep-fried foods, in favor of lightly steamed vegetables, soups, and rice. You don't have to be rigid, but do try to balance things out—eat a wide variety of foods. If you find yourself falling into the habit of eating light, no-fat "legal" meals during the day only to "make up for it" at and after dinner, relax a little at lunch. It is far better to take the middle road and improve gradually than to develop binge eating patterns.

Traditionally, the Chinese say that older people's diets should resemble an infant's more than a young adult's. Warming, well-cooked grains, legumes, and vegetables; broths; and simmered dishes will give the body stability and strength without burdening it with excess calories and added pounds. Many older people, having worked hard all their lives, feel they should be able to eat anything they like. Wise food choices can help prevent a dulling of the mind and clogged digestion, constipation, and the loss of appetite that often plagues older people.

Food's Role in Bringing the Body Back to Balance

Warming a Chilly Person

In diagnosis, a practitioner of Oriental medicine discovers where disharmony is located in the body; often the source of imbalance lies within the digestive system. One of the aims of this book is to elucidate the role of food in helping to correct minor imbalances, thereby preventing them from progressing to the point of becoming disease.

Recently Peter treated a woman with a cough and digestive difficulties: she experienced a loss of appetite, bloating after eating, a heavy waterlogged feeling in the legs, flatulence, loose stool, and fatigue. Her diet consisted principally of raw food; typically, she had fruit in the morning, a salad for lunch, and pasta with vegetables shortly before bed. She snacked on fruit and yogurt, and drank a few cups of coffee a day. She sometimes woke at night suffering physical discomfort, and felt tired and fatigued throughout the day. She had been raised on a typical European diet of meat, vegetables, and bread.

The diagnosis was Dampness in the Spleen, a condition that results from too much raw, cold food, excessive intake of liquid, and too many dairy products.

In cases like this, food can be used as an aid to strengthen the digestive system and clear the Dampness out. Raw food was eliminated from this person's diet, because it was forcing the already overworked Spleen to work harder. A regimen of Warming, nourishing foods consisting mostly of whole grains cooked to a gruel consistency, chicken broths, and root vegetables was prescribed, along with advice to cut back on fluid intake and Damp-producing foods such as dairy products and deep-fried foods. The patient was asked to substitute energy-nurturing herbal teas for cold water. Cold water exacerbates the lack of Fire in the Stomach, worsening digestion and contributing to the heavy build-up of Dampness.

The patient switched to a Japanese-style breakfast consisting of rice, miso soup, and perhaps some fermented soybeans (nattō) or an egg, which was more food than she was used to eating. In the early stages of treatment she had just the soup, sometimes with a few grains of rice floating in it. During these early stages she felt she still wanted fruit for breakfast, so she was asked to cook it with raisins and Warming culinary cinnamon. She was also asked to reduce her evening meal to soup, and to eat pasta, fish, and cooked vegetables at lunch. This change helped to increase her appetite in the morning and her energy level through the day.

Dairy foods can complicate Dampness in the Spleen by contributing to the formation of more Phlegm. Phlegm, a physical and energetic problem affecting the Lungs, stems from imbalance in the Spleen. When the Spleen is too weak, Dampness—not held properly in check—ascends into the Lungs, contributing to the formation of Phlegm there. Asthma, cough, or bronchitis is the result.

More specific foods could also be prescribed for the sufferer of Dampness in the

Spleen: naturally sweet, yellow or orange vegetables such as carrots, winter squash (i.e., buttercup, Hokkaido pumpkin, butternut, acorn, etc.), rutabagas, sweet potatoes, chicken, beef, and lamb; onions, green vegetables, and Warming spices—cardamom, coriander, cayenne, garlic, and fresh or dried ginger. Bitter foods and herbs—almonds, endive, and rye—would be used to eliminate the Damp and stimulate the pancreas's production of digestive juices; the rye would tone the Heart as well. This therapy is referred to as having the Mother Feed the Child. The mother in this case refers to the Heart, or Fire element, which is the mother of the Spleen/Stomach, or Earth element.

In the case of Peter's patient, after about three weeks she was noticeably stronger, her circulation had improved, and she could experiment with food on her own. She found that while salads were fine in summer, they didn't work for her as a main meal and were best eaten as a second course following warm food.

Cooling a Hot Person

At the other end of the spectrum, Peter once treated a businessman, a former rugby player, who was short and stocky. The man frequently overate at business lunches, washing lunch down with a couple of whiskeys. After such meals he suffered painful headaches that interfered with his job by preventing him from thinking clearly. His high-powered lifestyle required that the lunches continue, however, and at the time of his first consultation he was taking pain relievers for the headaches.

The patient had red eyes, a flushed, ruddy complexion, and a large belly. In addition to the headaches, he suffered from a sinus problem and constipation. He frequently had a stiff neck and shoulders, and if he got to bed after midnight, the time of day when the Liver is most active, he found it difficult to sleep. He had a strong voice and an abrasive personality, and breathed shallowly from the upper part of his chest. His pulse was strong and wiry, pointing to a Liver imbalance, and his tongue was red (indicating Heat) with a yellow coat.

The man was diagnosed as having primarily Liver Fire and Liver Yang Rising. His typical breakfast consisted of eggs, toast and jam, and coffee; a large lunch was washed down with whiskey, and for dinner, he either took his clients to an Italian, French, or Chinese restaurant, or he had an evening alone and ordered fast food, eating it while he worked.

This patient was reluctant to make any dietary changes; to be insistent would have driven him away. But, in fact, the Heat in his body had to be cooled down for the headaches to improve, and he needed to be persuaded to give up his passive "You fix me" attitude. He began by having cooked oatmeal with a glass of hot water and honey for breakfast to help move his intestines. He then began to work on improving lunches by reducing the amount of animal fat he consumed and by planning to have his meals at restaurants where he knew vegetables were readily available. Pasta with a light sauce and vegetables replaced steaks and chops. He ate the cooked food first and salads afterward. For his evening meal he switched to sandwiches on whole-meal bread.

The improvements were gradual, but as the change in eating, together with herbal medicine and acupuncture, began to take effect, the patient reported an increased appreciation for vegetables. He began to enjoy his food and to look at eating differently. As a matter of course he lost weight, began to take walks for exercise, and eventually lost the desire to drink alcohol. He also began practicing deep-breathing techniques. The headaches disappeared, but more importantly, by the end of treatment he was a vastly changed person: much more calm, balanced, and integrated.

One important point about this man's story is his unwillingness to make any changes at all in the beginning. But a sensitive practitioner can try to be understanding of this kind of refusal, work with it, provide the patient with a small lead, and hope that he will begin taking responsibility for his own health.

Food Influences and Energetics

Every food we eat affects our body in some way. Foods, like herbs, have Cooling and Warming properties. Foods also have Ascending and Descending energies. Foods that move energy upward are Yang, Warm, and Ascending. Foods that move energy downward are Yin, Cool, and Descending.

By now the concept of the medicinal or therapeutic use of food to balance our bodies may be clearer to you. Foods are chosen for their energetic properties to bring into balance the imbalances in the body. Since everyone's body and imbalances are different, the combinations of food needed will differ.

Knowledge of the properties of foods is important when we begin using food as a tool to bring our bodies back to balance. But first you need to know whether your imbalance is a Cold one or a Hot one, Deficient or Excess, Damp, Dry, or Wind. To determine this, please review Types of Bodies (page 46–47) and Types of Imbalances (page 47–49) in Chapter 2. Now refer to the information on food energetics listed below. If you are a person with a Hot constitution and a Hot imbalance, eat a few Cold and more Cooling foods in combination with lightly steamed vegetables, whole grains, and legumes—energetically Neutral foods that comprise a moderate, digestive-system-building eating plan. You don't want to eat *only* Cold foods; this diet is too extreme and can push the system further out of balance. Eating more Cool foods than Cold foods keeps the diet geared toward the Cool side of center to bring the body back to balance in general, with a little Cold influence to neutralize the Fire condition.

Foods to Cool the Body and Dispel Heat

Cold

alfalfa sprouts, bamboo shoots, banana, cantaloupe, clam, crab, grapefruit, persimmon, salt, sea vegetables, snow peas, Swiss chard, tomato, watercress, watermelon

Cool

apples, asparagus, barley, broccoli, buckwheat, burdock root, cabbage, celery, Chinese or napa cabbage, citrus fruits, dandelion greens, eggplant, lemon, lotus root, mango, millet, mung bean, pear, radish, sesame oil, soybean, spinach, strawberry, tangerine, tofu, water chestnut, wheat, wheat gluten (seitan), winter melon

Foods to Warm the Body and Dispel Cold

Hot

black pepper, cayenne, dried ginger, lamb, hot soybean oil (for Chinese noodle soup), trout

Warm

anchovy, arrowroot, barley malt, Chinese black bean, butter, cardamom, cherry, chestnuts, chicken, Chinese chives, chives, Chinese and regular culinary cinnamon, cloves, coconut milk, cooked carrot (Warm/Neutral), cooked peach, coriander, date, garlic, ginger, green bean, ham, kale, kuzu powder, leek, longan, maple syrup, molasses, mussel, mustard leaf, oats, onions, most orange and yellow vegetables, rice syrup, scallions, sesame seeds, shrimp, winter squash (i.e., buttercup, Hokkaido pumpkin, butternut, acorn, etc.) (Warm/Neutral), strawberry, sweet potato, sweet rice, turkey, walnuts

Neutral Foods

apricot, beef, brown rice, cabbage, carrot, celery, chicken eggs and gizzards, cooked carrot (Warm/Neutral), corn, duck, dried fig, grapes, herring, honey, kidney bean, lotus seed, milk, mushrooms (button and shiitake), olive, peanut oil, peas, pineapple, plum, pork, potato, Hokkaido pumpkin (Warm/Neutral), raspberry, rice bran, rye, saffron, sardine, shark meat, string bean, sugar, taro root, turnip, tuna, white fungus, yam

Tonic Foods by Organ

Lung

warming, easily digested foods to strengthen Qi. Soups, porridge, meat broths, strong broth of ginger, brown sugar (small amount lubricates Lungs), almonds, figs, ginger root, pork lung organ meat, molasses, olives (clearing), peanut, pine nut, white fungus (the silver ear clears Lung Heat)

Stomach/Spleen (and Middle Burner)

foods should be warm and easy to digest, including Warm and Neutral foods listed above. Also anise seed, azuki beans, barley, beef, black fungus (wood ears, elephant ears), brown rice (well cooked), brown sugar, chicken meat, cinnamon, fennel seed, ginger, honey, lentils, chicken and beef liver, molasses, papaya, peanut, Job's tears, peas, persimmon, potato, sweet potato, tangerine, tofu, white fungus.

Heart

celery (cools Heat affecting the Heart), black cherry, eggplant, heart organ meat, lotus root, rye, watermelon, wheat

Kidney

azuki beans, black sesame seeds, black fermented soybeans, celery, mulberry, pork kidneys, raspberry, string beans, sword beans, taro root, walnuts,[4] wheat. Chestnut, lotus seed, and potato nourish the Kidney Yin in particular.

Liver

black sesame seeds, Chinese black fermented soybeans, lemon, liver organ meat, raspberry

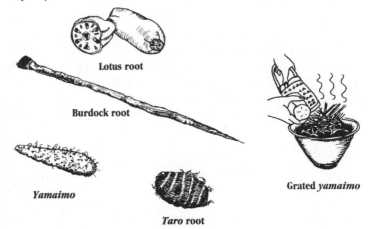

Lotus root

Burdock root

Yamaimo

Taro root

Grated *yamaimo*

Tonic Foods for Qi and Blood

Qi

foods that are Warming but not Hot, eliminating, or dispersing. Includes most vegetables, legumes, and whole grains.

Blood

beef, duck, grapes, honey, lamb, liver, milk, mugwort, oyster, red and black dates, shiitake mushroom, Chinese black fermented soybeans, spinach, strawberry, sweet-rice cakes (mochi). If there is lower back pain and dark circles under the eyes (Kidney Deficiency), include oyster, chicken livers, kidney organ meat, walnuts

The Five Tastes

The Five Tastes correspond with the Five Element Theory as described in two classical records on medicine in China, the *Nei Jing* and the *Nan Jing*. These tastes, or flavors, stimulate the movement of energy in the body. Each taste stimulates one of the organ systems more than the others.

In the *Neijing Suwen*, it says, "... Sour corresponds to the Liver, Pungent to the Lungs, Bitter to the Heart, and Salty to the Kidneys, sweet travels to the Spleen," and these are called the five entering routes.[5] The flavors enter and nourish the corresponding organs first. Once moving in the system, the flavors affect various parts of the body. The *Neijing Lingshu* says that "Sour travels to the tendons, Pungent travels to the Qi, Bitter travels to the Blood, Salt travels to the bones, and Sweet travels to the flesh."[5]

Although the flavors correspond to the organs and organ systems and these correspond to the seasons, the Chinese do not make—and neither should we—simplistic leaps in logic that would dictate, for example, eating Sour foods in spring (the seasonal correspondence to the Liver) to correct Liver imbalance, or eating more endive and dandelion in summer (the seasonal correspondence to the Heart) to stimulate the Heart. The interrelationships among the flavors, organs, and energy is more complicated.

Each taste, for example, is believed to have its own general action. Pungent foods are dispersing; foods that are Sour are astringent. The Sweet taste harmonizes and slows down the body's operating systems; Bitter foods are drying and dispensing; Salty foods have a softening effect.[6]

Each organ has a tendency to develop a particular set of imbalances that herbs, and to a lesser degree, foods, can address.

"...The Lungs disdain upward, rebellious movement, so we must administer Bitter herbs to purge and disperse. ...Lungs need to be converged or tonified with Sour herbs; Pungent herbs are used to sedate.

"...The Spleen disdains Dampness, so we must administer herbs to dry this Damp. One should avoid hot foods, overeating, and damp environments. ...The Spleen must be harmonized with Sweet herbs but sedated with Bitter herbs.

"The Heart disdains being scattered. One should consume Sour herbs to keep the Heart flow contained. ...One should avoid eating Hot foods. Heart disease should be cared for using softening methods. Salty herbs are utilized for this and for tonification. Sweet herbs are used to sedate.

"...The Kidneys disdain Dryness, so we must use Pungent and lubricating herbs to help mobilize and dispense the body fluids to lubricate the body. The Kidney requires solidifying. This is done with Bitter herbs, which tonify as well. Salty herbs are used to sedate.

"...The nature of Liver is to disdain constriction. Thus, one would consume Sweet-tasting herbs to soften it. ...Those who suffer from Liver illness respond to dispersing methods. One must therefore use Pungent herbs. If they need tonification, however, the Pungent tonics must be used for fortification. If they need sedation, Sour herbs should be used."[7]

Each taste is believed to have corresponding contra-indications as well. "Because the pungent taste disperses Qi, one should avoid eating Pungent foods in diseases of the Qi. Bitter taste purges the Blood. Thus in Blood disease one should avoid Bitter foods. Salty taste drains the bones and thus should be avoided in bone diseases. Sweet taste bloats the flesh. Thus, in diseases of the flesh, avoid Sweet foods. Sour taste contracts the tendons and should therefore be avoided in diseases of the tendons."[8]

A fairly overweight man under intense pressure at work may visit an acupuncturist for frequent pounding migraine and sinus headaches. Upon further questioning, this man would also admit he is suffering from a stiff neck, shoulder pain, and chronic constipation. His face is unusually ruddy, and his eyes are reddish. He would be diagnosed as having an imbalance called Liver Yang Rising, in which the Fire of the Liver organ and channel is fanned by the overconsumption of foods that irritate the Liver, such as coffee, alcohol, rich, fatty foods, and heavy red meats.

The condition is complicated by a blockage in the Large Intestine. In this case, acupuncture and herbs would be given to help Cool the Liver Fire, and the patient's practitioner would not only suggest Cooling, clearing foods (such as tofu, alfalfa, watercress, and lotus root), to Cool and lower the Liver Yang but also might suggest incorporating a small amount of Sour foods to sedate the Liver, such as vinegar, lemon, plums, and azuki beans. Foods that help unblock the Large Intestine, such as whole grains and cereals, lightly steamed vegetables (leafy greens and roots), oatmeal, and foods containing mucilage (such as taro, yamaimo, konnyaku, and nattō) would also be recommended.

Keep in mind that eating too much of any one flavor can throw the entire system off balance. And remember that while the Five Flavors can be used to stimulate an organ system that is out of balance, conversely, certain flavors should be avoided during these times of imbalance. *The Yellow Emperor's Classic* says, "Improper use of the Five Flavors may also injure the five...organs. Too much Sour taste may cause overactivity of the Liver and underactivity of the Spleen. Too much Salty taste can weaken the bones and cause contracture and atrophy of the muscles, as well as stagnate the Heart Qi. Too much Sweet taste can disturb the Heart Qi, causing it to become restless and congested, as well as cause imbalance of the Kidney energy, which turns the face black. Too much Bitter taste disrupts the Spleen's ability to transform and transport food, and causes the Stomach to digest ineffectively and become distended. The muscles and tendons may become scattered. Too much Pungent injures the pores and skin."[9]

In the case of a person suffering from PMS syndrome with abdominal cramps, dark clots in the menstrual blood, emotional depression, in addition to pain and distention under the ribs and sides, digestive disorders and a congested feeling in the chest, an Oriental medical practitioner would diagnose the imbalance as Liver Qi Stagnation complicated by a Deficiency in the Stomach/Spleen. To help correct the imbalance, Peter would suggest steamed greens (mustard Warming, Pungent green, or perhaps dandelion for its Bitter, Blood-tonifying properties) tossed with a dressing that has long been used as a Liver tonic—of olive oil, cayenne, and lemon. Digestion problems caused by a weak Spleen would benefit from simmered rutabaga, yam, or turnip, energetically Sweet and Warming vegetables, topped with slivered scallions (Warming, Bitter, activate Qi). These dishes can be accompanied by fish, chicken, soup or stews that include root and green, leafy vegetables, legumes, eggs, and a whole grain.

Eating with food energetics can be beneficial, but don't go overboard; the other systems in the body need to be nourished energetically as well. Keep balance in mind; eat from all the food groups; and listen to your own body—often, if you open up to its urgings, your inner intelligence will tell you what the body needs.

Ascending and Descending Foods

Food can help raise or lower energy in the body, as herbs can, but food has a somewhat less direct effect than herbs. How can this be of benefit to someone trying to rebalance his or her body? Imagine you have the flu and a cough that settles in the Lungs. Eating Ascending foods will help disperse and unblock the settled cough, excrete it through the pores, or raise it so it can be coughed up. Once the condition becomes chronic, however, you need more than food and self-help remedies to treat it. Please see a practitioner in that case. Examples of Ascending foods are: basil, bay leaf, cabbage, capers, carrot, cayenne pepper, dill and fennel seeds, garlic, ginger, mustard greens, onion, scallion, shiitake mushroom, and yam.

You can encourage clogged intestines or energy stuck in the lower abdomen to clear out by eating some foods with Descending energy. Descending foods push the block downward and facilitate its expulsion through the stool, urine, and menses. Some Descending energy foods also help lower fevers. Examples are: apple, bamboo shoots, banana, barley, buckwheat, celery, cucumber, eggplant, fig, kasha, kohlrabi, lettuce, lotus root, mung bean, muskmelon, common button mushroom, spinach, strawberry, Swiss chard, tofu, tomato, vinegar, watermelon, and wheat.

Five Tastes		Pungent	Sweet	Bitter	Salty	Sour
Directions of the Five Tastes	Entering Route	Lungs	Spleen	Heart	Kidney	Liver
	Travels to	Qi	flesh	Blood	bones	tendons
Tastes Indicated	Element	Metal/Lung	Earth/Spleen	Fire/Heart	Water/Kidney	Wood/Liver
	Functions	expels Cold and toxins, disperses, opens the pores, stimulates circulation	nourishes, warms, tonifies	hardens, dries, purges, cools	softens lumps, lubricates, draws energy downward, regulates fluid[11]	constricts, absorbs
	Symptoms	a cold, the flu, mucus congestion, blockage of fluids; need to sweat, secrete, or get your digestion moving	the body is weak, the extremities are cold; need to build and strengthen	weak digestion, high cholesterol levels, diarrhea, excessive clear vaginal discharge; need to protect the system from parasites, or stop a sweet craving	hardened, swollen lympth nodes, cysts, constipation, sore muscles; need to regulate fluids in the body	mucus, excessive perspiration and other fluid loss, clogged digestion; need to stimulate bile or digestion, drain Excess in the Liver
Excessive Intake		Injures the pores, skin, and hair	Disturbs Heart Qi Causes imbalance in the Kidney Qi	Disrupts Heart Qi Disrupts Spleen's ability to transform and transport Causes Stomach distention Scatters muscles	Weakens bones Contracts, atrophies muscles Stagnates Heart Qi Can harm the Blood	Makes tendons flaccid Results in overactivity of Liver Results in underactivity of Spleen
Contraindications		avoid in diseases of Qi and Qi Deficiency	avoid in diseases of the flesh	avoid in diseases of Blood and Blood Deficiency	avoid in diseases of the bones	avoid in diseases of tendons

Foods of the Five Tastes

Pungent
basil, bay leaf, black pepper, capers, cayenne, coriander, dill seed, fennel seed, garlic, ginger, kohlrabi, leek, marjoram, mustard greens, nutmeg, onion, peppermint, daikon/radish, rice bran, rosemary, safflower, scallion, soybean oil, spearmint, taro, turnip, watercress, wheat germ, white pepper
Sweet
most meats, fruits, vegetables, legumes, fish, dairy products, and oils
Bitter
alfalfa, asparagus, capers, celery, kohlrabi, lettuce, romaine lettuce, rye, scallion, turnip, vinegar, white pepper
Salty
barley, clam, crab, millet, mussel, octopus, oyster, pork, pork kidneys, salt,[10] sardine, sea vegetables, shark meat
Sour
azuki, cheese, grapes, litchi, mango, olive, papaya, peach, plum, saffron, strawberry, tangerine, tomato, trout, vinegar

If you are seeing a practitioner for any health problems, discuss food and the role food plays in imbalances with him or her. The practitioner will most likely make food recommendations, based on the principles of Yin and Yang, the Four Phases of growth, the Five Elements, and the seasons, to aid your recovery. It is also likely that he or she will advise you to stay away from foods that could aggravate your condition. Your practitioner should guide you in your search for the best diet for your condition and should not let personal dietary biases influence his or her advice.

Endnotes

*1 *The Yellow Emperor's Classic of Medicine*, Chapter 23, trans. Maoshing Ni (Boston: Shambhala Publications, 1995), p.12.
*2 Story is included in text by Shizuo Ōta and Tetsukan Shigeno, *Kampō wo Taberu* (Tokyo: Sanichi Shobo, 1985), pp.104–108. (Personal translation.)
*3 *I-Ching, The Book of Changes*, ed. & trans. John Blofeld (New York: Arkana/Viking, 1991).
*4 An interesting aside on nuts, and walnuts in particular: they are often associated with the Kidneys in Oriental food therapy because they physically resemble the Kidneys, the House of Jing. Jing is the "concentrated essence" of life that we receive from our parents, the seed quality of our inherited constitutions. The "concentrated essence" of a plant is found in the nut. In addition, the walnut is also similar in shape to the brain, which in Oriental medicine is said to be ruled by the Kidneys.
*5 *The Yellow Emperor's Classic of Medicine*, Chapter 23, p.95.

*6 Ibid, Chapt. 22, pp.93–94.
*7 Ibid, Chapt. 22, pp.90–92.
*8 Ibid, Chapt. 23, pp.95–96.
*9 Ibid, Chapt. 5, pp.12.
*10 Eat salt in small amounts. Too much salt causes fluid retention, high blood pressure, and/or Blood complications. Sea vegetables, rich in mineral salts, do not cause these problems.

C H A P T E R 4

The Therapies

Sleepless night.
Diet, mind, conditions
Hold the possibility of correction.[1]

Deng Ming-Dao

In the United States, Oriental medicine is equated with acupuncture. This is an accurate image, because acupuncture is the primary form of treatment in many clinics. But Oriental medicine's therapies include a rich, interesting collection of other techniques: massage, bone-setting, moxibustion, qigong, and a herbal and dietary therapy, all of which apply the same basic theories and premises as acupuncture to the same end—the regulation of energy and restoration of balance. But the techniques approach regulating that energy in different ways.

Acupuncture

"I could never have those needles stuck into me!"
How many times have we heard it? This is probably the most frequent response when I suggest to friends, family members, or acquaintances with chronic health problems that they try Oriental medicine. They shudder and dismiss the thought. The images of acupuncture that most of us have been exposed to generally include a body lying prone on the table with hundreds of foot-long needles piercing the skin, like a human pincushion—not exactly the kind of picture that would encourage one to rush out and try acupuncture.
The drama of the human pincushion rarely occurs, however. Of all the treat-

Acupuncture Method

ZHĒN LIÁO FĂ
SHINRYŌHŌ

ments I have had, ten is the most needles the acupuncturist used at any one time. Ten tiny, stainless steel needles (they can sometimes be made of gold or silver) that were discarded after use. Peter, and many practitioners like him, keep a set of needles for each client. Even though the needles are properly sterilized and reused, no client is ever touched by a set of needles used on someone else. (In the aftermath of AIDS, reusable needles may soon become obsolete, however.) Insertion of the needles is not painful. Practitioners undergo extensive training to perfect their insertion technique.

The patient usually feels something, though, particularly if the acupuncturist was trained in a Chinese technique. In China and sometimes in Japan after a needle is inserted, the acupuncturist delicately turns it until the client nods or hums a sign of acknowledgement that the energy channel has been tapped. There is a definite feeling associated with this experience. Most Japanese-trained practitioners insert very short, thin needles barely breaking the surface of the skin. These insertions are practically imperceptible.

Attaining Qi

得
気

DE QÌ
TOKKI

How, as a patient, do you know when the meridian has been tapped? It depends. Sometimes when the needle pierces there is no sensation; you may not even realize the needle has gone in. With Chinese-style acupuncture, as the practitioner manipulates the needle, suddenly you "get" it, a sensation of movement under the skin, the *De Qi*, or the "coming of the energy." Depending on the level of energy at that point in the body, the sensations range from a feeling of reverberation to a racing blaze of energy moving up or down the meridian. There may be a ringing or a tingle in another part of the body as the energy travels. Sometimes blocked energy takes a few minutes to pass, but the actual sensation is, again, very light. The few controlled clinical tests that have been done on Chinese and Japanese styles have not shown any one form of acupuncture to be clearly more effective than the others.[2]

Once the needles are inserted, they will be left in the skin for an average of 15 minutes to half an hour; during this time the patient, covered with a light blanket or sheet, may relax, meditate, or sleep. When a needle is removed, there may be a red mark in its place, which will fade momentarily. It signals that the needle was "on target" and its influence should affect a shift toward balance and health.

The points, found according to the measure of the patient's own thumb, a measurement called the *cun*, are gateways to the meridians, Qi, and Blood. Stimulating or unblocking this energy can have wide-ranging effects; pain can be alleviated or sensation completely blocked. Moods can be improved: anxiety lifted, fear quelled, anger soothed. Neuralgia, muscle, joint and tendon pain, cramps, headaches, and eyestrain can melt away. The effects depend on proper diagnosis and the combination of points chosen by the practitioner to correct imbalance.

Acupuncture treatment for chronic, long-term problems often takes a while.

"It didn't take you a week to get sick; it's not going to take a week to get better," Peter often says. My first experience with acupuncture was to correct my menstrual cycle that had been suppressed for nine years. Treatment consisted of weekly treatments with Peter for about six months. Patience pays off—the time during the course of treatment can be constructively spent making lifestyle and dietary changes to foster balance and bring one closer to homeostasis.

Moxibustion

Moxibustion Method

JIŬ FĂ
KYŪ PŌ

Moxibustion is a form of heat therapy that warms and stimulates the body's Qi and is recommended for imbalances of a Cold, Cool, or Deficient nature. Cold hands and feet, cramps in the lower abdomen, pain in the lumbar, and digestion difficulties are problems typically treated with moxibustion. The moxa itself is a dried herb (Chinese mugwort), rolled into a small ball and placed over a slice of garlic or ginger, which acts as insulation between the skin and the burning herb. The garlic and ginger have healing and warming properties of their own that aid the treatment. The mugwort may also be packed into a long cylindrical stick, which is lit at one end, held over a point and gently rotated in circular movements, or rocked back and forth over the area to stimulate and warm it.

Moxa sticks can be used frequently, particularly in winter, to relieve local pains such as sore muscles or shoulders that signal the onset of a cold, back pain during PMS, menstrual cramps, sciatic and rheumatic pain, and constriction under the rib cage. Sometimes distal points—those points further down the related meridian—are added, such as a Stomach point on the lower leg, to augment the treatment. You can learn to do this for yourself, and the sticks can be purchased by mail or at pharmacies that sell Oriental medicine equipment. Moxa sticks make an excellent addition to your Emergency Self-Help Kit. (See the sections on salt ring and ginger moxibustion on pages 94–95 in Chapter 6. See also ordering information in the Appendix.)

A caution: be careful using the sticks. They are hot, and the rocking motion of the treatment can lull even an old professional into a stupor. Once in China, a doctor applied a moxa stick treatment to my belly and kept nodding off into sleep, nearly touching the lit stick to my abdomen several times. He caught each slip just in the nick of time, and I wondered if he were teasing. At any rate, play music or keep someone nearby to talk to while treating yourself to avoid similar near-heart-attack situations.

Moxibustion is *not* to be used for conditions of Heat, including fever, inflammation, high blood pressure, and heart problems.

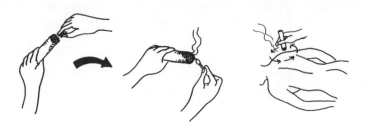

Massage

AŇ MŌ
AN MA

Massage Therapy

The patient's particular set of imbalances dictate the therapies that will be used in treatment. *Tui na* (Chinese massage) and acupressure are widely practiced as an accompaniment to acupuncture. By themselves they constitute far-reaching preventative treatment, physical therapy, and an effective means of self-treatment.

Tui na (pronounced too-ee *nah*), or *anma* (in Japanese), dates back to about 2,000 B.C., says Master Share Lew, a Taoist priest in his 70s who was the first person, to our knowledge, to openly teach *tui na* techniques to Americans, in the early 1970s. Lew's style of *tui na* includes 13 different hand techniques that resemble acupressure, French and Swedish massage, chiropractic manipulation, and Rolfing. The ancient Chinese method of bone repairing is also a form of *tui na*.

Acupressure (or shiatsu, as it is called in Japanese) is closely related to acupuncture in that it involves direct stimulation of the same points. The difference is that acupressure does not penetrate the skin. The acupressure practitioner may use a small wooden stick to stimulate points, but generally pressure is applied with the fingertips, the knuckles, and the elbow.

All forms of massage stimulate the Qi and Blood through direct contact with the skin, promote blood circulation, and stimulate nerves, muscle, skin, and bone. Massage is often given before acupuncture in Oriental medicine clinics. It is also a common feature of martial arts practice-rooms, where banged and bruised limbs are treated to a deep and rough massage with Dit Dat Jao (kung fu lotion, see Glossary), Tiger Balm, or a commercial massage cream containing camphor or eucalyptus.

Acupressure

ZHĬ HOU
SHI ATSU

Acupressure

Many of the Self-Care sections of Part II of this book include a combination of acupressure points that have been commonly used in Oriental medicine to help alleviate a syndrome and its symptoms. The points are illustrated on the BodyMap, page xx. Names of points are in English, Chinese, and Japanese. A written description of the location of each point is also included.

The amount of pressure applied to the points depends on the individual's comfort and tolerance level. Different schools of massage suggest different amounts of pressure, but in general it is safe to let your body's natural intelligence dictate.

Look for a sensitivity at the acupressure spot; press and rub or warm with moxibustion (except in cases of inflammation) until the sensitivity diminishes, or the bump or hard spot under the skin begins to dissipate. We indicate instances where intense pressure or moxibustion may actually be detrimental.

Herbal Medicine

Herbal Medicine

HÀN FĂ
KAMPŌ

The Chinese pharmacopeia includes some 6,000 substances, of which about 300 are commonly used in over 800 formulas. Chinese herbalism is a rich school of study in itself. Properly diagnosing imbalance and prescribing the right combination of herbs in the correct proportions is nothing less than an art. Years of study are required. Nigel Dawes, a Japan- and China-trained herbalist from Britain, and the director of the New Center for Holistic Health's Herbology Department in Long Island, New York, describes three stages in the study of herbal medicine. Traditionally, he says, students get to know the individual herbs, a two-year study. This is followed by a year of memorizing herbal formulas. After a minimum of three years of study, students are allowed to begin to see patients, diagnose, and prescribe herbs, but this is only the beginning of a path that could take a lifetime to tread, if one aspires to understand the complexities and nuances of this field. And only after many years of practice, he adds, can an herbologist attain complete command over the herbs and formulas and fully understand the synergetics of the combinations and how they will affect each patient—the true art of herbology.

The Japanese version of herbology, called *kampō*, has existed for over a thousand years, but seemed in danger of obsolescence with the introduction of Western allopathic medicine in the second half of the nineteenth century. It was Keisatsu Otsuka, the founder of the Kitazato Hospital in Tokyo, who rescued it from that fate. He organized patterns of symptoms into syndromes treatable by *kampō* formulas that allopathic doctors, who did not have the time to study Oriental medicine deeply but who were interested in combining the benefits of modern Western medicine and traditional Eastern medicine, could easily employ.

This approach revolutionized health care in Japan, where *kampō* is a popular and widely used branch of medicine today. There are dozens of books that help lay people identify symptoms and diagnose imbalance by themselves. Some pharmacies that stock herbal medicine also employ a trained herbalist to interview customers and help them choose an appropriate herbal medicine. Allopathic medicine and *kampō* exist side by side, maintaining a surprisingly harmonious and complementary relationship. In major metropolitan areas, at least, it is relatively easy to find a doctor of Western medicine who has studied Oriental medicine. My gynecologist in Tokyo offers her patients the choice of Eastern or Western therapy. Odd for a gynecologist—at least in my experience—one minute she would analyze mood swings in terms of my estrogen/progesterone imbalance, and the next, tell me to sing happy songs to buoy my spirits (a common Chinese remedy for the blues).

You will find a number of herbs from the Oriental medicine pharmacopeia recommended in *Back to Balance*. These commonly used herbs function primarily as tonics—strengtheners that increase energy levels, vitality, and longevity. Tonics (or Superior Herbs as they are also called) have been used in China for thousands of years. The legendary sage Shen Nung is said to have discovered and consumed dozens of them about four thousand years ago. Tonic herbs possess Warming or Cooling properties and have direct effects on the meridians, blood circulation, and the body's orifices. Some tonic herbs are detoxifying while others are anti-inflammatory, drying, moistening, or nourishing. Some herbs quiet a specific organ while others are stimulants or have aphrodisiac qualities.

Tonic herbs may be taken for prolonged periods without side effects, but contraindications are listed when they apply. Tonic herbs should be used only when the body is in relatively good health. It is important that tonics not be taken when you are sick. Don't take a warming herb, such as astragalus, for example, after cold and chills have broken out—this can weaken the body further by driving the illness deeper into the system. Two herbs to use with discretion are *ma huang* and Korean ginseng. *Ma huang* is a Lung and Kidney tonic, a stimulant, and a common asthma remedy. It can be very drying and can weaken the Yin energy if used for a prolonged period of time. Korean ginseng can be too strong, producing an uncomfortable nervous "high" similar to that of caffeine in people with Hot constitutions. Please speak to a practitioner before taking either herb, particularly if you have a heart condition.[3]

Folk Remedies

Folk Remedies

民
間
療
法

MIN JIĂN LIĂU FĂ
MINKAN RYŌHŌ

Folk cures make up a large portion of this book and they are the medicine of the common people, truly the oldest form of medicine on earth. In the West there exists an extensive body of folk medicine that incorporates indigenous fruits, vegetables, trees, bushes, and common weeds. As Oriental foods and medicine continue to make their way across the world and into the American marketplace, more and more of us will have access to the fruits, vegetables, legumes, wines, spices, and herbs that make up the Oriental home remedy kit. The medicinal value of some vegetables is simply astounding. The lotus root, for instance, works to heal hemorrhoids and cough. The daikon radish is an excellent food for a cold sufferer, helping bring down a fever and dispel a nagging cough.

When folk remedies work, a quick look at the food's energetic qualities, flavor, and function often reveals why. The lotus root, for example, is Sweet and Cold; it affects the Spleen, the Stomach, and the Heart. Congestion in the Lung is Damp Heat that can be caused by an imbalance in the Spleen meridian, which the lotus root would help rebalance. The lotus root also has hemostatic (stops bleeding) properties that help relieve hemorrhoidal bleeding. It can be ingested or applied externally for that purpose.

The daikon radish, similarly, is Cool, Pungent, and Sweet. Its primary effects are on the Lungs and Stomach. Its applications are internal and external, meaning the radish can be eaten as well as applied in compress form over the skin. When applied as a compress, the skin acts as a digestive organ, absorbing the energetic properties of the daikon essence and transporting them to where they are needed.

Dietary Therapy

Dietary Therapy

YAŌ SHÀN
YAKU ZEN

Dietary therapy is a very helpful and accessible branch of Oriental medicine that can be used to prevent illness and rebalance the body. Many practitioners of Oriental medicine find that much illness results as a repercussion of digestion or dietary problems. Cleaning the system and eating foods appropriate to one's body type and condition can have tremendous health benefits. The energetics of food and general dietary guidelines are discussed in greater detail in Chapter 3.

A note: Although we have written extensively on food's therapeutic benefits, it should be emphasized that there are no absolutes concerning food. Healthy adults ought to be able to eat anything in moderation, and even foods whose nutritive value is questionable are, at times, okay. Fat, for example, though its reputation is currently suffering, is not intrinsically bad for us and is necessary in small amounts, yet current studies of Americans with blocked arteries show that the elimination of fats completely from the diet, in conjunction with lifestyle changes, reverses atherosclerosis. The therapeutic use of food is relative and depends very much on the background and current health situation of the patient. Conversely, the avoidance of foods that do have nutritive value can also, at times, be beneficial. Spicy foods, for example, activate Qi, promote sweat, and are appropriate in hot weather. A person with a Spleen, Liver, or Heart imbalance, however, might be advised to avoid spicy foods until he or she had recovered completely.

Furthermore, the Chinese believe that one's emotional state at the time of ingestion is nearly as important as the nutritional and energetic qualities of food. Genuine pleasure derived from eating a certain food makes that food beneficial for that body. Eating when angry, on the other hand, can prevent the smooth and efficient digestion and absorption of food, no matter how nutritious it is, objectively speaking.

Hands-on Self-Help Techniques

Decocting and Infusing Herbs

Many remedies in the Self-care sections are medicinal teas. We suggest you purchase the bulk herb and make the tea yourself by decocting the roots and berries or infusing the fresh or dried leaves. Prepackaged herbal tea bags are fine as alternatives to caffeinated beverages, but they do not contain enough herb to be of use medicinally. The average tea bag contains 2 to 3 grams of herb, while a medicinal infusion, to have any real effect on the body, calls for at least 10 grams per $^3/_4$ liter of water.

Decoctions

Herbal decoctions are made by cooking about 5 to 10 grams of roots, barks, berries, twigs, and other hard parts of the plant in a cup and a half of water. They are boiled in a fireproof ceramic pot or a Chinese herb cooker for one minute and then simmered for 10 to 20 minutes, or until the liquid is reduced by a quarter to one-half, depending on how strong a decoction is desired.

Chinese herb cookers are porcelain or earthenware pots with two lids: a flat lid and a dome cap over that. They come in several sizes; the smallest size holds about two cups of water and herbs. The herbs are added to water, covered with both tops, then placed in a metal pot of water, which is brought to a boil, then turned down to a simmer, to cook the herbs for the next 10 to 15 minutes. The cookers can be purchased in Chinatowns.

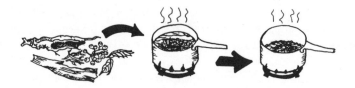

Infusions

Herbal infusions are teas made from the fresh or dried leaves of herbs. Slightly crush or bruise fresh herbs to release the volatile oils before pouring hot water over them. Use about 2 rounded tablespoons for a pot if you are drinking the tea for its medicinal value. A ceramic teapot makes the best container. Infusion time is 3 to 5 minutes.

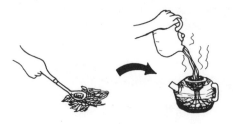

Compress

A compress is a warm herbal fluid applied to a bandage or cloth and fastened to the body. The body absorbs the healing properties of the herb or food through the pores as if the skin were another organ of digestion. Keep the compress warm by placing a hot-water bottle or heating pad over it. Ginger, daikon radish, and burdock root are commonly used for compresses. The root or herb is grated and boiled, then a clean towel, piece of muslin, or cotton cloth is soaked in it and applied over the affected area. A compress can help relieve swelling, cramps, spasms, energy blocks (pain), and muscle aches.

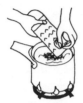

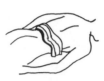

Hydrotherapy

The Bath

FU RO

Herbal Baths

The bathing tradition is highly regarded in Japan. Bath-taking has very tangible effects: it can stabilize emotions, increase circulation, and reduce stress. Bath salts from hot springs, floral salts, dried herbs, fresh fruit, flowers, branches, and leaves have been added to baths in Japan for hundreds of years. Some of these fragrant baths have become national traditions. The distinctive citrus, yuzu, a frequent ingredient in winter stews, is added to the tub at New Year's to improve digestion, strengthen the Stomach, increase the body's intake of vitamin C, support the function of blood capillaries, prevent frostbite, warm the body, give relief to aching joints and tendons, and uplift and refresh the spirit.

Sweet flag leaves (*shōbu*, sometimes misleadingly translated as Japanese iris) are said to help warm a Cold constitution, alleviate neuralgic, rheumatic, muscular, and lumbar pain, and lower the blood pressure. Traditionally, they are added to the tub on May 5th in recognition of the national holiday Children's Day. The fresh or dried leaves of the daikon radish are circulation-stimulators and are used to regulate mood swings, alleviate neuralgia, neck, shoulder, and head aches, and stimulate circulation in the lower abdomen. *Cryptomeria* branches, which are kept in the glass cases of sushi bars for their antibacterial properties, can be added to baths in spring for a toning, rejuvenating, skin-tonifying hydrotherapeutic experience.

To use fresh plants in the bath, put the whole flowers in, or scatter the petals onto the water's surface. If you are using the flowers and stems, as could be done with calendula, or only the stems, as with the sweet flag, tie them together with string or rubber bands. Bruise the stems and flowers slightly before adding a bunch or two to the water. Or, if you are using branches, you can make a decoction of the branches, strain it, and add the liquid to the bath before you get in. To use the dried herb, put it into a fabric bag, tie the bag shut, and infuse in hot water. Add the infusion and the bag to the bath. Let the bag float in the tub while it fills and keep it in as you soak. To make a ginger bath, grate a 2-to-3-inch-long piece of ginger, cook it in a liter or so of water for 10 to 15 minutes, and add that to the bath. Or place the grated (or sliced) ginger in a bag and add that directly to the tub water as the bath fills. Leave it in as you soak. The second method produces a lighter solution. Directions for other baths are included in the Self-Care sections.

Sitz Baths

A sitz, or partial immersion, bath is taken to stimulate the circulation and tone the smooth muscles of the lower body. Sitz baths are classified according to temperature. In general, they are good for imbalances involving the Liver and Kidney organs and meridian systems, and for problems involving the reproductive, circulatory, digestive, and eliminatory systems. The contrast sitz is the most beneficial and works best if the feet soak in one temperature while the pelvic area soaks in another. The *Encyclopedia of Natural Medicine* emphasizes that the water level of the hot bath should be at least an inch higher on the body than the level of the cold water. A higher hot-water level ensures adequate warming of the area.[4]

Hot sitz bath—can be taken for 3 to 10 minutes at a temperature of 105 to 115°F or 41 to 46°C. Sponge the pelvic area with cool water afterward. The hot sitz bath is contraindicated if there is acute swelling or infection. This type of sitz bath relaxes and opens the passages of the lower body.

Cold sitz bath—is used to tone the smooth muscles of the lower abdomen following a hot sitz bath. Immerse the pelvic region in cold (55 to 75°F, 12.5 to 24°C) for 1 to 3 minutes. Rub the hips while immersed. The cold water level should be lower than the hot to prevent chilling.

Contrast sitz bath—is what we refer to in the Self-care sections of the book when a sitz bath is mentioned. It requires two tubs large enough to sit in and have the water cover the lower abdomen up to the kidneys or navel. Fill one tub with hot water and the other with cold, taking care to have the water level of the hot tub higher than the cold. Soak in the hot for three minutes, then switch to the cold for one minute, rubbing the hips and lower back as you sit. The feet can be held in the opposite temperature for a stronger effect. Switch from hot to cold three times (six changes total). Keep a towel over your shoulders to prevent chill.

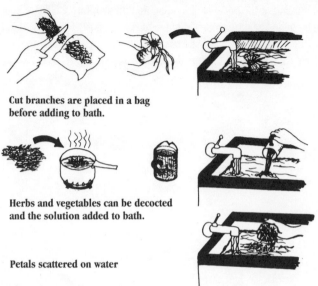

Cut branches are placed in a bag
before adding to bath.

Herbs and vegetables can be decocted
and the solution added to bath.

Petals scattered on water

Herbal Wines

Great for conditions of Deficiency and/or general toning and strengthening,
herbal wines can be kept for a year or longer. The alcohol preserves the medicinal
properties of the other ingredients and has Warming properties of its own. In traditional Oriental medicine the wines became very complicated affairs, with recipes
including sometimes 10, 50, even 100 different herbs. Generally, the more herbs in
the formula, the more diffuse and widespread the effects are. We include very simple recipes using common plants and herbs. Use a liter of 45° alcohol (Japanese
shōchu, vodka, or even brandy). Also, keep to the amount of sweetener listed in the
recipes, even when it may seem to be too sweet for your taste. Alternative natural
sweeteners, such as honey and dehydrated cane juice, may be added rather than
white granulated or rock sugar.

Rice Porridge

In Asia, rice porridge is considered to be one of the most nutritious of foods. It
warms the entire body and is indicated in many Deficient conditions described
throughout this book. To make porridge, see under Recipes in the Appendix.

Plasters

Plasters, also called poultices, are made with ground or grated plants or vegetables, which are wrapped in gauze or a cloth—either by themselves or in a base
of cooked rice or flour and water—and placed over the skin. Plasters are messy
and take time to prepare, making them nearly obsolete; however, they are one of
the oldest forms of traditional medicine and they work. Plasters, like compresses,

Medicinal Wine

YAÒ SHÀN ZHŌU
YAKU SHU

Porridge

YAKU ZEN GAYU

take advantage of the power of absorption that the skin has; the active ingredients or energetic and healing properties of the food or herb enter the body through the pores, travel through the body, and reach an affected area that may be difficult for a medicine or tea to reach through the digestive system.

poultice

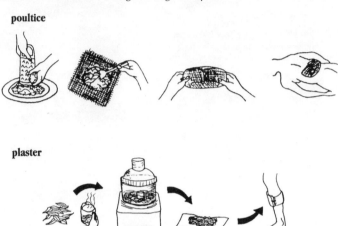

plaster

Endnotes

*1 Deng Ming-Dao, *365 Tao Daily Meditations* (San Francisco: HarperCollins, 1992).
*2 "The Nuts and Bolts of Needling," *Consumer Reports*, January, 1994, p.58.
*3 See the Warning note in the Appendix.
*4 Michael Murray and Joseph Pizzorno, *Encyclopedia of Natural Medicine* (Rocklin, Ca.: Primo Publishing, 1991), p.485.

C H A P T E R **5**

Seasonal Balance

Life is a rhythm: a heartbeat, a breath, a pace. Life is phases: childhood, youth, adulthood, old age. Rituals—initiation, marriage, childbirth, harvest—mark the phases. Passages—birth and death—define life's cycle, just as the tides, the moon, bursting energy in spring, fullness in summer, bounty in fall, and closing for the winter reflect the turnings of the cycle.

The seasons are natural markers for the rhythms and passages of time. The ancient Chinese considered them so important that they assigned each season an element—Wood, Fire, Earth, Metal, Water. They carefully documented the characteristics of each season and the ways in which the seasons affect us. The ancients respected the seasons with good reason; their lives depended on them much more than ours do now. We, on the other hand, live life far removed from nature and think it hardly affects us.

Journeying back to balance means honoring nature and the seasons as a model for balance. Nature's constant state of flux reflects the constant motion of our own existence. At times nature rages and creates all sorts of havoc, but these times pass just as they do for us on a personal level. The calm returns and the sun shines again. It is important to remember this, particularly when we are involved in healing ourselves. Nature always, sooner or later, moves back to center, to homeostasis. Things tend to go better when we follow that model, return to center frequently, and do our best to stay there.

It is easy to alter one's life to become a conscious participant in the movement of the seasons, but participation requires a shift in priorities. To do this, sometimes we need to give ourselves permission to live in less than high gear all the time. Simplifying life, cutting back on obligations, building in fewer tight deadlines and more unstructured time into one's schedule will provide the time to participate in the changes of nature. Honoring one's bond with the natural world can help dissolve the hubris and sense of separation that living in the modern world encourage.

We are most vulnerable to catching colds and other infectious illnesses during the changes in season if our bodies are weak, tired, run-down, and stressed-out. To prevent falling prey to the vicissitudes of seasonal change, we can fortify ourselves with rest, de-stressing techniques, proper nutrition, and by increasing our intake of adaptogenic supplements and tonics. The following sections provide tips on moving with the flow and impetus of seasonal changes gracefully.

Seasoning and Localizing the Diet

Conceptually in Oriental medicine there are either four seasons, corresponding to the Four Phases used in diagnosis, or five, corresponding to the elements of the Five Element Theory. In reality, there are four, five, even twelve seasons of the year, depending on where one lives. Personally, I am inclined to think of Japan as having two seasons, rainy and not rainy, rather than the usual four (or the traditional twelve). Whatever the case, in every country each season is marked by particular vegetables, fruits, or fish that reach maturity at that time. The Japanese still honor this coming into season at the market and at restaurants by offering the very first ripe produce, the first baby eggplant, or the very first deluxe *matsutake* mushrooms, at a premium. They are served to important guests or given away as impressive gifts.

Traditional Asian cultures emphasize the importance of eating with the seasons—a point we are forgetting. Think about it. Do you know when potatoes are harvested? What about asparagus? Spinach? Peaches and plums? Mushrooms? Slowly people are forgetting what is grown locally and what is not, and what ripens when. This kind of cultural and culinary amnesia affects the body, which is highly attuned to the foods, water, and soil surrounding it. Eating locally and with the seasons cultivates the body's connection to its habitat and brings it into greater harmony with its environment.

Becoming aware of how the change of seasons affects our health is helpful. Each season brings out weaknesses in individual constitutions. Chilly people, for example, feel uncomfortable in winter, and people with naturally Hot constitutions tend to feel an aversion to summer. Damp people cringe inwardly with the approach of the rainy season. Gearing up for these times by using food, herbal wines, and tonics to balance and counteract the effects of weather helps maintain health. Since a cornucopia of foods has become available throughout the year in supermarkets, it may be helpful to become familiar with types of food more appropriate for you during each season so you can learn to choose the right foods almost instinctively.

To do this, keep in mind a rough outline of food energetics based on your personal needs. As we discussed in Chapter 3, a Cool constitution will find root vegetables such as yams, turnips, rutabagas, and other orange and yellow vegetables nurturing and warming. These could be cooked with Chinese herbs—astragalus, dang gui, codonopsis, wild mountain yam, and Chinese red dates—the root vegetables could also be cooked with lentils or tofu and served with well-cooked brown rice. Conversely, several consecutive salads with fresh tomato, cucumber, and lettuce, too many slabs of cold tofu, or quantities of chilled diet sodas or ice cream will result in a slowly growing chilliness and decreased circulation in a Cool person, even in summer. A rough outline for this person could look something like this:

When I need to feel warm and full, I should eat: root vegetables, yellow and orange vegetables, red meats, dairy products, whole grains, beans, legumes.

A mental list of foods for a person with Excessive Heat tendencies could look something like this:

When I need to cool down or clear out, I should eat: tofu, soybean products; green leafy vegetables, such as fresh coriander, spinach, Swiss chard; sprouts—mung bean, daikon and alfalfa—and daikon radish root.

It is possible to keep it simple. This is the practice of balance for everyday life. If you have a serious imbalance or problem, please see a practitioner you can work with to create a comprehensive plan of action. Also see Chapter 3, where we discuss the energetics of food in greater detail.

Surviving Spring

Spring is ruled by Wood. In spring, energy rises from deep within the earth out toward the tips of trees and buds that are becoming ready to burst and expand. Crocuses push out of the ground, up through the last vestiges of snow. Spring is the time of planting, the turbulence of growth, easily changeable weather, the greening, the bursting into new life: the life force at its most insistent.

Spring's energy is Yang, it moves upward, and it is the natural time for elimination. Begin to incorporate light, eliminating foods into your diet in spring—cucumbers, tofu, and citrus fruits—but keep eating the heavier winter foods—brown rice, beans, meat, and other whole grains—for needed warmth. Eating the appropriate foods at the appropriate time ensures the appropriate body response during each season.

Wood controls the Liver, a sensitive organ. The Liver, as mentioned earlier in Chapter 2, is in charge of storing and cleansing the Blood, which it releases when the body moves. If you are careful not to let the wildly changing patterns of wind, rain, sun, and temperature affect the Liver, and take special care to tone the Liver in spring, you will be on your way to keeping healthy the entire year.

Regulating your habits, practicing ways to keep calm and on an even keel, avoiding foods that congest the Liver, and eating to tone and cleanse the Qi and Blood will help keep the Liver in balance.

Dressing for spring depends on the climate, but spring in many climates is characterized by sudden changes in weather. Dress in layers and wear natural fibers close to your skin. They rarely irritate the skin, allow ventilation, absorb moisture well, and feel good. Keep rain gear handy and within quick reach but avoid sunglasses whenever possible.

Change of Season Tea

Protect yourself from colds and flu during seasonal weather changes with an ancient Chinese tonic brew called Change of Season Tea. The tea can be drunk whenever stress levels reach uncomfortable highs.

3–5 g codonopsis
3–5 g lycium berries
3–5 g astragalus
3–5 g dioscorea

Add equal amounts of herbs to a fireproof earthenware pot with 2 cups of water and decoct, cooking for about 20 minutes on low heat, until the water is reduced by about a third. Divide the tea and drink half in the morning and half in the evening. The tea can also be refrigerated, then heated up and drunk warm the next day. The herbs can also be saved and reused once.

Surviving Summer

Summer is lush, growing, alive, and expansive. The light fresh greens of spring take on deeper hues, the lushest roses bloom profusely, tomatoes, eggplants, pumpkins sprout and ripen on the vine. Heat is sultry, filling the air like a vamp's perfume.

You have a better chance of staying healthy and avoiding a summer cold by taking precautions against the sudden cold that air conditioners produce. Scorching heat alternating with frigid air conditioning can lead to dehydration, fatigue, and colds. To deal with these conditions, it is important to avoid dehydration. If you don't feel thirsty, cultivate the habit of drinking regular amounts of water at set times. Drink small amounts at intervals rather than a liter all at once, and avoid iced drinks at any time of year.

Acupuncturists say that iced drinks weaken the Kidneys in winter. In summer, as the hot body receives the ice, the strong reaction that follows weakens the digestive system. Drink only warm or room-temperature drinks. In China mainly boiled water and tea are drunk, although this is changing. The civilized custom of drinking warm beverages is said to satisfy the body's needs faster because the temperature of the liquid is closer to the body's temperature, allowing the liquid to be absorbed more quickly by the system.

According to Chinese tea lore, not all teas are appropriate for summer imbibing. In hot weather, provided you are in general good health, a Cooling tea is recommended. Try Long Jin Cha (Dragon Well Tea), Chinese green tea, or chrysanthemum tea (called roku-cha and kiku-cha, respectively, in Japanese). All three can be found in Chinatowns on both coasts of the United States, or can be ordered from shops listed in the back of the book. In Japan, Japanese green tea, brown rice or "popcorn" tea (as it is sometimes sold in the West), and roasted barley tea, respectively known as bancha, genmai-cha, and mugi-cha in Japan, are popular and refreshing summer beverages. Oolong tea and black tea are less appropriate for summer because they have a Warming effect on the body.

Fruit juices have a high sugar content and increase thirst. Dilute juice 50–50% with water for a more thirst-quenching drink. Lightly steamed vegetables are preferable to salads and raw vegetables in summer because in Oriental medicinal theory, uncooked foods lack balance and, eaten to excess, create Damp in the body, which could manifest as illness or imbalance in fall or winter. If you must have a salad, eat it at the end of the meal as the Italians do, after the warm food has reached the stomach. Eat less meat and avoid fried and fatty foods which are Heat and Dampness instigators that create digestive difficulties in hot, humid weather. Pasta served under a light vegetable sauce, or a grain salad such as tabouli (prepared with digestion-promoting herbs: parsley, mint or coriander) make deliciously cooling summer meals.

Ice cream is triple trouble: cold, ice, and fat. Women with menstrual cramps should especially try to avoid ice cream. Watermelon, another summer favorite, is very Yin but it is fine with a little sea salt sprinkled on top. Traditionally the Japanese eat grilled eel in summer and swear by its rejuvenating powers. Try it.

Older Japanese often wear tummy warmers, or haramaki, to protect the digestive system from the hazards of moving in and out of alternately hot and cold environments. If you use air conditioning, adjust the temperature so that it is just under the temperature outside.

Summer is a time to conserve energy; yoga, swimming, and water sports are perfectly geared for the season. Hot weather tends to affect the Heart meridian and we become irritable, upset, and impatient in summer. Take time out to relax and mentally "chill."

The Chinese have one more tactic to deal with the hot weather. *Jōsan (Shang Shan)*, literally "ascend a mountain," means visiting a cooler place in summer to rejuvenate. Many city dwellers like to get out of the city in August, and they are quite right to do so. There is a theory that negative ions abound in country air and near natural water sources. Positive ions, said to be very draining, saturate urban air in summer.

Ascend a Mountain

SHÀNG SHĀN
JŌ SAN

Surviving Autumn and Winter

Leaves change color, dry, and drop in autumn. Grasses and weeds release pollen that scatters and falls. Temperatures become lower. Birds fly south. Vacationers close summer homes, homeowners put up the storm windows and increase insulation. As nature's energy begins to slow and turn inward, people prepare for the winter.

As in spring, what one really wants to watch for in fall is being caught unprepared in unexpected weather. A morning that starts off warm can turn into a cold evening. Cold breezes have a way of sneaking in on us, wriggling in behind uncovered necks or down inadequately covered backs. The area most vulnerable to cold, the Chinese say, is the Gate of Life, an area on the back that lies just between the Kidneys. Wear woolen undershirts and scarves, and when in doubt, carry an extra sweater.

Frigid air, frost, snow, a cessation of growth—winter's energy moves inward and compels our bodies to follow suit. We cover ourselves in layers of clothes while the body heat goes deep within. Emotionally we tend to hibernate with books, warm soups, plans to hatch for the coming spring. Some people find winter, when the demands of the world are at a low ebb, a good time of year for making an inward journey.

As it grows colder, eliminating or cutting down on iced and cold foods and drinks will maintain the strength of the Kidneys. Oolong tea and Tei Kuan Yin (literally, Iron Goddess of Mercy) tea are warming, and you will want to incorporate more warming, energetically inward-moving foods into your diet: whole grains—brown rice, millet, oats, buckwheat groats, and barley, more root vegetables, and soups and stews with meat or fish. Grains, seeds, and nuts have an inward action as do pickled and salted foods, which traditionally made up a large portion of the food on the Japanese table in winter.

In autumn and winter, the Japanese eat many long-simmering dishes made with burdock, daikon radish, lotus root, carrots, chrysanthemum leaves, butterbur (fuki), shiitake, tofu, chicken, pork and beef, sweet potatoes, leeks, devil's tongue, ginkgo nuts, chestnuts, and miso. In China one finds hot soups cooked at the table and more meat. In winter many Chinese still follow the satisfying custom of making warming herbal wines for themselves and their friends and imbibing a small glass after dinner to warm themselves for the cold evening ahead.

C   H   A   P   T   E   R   6

Pain and Vitality

Flip sides of the coin of feeling alive—pain and vitality are the Yin and the Yang polarities of our experience in the body. Just as the terms Yin and Yang are sometimes misinterpreted to stand for rigid, unmoving polarities, such as "bad" and "good," some people block out the significance of pain to make it mean, simply, the "enemy." They spend money readily on medications to numb pain, and often ignore its message that something is wrong. Particularly when pain's appearance is sudden and unannounced, our natural impulse is to fear it, the uncomfortable and the unknown, and we try to suppress it in the hope that it will just go away. Many of us live in chronic pain and are afraid of seeking treatment that, if it doesn't help, could make a bad situation worse.

We make vitality out to be the good guy, the ideal state; everybody wants life to be full of vitality. But our definition of that state is limited and limiting. As we see it on television and in the movies, vitality and sex-appeal are indistinguishable. "It" sells—everything from Coca-cola to cigarettes. But this media-inspired brand of vitality is by no means the only type of mental and physical well-being we experience. The state is different for each person. The way I feel vital and alive today is different from the way I will feel vital and alive next year, or the way you feel vital and alive today or next year.

This chapter is a contemplation on several different aspects of pain and vitality: how to use pain as a tool for healing and transformation, how to alleviate pain by yourself, and how to live in ways that will develop the potential for vitality in your own life.

Pain

It was pain that brought us, the authors, to the doors of Oriental medicine, and it was the successful alleviation of that pain that drew us in. Yes, pain hurts, but it serves several extremely important, life-preserving functions in the body. First, it alerts the central nervous system to damage or destruction in the body's tissues. Without this response, everyday life would be a dangerous proposition. The body would never learn to fear fire or recognize when to rest strained knees from jogging. It would never know when to stop eating, reading, or working. It can tell us when to run, when to escape, when to stop, and when to pull away. Pain can prompt pivotal life changes and lead us to momentous discoveries. Learning to cope with pain is one of the greatest challenges that life presents us with. Surely it is no coincidence that the Buddha cast pain as one of life's Four Noble Truths.

We experience two types of pain: acute and chronic. What happens during the course of pain's stimulus and our response to it? In Western medicine terms, the sensory nerve picks up a pain signal and releases chemicals that travel to the brain on two different types of pathways, a fast one and a slow one. The faster message arrives at the cerebral cortex on the brain's surface and sends out a piercing neural message. The slower message is answered with an aching, lasting pain, the pain that provides the damage report. This mechanism has been shown to be the same for everyone, transcending race, class, education, and experiential divisions.

The brain's response to pain varies for everyone, although there is overwhelming evidence in Western and Eastern medicine that suggests we have much more control over that response than we think. Research shows that by feeding our central and peripheral nervous systems with certain stimuli or information, we can decrease activity on pain pathways and diminish our fear of pain and our emotional responses to the pain stimulus.

Pain's psychological component cannot be underestimated. In fact, our emotional experience of pain has been shown to be closely related to the "fight or flight" mechanism, and it seems that just the anticipation of pain triggers the release of adrenalin and cortisol, the active components of that mechanism. Painkillers such as morphine act not on the local tissue of the painful area itself, but on the brain's emotional and reactive centers. Incredibly, the patient feels the same pain—only his or her responses are altered.

Allopathic painkillers, tranquilizers, and muscle relaxants can actually help people deal with pain and even facilitate its cure by allowing spasms to subside; healing takes place as muscles relax, circulation increases, metabolism decreases, and oxygen levels in the body increase. Painkillers, however, are sometimes addictive, others are narcotic. Some make the patient feel muddled, others have a numbing effect. Prescription and over-the-counter drugs tax the body's filtering systems, primarily the Liver, and in this way stress the body even more, taking energy that could be used to disperse the pain away from the function of healing. There are alternatives to drugs which we will briefly explore in this chapter.

The Oriental Medical View of Pain

In Oriental medicine, whenever there is pain, there is blockage. Headaches, eyestrain, sore throats, stiff shoulders, a constricted heart, a bellyache, menstrual cramps, an aching or pinched nerve down the leg—whatever and wherever that pain resides, the root cause is understood to be some sort of block or obstruction.

Just what becomes blocked, and what carries out the blocking in the pain scenario? Oriental medicine explains blockages as Excesses or Stagnant Qi and Blood. Qi and Blood can become "stuck" or lodged in the organs or along the pathways—meridians, lymph and blood pathways, and nerves—through which the body's energy and fluids flow. We do not have a corresponding terminology in Western medical terms. This is one area in which the gap between the Oriental and Western approaches has yet to be overcome. Try to stay open to the terminology and allow yourself to use the images as metaphors. They are your building blocks to learning how to alter your pain response.

Remembering the simple rule of blockage provides us with an alternative scheme for understanding and experiencing pain beyond the visceral reality that it hurts. Instead of reacting to pain, we can learn new responses to it. We can learn to work with it rather than run from it, to accept it, relax with it, and even enter it rather than hide from it. This is a powerful position to hold regarding pain; we can learn to use our faculties to dispel it. Though at the moment you may not believe it, anyone can learn simple techniques to alleviate pain.

But first, an outline of some pain palliatives and forms of relief Oriental medicine can provide.

Administered Treatment for Pain Relief:

Acupuncture, Moxibustion, Acupressure, and Herbal Medicine

Acupuncture is best known in the United States for its anesthetic qualities. It can provide immediate and immense pain relief, particularly if the problem is stagnant energy lodged deeply within the body. It does this by stimulating the blocked Qi and Blood that lie deep inside. Not that long ago, I experienced a migraine that began as heat at the base of my spine and crawled slowly up my back over the course of an extremely tense work day, until it crept up my neck and firmly held my head in a serious clamp, complete with flashing lights and almost unbearable pain. By the time I got to Peter's, I was nauseated from the pain. Peter began the treatment immediately and within half an hour the clamp around my head released, the lights were back to normal, the nausea a memory.

Moxibustion can move Stagnant Qi and Blood and also provide valuable heat treatment that warms the affected area and increases circulation, bringing noticeable pain relief for many conditions of constriction and tightness within a matter of minutes. Oriental massage is also capable of unblocking energy stuck along the meridians. Herbal medicine can also move Stagnant Qi and Blood to offer effective pain relief.

Acupuncture and herbal medicine require another's assistance; and although acupressure can be self-administered to treat specific points for specific problems, a complete acupressure treatment also requires the care of a professional. We should add that in the case of massage, you certainly don't need to see a professional for some warming, energy-circulating, hands-on aid. A caring pair of hands and a little sensitivity can go a long way in relieving a sore lower back, stiff neck and shoulders, or even a headache. Sensory pleasure in the form of massage is "astonishingly potent" in overcoming anxiety and pain, says Deane Juhan, author of *Job's Body*, a highly praised manual on bodywork. Touch sensation is carried to the brain on thicker, faster, and more numerous pathways than pain is, he explains. When the painful area surrounding an injury, for example, is gently rubbed, the brain is inundated with pleasing touch stimuli that drown out the acute pain signals. The massage lotion can make a difference. Tiger Balm or lotions that contain camphor or eucalyptus cool the skin and create a tingling sensation that also works to counteract the pain. A less stimulating almond oil with lavender can effectively treat an aching pain that is the result of exhaustion or a cold; it will induce relaxation and sleep.

While acupuncture, moxibustion, acupressure, and herbal medicine are put to use to stop pain, they are simultaneously administered to correct imbalance, and are therefore aimed also at reaching the root of an illness. The self-administered pain relief methods in the following section are symptomatic. They help temporarily, until professional assistance can be secured.

Self-Treatment:

Heat (including Baths and Moxibustion),
Acupressure, Deep Breathing and Visualization

Heat is commonly directed toward pain to warm and loosen tight, constricted areas, and get the Blood and Qi flowing again. A hot ginger compress is one form of heat that is effective in treating pain. Holding a blow-dryer on tight shoulder muscles can help loosen them, while a hot-water bottle can do wonders for abdominal cramps. (Cold application, i.e., ice pack, provides temporary and local relief of painful inflammation.)

Pain-relieving Baths

Taking warm baths with various herbs can help alleviate different types of pain.

Herb	Function
Beefsteak leaf/flower	relieves rheumatic, lumbar, and shoulder pain, anxiety, and headache.
Togarashi chili pepper	warms and soothes rheumatic pain and stiff shoulders. Cut 10–11 2-inch-long dried togarashi chili peppers into thin rings and decoct in 1 quart of water until reduced by a third. Add to a full bath with tangerine peels. Contraindicated for sensitive skin and for children.
Daikon leaves	affect lower-back, rheumatic, and nerve pain. Use a handful, dried or fresh.
Garlic	relieves neuralgia, hemorrhoid pain. Steam 3–4 peeled cloves to remove smell, rinse, wrap in gauze, fasten, and add to bath.
Ginger	warms painful rheumatic joints, eases headache, neuralgia.
Hatomugi (roasted Job's tears)	affects rheumatic pain, anxiety. Decoct 30 g and add to bath water.
Lavender	reduces anxiety, headache, provides general pain relief.
Parsley	soothes anxiety, restlessness, irritability.
Rock salt	relieves neuralgia, pain in joints and tendons, back and shoulder pain. Add about 30 g per bath.
Rosemary	is for general pain relief.
Sake	lessens the pain of sore knees, Achilles tendon pain, sports injuries. Add 720 ml to bath water that is just 1 to 2° above skin temperature.

Leaves in bath

 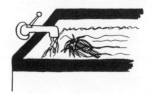

Moxibustion

Moxibustion can be used by the layperson for general pain relief. Apply it directly over tired, sore muscles, spasms, and painful or blocked organs to clear the pain. Moxibustion is not appropriate where there is inflammation. Use cold packs and ice instead.

Stick-on moxibustion is simple to use (Kamiya Mini is one popular Japanese brand). First rub Tiger Balm over the painful area. Push the dry herb stuffed into a small cardboard cylinder up to the tip of the cardboard using the plastic wand included in the box, then light it by rolling an incense stick on the top of the herb (but be careful because the incense can sometimes stick to the moxa). Place the cardboard holder onto the skin, and wait for the herb to smolder down. The actual smoldering heat never touches the skin, but the cardboard cylinder provides a tunnel that maximizes the effects of heat by funneling it to the point.

As the herb burns down, heat will begin to penetrate the skin. Most people can tolerate this heat without removing the moxa before it has burned all the way down. If you are sensitive to heat or have sensitive skin, remove the moxa when it becomes uncomfortable. Moxa sticks work just as well. (See the Appendix for ordering information.)

Salt Ring Moxibustion

The salt ring method of moxibustion treatment is particularly effective. It can be used on the lower back for lumbar pain, lower abdomen for abdominal and menstrual cramps, and upper abdomen for digestive difficulties. To use:

1. Cut a 2"-diameter round, 2" deep piece of cardboard tubing and place over a piece of Japanese washi paper or muslin. Fold the sides of the paper or muslin down over the tube and secure in place with a rubber band. Make sure the bottom is flat and secure.
2. Now fill the tube $^1/_3$ of the way full with sea salt.
3. Roll dried mugwort herb commonly used for moxibustion into a ball the size of a walnut, place the ball on top of the salt, and light it with a stick of incense. The salt will get hot.
4. Move the tube over the entire painful area, adding more moxa as it burns down, for a total of 30 minutes.

Ginger Moxibustion

Ginger is a warming root. This moxibustion combines the Warming effect of the ginger base with that of the moxa for a "double whammy" of heat. To use:

1. Take a slice of ginger 1" in diameter and $1/8$" thick and prick holes in it with a fork.
2. Rub Tiger Balm over the painful area and place the ginger section on it.
3. Take a piece of moxa about the width of your fingernail and light it. Put it over the slice of ginger. You can also place a piece of tissue paper over the ginger before this step if you think the plain ginger will get too hot. Stick-on moxa over ginger works well too.

Acupressure Points for Nonspecific Pain

In Oriental medicine there are some points on the body that are regularly stimulated for treatment of pain in the body. These areas are points of sensitivity along organ channels where energy accumulates and become blocked. By rubbing, pressing, massaging, and warming these points, you can stimulate the energy's movement and clear blockage, which, in turn, clears pain. The points are listed below using their English names. L.I.4 refers to the fourth point along the Large Intestine channel; LIV.3 is the third point along the Liver channel; ST. stands for the Stomach organ and meridian system, while SP. stands for the Spleen. You can stimulate these points yourself in combination with any other treatment you are receiving for a painful condition, but talk to your practitioner first if you are unsure about combining treatments.

Opening the Four Gates

This treatment is composed of four points that are useful in clearing pain for a number of diagnoses. Generally, the top two points can be used to clear pain in the upper half of the body (e.g., heartburn, shoulder and neck pain, and headaches), and the lower pair of points can be used to clear pain in the lower half (e.g., menstrual cramps, pain in the lower abdomen, rheumatic or arthritic knees and ankles). The four points balance the Yin and Yang energies and increase the circulation of Qi in the body. (See the BodyMap for the exact location of and an explanation of the points.)

L.I.4—Activates Qi in the entire body, is used for headaches, red and swollen eyes, nosebleeds, sore throat, arm pain, and cardiac pain.

LIV.3—In combination with L.I.4, activates Qi in the entire body, helps relieve pain in the lower body, hips, and abdomen, calms and soothes the Liver, also treats headaches and fullness in the abdomen.

Stomach Pain

ST.36—Tonifies central Qi and whole body; a salt moxa treatment on this point in conjunction with moxa applied directly to the painful area works best.

SP.6—Combines well with ST.36 to relieve abdominal pain with bloating, loose stool, and nausea. Combined with LIV.3 and a salt ring moxibustion treatment to the lower abdomen, it alleviates menstrual pain. This point also invigorates the movement of Qi and Blood, especially in the legs.

Knee Pain

ST.36—Tonifies entire body; see above.

ST.35—Lies in the eye of the knee (the indentation on the outer surface of the knee). If the sides of the knees hurt, spread Tiger Balm over the painful area and place 3 to 5 balls of moxa on it. Light the moxa with a stick of incense. The area should feel warm and turn slightly red.

Deep Breathing and Visualization

All of the treatments listed above are more effective if done while practicing deep abdominal breathing. But in any painful situation, even if you do nothing else but breathe deeply, you will begin to loosen muscles and stop the contractions and spasms.

> Imagine taking your breath to the point of pain and allowing the breath to penetrate the contractions, the pounding, or the piercing stabs—however the pain is being manifested. Allow your imagination to carry the pain out as you exhale. You can also visualize your breath as white light.

Many kinds of pain respond well to visualizations. Here is another:

> Picture the painful area as a block of ice. Take some time to feel how cold and solid this ice block is. Let your mind fully define the borders and edges of the block. Now imagine the sun beating down on the block and beginning to melt it. Allow the melted ice to run down your nearest limb like water out a drain pipe, flowing out of your body, while clean water enters through the crown of your head or through the nasal passages with the breath, flushing and cleansing the area.

This visualization works extremely well when it accompanies massage, acupuncture, or other forms of bodywork.

An old college friend who says she "rarely does these sorts of things," tried this for a sinus headache:

> I sat down and imagined my body was a house, my feet being the first floor and my head the attic. I started at the first floor and imagined myself climbing stories of my house, opening the windows as I went up, until finally I came to the attic, opened those windows, and imagined that the pain flew out—and it did!

These visualizations are very simple techniques that help alleviate pain by changing the body's response to it. Anyone can use them. Breathe deeply and relax your body completely before launching into the visualization. Developing images with which you resonate is also helpful. In my own visualizations with pain, the pain often takes the form of rocks, stones, or nuts that I imagine become entwined by and pervaded with light, which bursts them or melts them away.

One word of caution: at times the pain refuses to "melt" or "burst" away. Do not force the image. At these times you may wish to experiment by creating a dialogue with the pain and asking it why it is there. Write out your questions for it, and write down its answers in another color pen. Do not censor these answers, and write down exactly what comes into your mind in response to your queries. Questions such as "Who are you?" and "What are you trying to teach me by being here?" can lead to surprising clues concerning the root of the pain and how you may go about resolving it.

Working with images that come naturally to you will bring strength and greater efficacy to your visualizations. However, you don't have to work with pictures. Sometimes that will be effective, at other times, sensing the flow of energy coursing through the body will bring the sought-after relief. Some people work with color rather than pictures; others give pain a voice and dialogue with it. Whatever works for you is right for you, so give it a try.

The Elements of Vitality

Three Treasures

SĀŇ BĂO
SAN BŌ

Vibrant health—a sense of well-being in mind and body and enthusiasm for life—reflects balance among all the organs and channels of the body. In Oriental medicine, vibrant health depends on an abundance of three types of energy called the Three Treasures, which reside in the body. These are Jing, Qi, and Shen.

Jing is generative, creative energy, the body's essence that is stored in the Kidneys. It determines the sexual, genetic, and hormonal biochemical character of the body. All other energies of the body are dependent upon Jing. As it interacts with the vital organs, Jing is transformed into Qi. The conservation and nurturing of Jing can be accomplished through Chinese health exercises collectively called qigong (pronounced chee-GUNG).[1] Illness, overwork, nervousness, stress, poor nutrition, worry and obsession, drugs, liquor, alcohol, lack of sleep, and excessive sexual indulgence can exhaust supplies of Jing. It is best to guard it like the jewel it is. Taking care of Jing can significantly slow down the aging process.

Qi is present in all physical aspects of life. It is everywhere, "matter taking shape."[2] We breathe great amounts of this second treasure whenever we go outside and fill our lungs with deep, lust-for-life-filled breaths of air. Qi is flowing and moving, it lives in every action, every gesture, every food, every animal's instinctive behavior, in every child's conception, in every adult's death. A tree's rings grow

JING
SEI

QI
KI

SHEN
SHIN

thick with the movement of Qi, its leaves, buds, and fruit ripen with it. All physical life, living and nonliving, is a manifestation of Qi.

Qi in the body originates from the air you breathe, your own Jing, from food that is broken down in your body. You also inherit Qi from your parents. Deficiencies in any of these sources will result in diminished Qi. Strong Qi brings immunity to disease, increased stamina, and longevity.

Each time you take a breath, particularly when you are deep-breathing or practicing relaxation exercises, yoga, meditation, or qigong, you alchemically stir Qi, allowing it to transmute into Jing and Shen—the third Treasure, the body's spiritual energy. The Shen is said to reside in the Heart. Worry and stress can drain Shen, leaving behind confusion, forgetfulness, and distress. People suffering imbalances affecting the Heart meridian are particularly vulnerable to problems with the Shen. A broken marriage, a deep disappointment, the loss of a loved one—these can drain your higher light, leaving in its wake depression, anxiety, and the feeling of being lost in a black hole.

An Oriental medicine practitioner looks for the balance of these three types of energies in the condition of the skin and hair, the luster or lack of it in the eyes, and in the way the client speaks. Clear, healthy-colored skin, a rich, abundant head of hair, brightness in the eyes, and clear speech indicate a vital, healthy person.

All the organs and meridian systems are important in insuring our health and vitality, but three of these play especially significant roles. The Kidney is a primary player on the vitality circuit in that it stores Jing. The Yin and Yang balance, or the Hot and Cold energy of the entire body, depends on the Yin and Yang balance of the Kidney. The Kidney's generative energy is essential to nourishing the brain and spinal column, helps to build bone and Blood, and is necessary for proper sexual maturation. A deficiency in Kidney Jing results in muddled thinking, poor memory, weak bones and muscles, and a weakened or immature sexual function.

The Spleen's transforming function of changing food into Qi and Blood makes the health of this organ a primary concern. The action of the Spleen strengthens and nourishes muscles. It is said to "control the four limbs." When the Spleen is dysfunctional, the nutrients from food are not synthesized and distributed properly throughout the body.

The Lungs take in Air Qi (oxygen) and refine it into usable energy for the body. When Air Qi meets Yuan Qi (the spark that ignites metabolic changes in the body), the Air Qi is converted into generative energy, which in turn nourishes the other organs and Blood.

Vitality is the ideal, a state of grace that we move toward and away from, depending on current circumstances. There are also people who do not immediately strike one as being healthy, but who are full of vitality. Many people whose bodies are diseased maintain a joy in living that is full of compassion and understanding.

If you are ill and reading this, please remember that it is important to avoid getting caught in mental blaming exercises and that you have not consciously chosen to become ill. Although most of us can safely assume some responsibility for becoming ill, you are not to *blame* for being sick nor are you a failure as a person because you are ill. The old adage, "Healthy body, healthy mind" does not always apply.

No matter how hard we strive to preserve life, there are times when no amount of effort will effect a cure. This does not mean, however, that healing in those situations is not taking place. Healing's definition depends on your point of view. Terminal illness often results in bringing families, friends, and community members together in deeply bonding ways. Although as a health practitioner and as one who has been healed we are committed to the improvement of the physical condition, we see that kind of bonding through illness as a significant form of healing that extends beyond one person's physical condition. The days when healing referred only to the physical body are over; and for holistic and allopathic medicine to truly become complementary systems, this is one area where a bridge is needed.

Vitality, in the sense of an abundance of Shen, an upholding of the life principle, and the possession of a positive attitude, is seen not only in the living but also in the dying. Acceptance of dying is an aspect of vitality. This is a paradox in life that seems more readily recognized by Eastern spiritual and medical traditions than by Western ones, although many people in the West have certainly woken up to this paradox by themselves.

Vitality Builders

Once you decide you want to feel that *joie de vivre* mentioned earlier, you have taken the mental leap toward that goal. It is not necessary to make all the changes at once, however. Take your time and be gentle on yourself.

When Peter was working as an intern, one of the first cases he observed was an older man, a roofer by occupation, who was suffering from a bad ulcer. He had been prescribed new medication and said that shortly after taking it he began to experience excruciating back pain. In Oriental medical terms, the medicine was exacerbating the man's already weakened Kidneys. Upon further questioning, the patient revealed that he drank 20 cups of coffee a day with three spoonfuls of sugar in each! He was asked to cut down on the coffee, to slowly eliminate the sugar, and to begin exercising routinely. Instead, he chose to cut coffee out altogether and to drink tea with no sugar. He also began taking walks at night but didn't want to do any more exercise than that.

While receiving treatment, the client carried out those changes only. In the course of treatment his back pain disappeared and his ulcer cleared up. In addition, he lost thirty pounds and began to appreciate his healthier body. He eventu-

Air Qi

KŌNG QI
KŪKI

Original Qi

YUÁN QÌ
GEN KI

ally began to take more interest in what he was eating and quit smoking on his own initiative.

Health professionals and those seeking healing will find the last part of the man's story helpful. Seeing a health practitioner with the intention of getting better and investing a small amount of effort begins a chain reaction of benefits that takes on a life of its own. The rewards far outweigh the initial investment.

Movement Generates Vitality

Traditionally, the Chinese recognize the need for exercise in their formula for balance. Exercise is a good place to begin honing your potential for vitality. Regular physical activity may not be the easiest step toward that goal, but it significantly contributes to the feeling of well-being. Tailor the type and amount of exercise to your own needs. A young man we know recently gave up weight lifting to practice yoga. He finds the yoga pleasant and the meditation meaningful, but it doesn't provide him with adequate aerobic output. Jogging and swimming turn him off, Nordic Track is too trendy, and hiking, his exercise of choice, is impossible half the year. So he bought a trampoline and bounces off his tension at the end of the day until he works up a good sweat. A zany solution, perhaps, but for him it works.

Begin sensibly. If all you've done for the last fifteen years for exercise is carry groceries from the car to the house, don't try to run a mile around the track tomorrow. Check around, try finding a once-a-week yoga class. Qigong and tai'chi (Chinese movement that is more complicated and less repetitive than qigong) are ideal for people just starting out.

TÀI JÍ QUÁN
TAI KYOKU KEN

Exercise can be broken down into two types. External exercise requires that you use your body in some form of aerobic activity, expending large amounts of energy in the process. It builds musculature and strengthens the body's frame. Jogging, working out at the gym, biking, swimming, rock climbing, canoeing, and playing squash all fall under this category. Internal exercise, such as yoga, tai'chi, and qigong, builds up the energy supply rather than depleting it as external exercise does. As we age and our supplies of inherited Qi decrease, ancient Taoists and martial arts masters believed, the balance should shift from external to internal exercise to maintain the body's physical power while supplementing its Qi resources. In kung fu, for example, physically strenuous fighting forms are taught to youths from the beginning of adolescence; as the youth matures, forms that train the internal energy are introduced. Older, accomplished kung fu masters rarely exert much physical power. Instead, they exude highly developed Qi that can, if they desire it to do so, vanquish an opponent. With the development of internal forms of exercise, the cultures that contributed most to their development—China, Japan, and India—shatter the typical Western conception that the higher the expenditure of calories, the better an exercise is for keeping one fit and trim.

Internal exercise does require that the body move, which makes the muscles strong yet supple. It improves posture, increases the intake of oxygen, and enhances the functioning of the respiratory, digestive, endocrine, reproductive, and elimination systems. Its effects on the emotions are equally beneficial, calming the mind, attuning us to the environment, and diminishing insomnia caused by mental restlessness. Internal exercise is highly recommended for people in competitive, stressful working environments, for those who suffer from headaches, back and shoulder aches, allergies, and asthma, and for anyone over the age of 40 (although the younger, the better).

Another benefit of internal exercise is that it works to unite the split between the mind and the body. Anyone with a compulsive behavioral disorder knows firsthand what agony this split can cause. Anyone who has ever had a nervous breakdown, suffered manic depression, or has only felt himself or herself functioning on "half-power" understands this as well. There is a feeling that one is not all there, that one's behavior is not under one's own control. The regular practice of yoga, qigong, or tai'chi helps us to accept whatever physical and mental conditions we might be suffering from by increasing our immediate sense of well-being, concentration, and calm. In that space the mind becomes clearer, we feel more grounded, closer to nature, and nearer to the realization that there is no "real" separation between body and mind. Much healing can be done from the starting point of internal exercise. But it takes practice and consistency.

Regularity is the key to allowing exercise to have a real effect on the body. The main point about exercise is that you keep it up until it becomes a habit, as automatic and matter-of-course as brushing your teeth or combing your hair. If possible, try to include a variety of movement in your exercise routine. Ideally, for the optimum effect on health, breathing exercises, stretching, aerobic exercise, and strengthening are practiced on an alternating schedule.

Too little physical exercise can lead to poor circulation of Qi and Blood, resulting in weakness, muscle wasting, shortness of breath, and obesity. Excessive exercise or too much of one form of exercise, particularly if it is unsuited to your body or your needs, can lead to weakness, stiff joints and tendons, excessive sweating, and insomnia. While almost all exercise can be beneficial depending on the amount and body condition, yoga, tai'chi, and qigong ultimately lead toward long-term health and well-being.

Acupressure for Vitality

The following acupressure points are commonly used to maintain health and vitality. Vigorously rub and press the points on both sides of the body or use moxibustion to stimulate and warm them. (See the BodyMap for the exact location of points.)

L.I. 4—Activates the flow of Qi in the whole body.

気功

QÌ GŌNG
KI KŌ

ST. 36—Tonifies energy in the entire body.

Stimulating these points regularly vitalizes and invigorates the system. In addition, they incite the body's immune response and help to fight off infection. They also increase the function of the Lungs and digestive system, so that we can take in greater amounts of nutrients and oxygen and transform them more quickly into usable Qi.

C.V.4—Strengthens the primary body fire or Yang energy.

C.V.12—Tones the digestive system and the Middle Burner, the energy center in the mid-thoracic trunk that include the digestive functions of food breakdown, transformation, and transporting to the Lungs; the nutrient then combines with oxygen and is distributed throughout the body.

Moxibustion applied to these points strengthens the Congenital Qi, tonifies the Kidneys and digestive system, and revitalizes depleted energy.

Regularity and Quiet Time

Vitality results when you take care of yourself in other ways as well. Regularity in sleep, for example, is important to nurture the body. We highly recommend going to bed at the same time nightly to create a natural rhythm in the body that enhances metabolism and well-being. Ideally, try to get to sleep by 11 P.M., the hour the Liver enters its most active phase, cleansing and tonifying itself. Eating late and digesting while you sleep strains the Liver's self-regulating function. Activity late at night robs the Liver of energy it needs to complete this function thoroughly.

Building quiet time into your daily schedule is another often overlooked vitality secret. You don't necessarily have to meditate. Just sitting and taking stock of the day or your state of mind, or better yet, letting go of the day and that state of mind, can do wonders. People full of love for life are generous with themselves. Find the right moment in the day or the week to give yourself a special treat: a hide-out at the movies, a hot aromatic bath, a pedicure, or a massage. Affirm yourself! Pat yourself on the back and congratulate yourself for taking active steps to change your life for the better. These small actions go a long way toward building a positive attitude, which is truly the hallmark of those with verve and a zest for life.

Balance in the Bedroom

In Oriental medicine, sex plays just as important a role in one's health as correct diet and exercise do. As in the case of diet, guidelines have been laid down, but these are adjustable to individual needs. Regular sexual intercourse is seen as being beneficial to health.

1. Abstain from sex if you are feeling tired or unwell.

2. Abstain if you are under the influence of alcohol or drugs.

   (The two preceding conditions are considered to be particularly detrimental. If sex is performed on a regular basis during those times, it can lead to a loss of Jing and can result in weakness, lower back pain, dizziness, an inability to concentrate, premature ejaculation, and impotence.)

3. Abstain from sex when being treated for problems related to the Kidneys or urogenital system.

4. For women, too many births or abortions can lead to weakness of Blood and Jing, manifesting as menstrual problems, lack of energy, and dry hair and skin.

5. It is advisable for the male not to ejaculate every time he has intercourse. The older he gets, the less frequent this should be. Ejaculation can be timed to days he is feeling healthy and robust.

6. It is important for both men and women to engage in some kind of training or exercise that builds rather than spends energy.

The guidelines listed here are meant to be just that, guides to maintaining balance and equilibrium in regard to your sex life. They are not hard and fast rules. Maintaining balance includes avoiding the trap of rigidity in every facet of life.

Care of Injuries

In ancient times the practitioner would mend broken bones and use various herbal poultices and ointments. Today, for broken bones, severe burns, and other acute cases, go to an emergency unit at the nearest hospital. Oriental therapy can be used as a complementary therapy to facilitate a speedy recovery, however.

Over the years, Peter has noticed in his practice that accidents among his patients often occur during periods of imbalance in certain organs or meridians. For example, when there is a problem in the Kidney organ and energy system, which runs through the back of the knee and the ankle, knee or ankle injuries tend to happen more frequently.

Peter treated a nurse in her mid-50s who complained of knee pain that had started two days before as she was hiking in the hills of Kamakura, outside of Tokyo. This woman had no prior history of knee problems and could not understand where her painful, weak knees came from so suddenly. The pain was located in a band around the area just below the knee. Two main points of the Spleen and Stomach meridians, which run along the inner and outer sides of the knee, are located in this area (ST.36 and SP.9). As Peter questioned the woman, she revealed that she had been suffering from indigestion, nausea, bloating, flatulence, and intermittent diarrhea—all signs of disharmony in the Stomach and Spleen organ systems—the week before. Her pulse and abdominal diagnosis confirmed this. She received local treatment for the knee pain as well as treatment for imbalance in the digestive system. The digestive problem had caused a disruption of Qi through the

Stomach and Spleen channels, making knee injury more likely. If only the knee pain had been treated, therefore, the problem may not have cleared up as well or as quickly.

Bimonthly, or even monthly, holistic or Oriental medical checkups can help prevent serious imbalance. Many of Peter's patients visit him regularly for checkups whenever they feel "off," thereby preventing serious illness by nipping disharmony in the bud. The body shows subtle signs of imbalance before illness actually occurs, and a competent practitioner is able to pick up on them and act to rebalance the body and advise the patient. If this sounds expensive, consider that you are investing in the most practical health insurance money can buy.

Dissipating Vitality

All of us, no doubt, are in agreement that we cherish vitality, hold it up as our ideal way to feel, and many of us probably take measures to realize our vital potential. But becoming stuck in draining habits, work, or relationships can prevent us from feeling as well as we could.

One common obstacle that prevents us from realizing the vitality locked inside of us is worry. Worry weakens the Spleen and the digestive system. It drains our energy and accomplishes nothing. In particular, try not to worry about getting old. The fear of aging and dying obsesses denizens of the modern world to the point that magazines on longevity are filled with mail-order health tests and ways to measure our H.Q.'s—"Health Quotients." Who has to take a test to know whether he or she is healthy or not? Each of us has that knowledge inside us. Instead of focusing on the negative aspects of aging, begin feeding your mind positive information about becoming older; aging and death are natural parts of the life cycle. Worrying about them dissipates energy we could be using to focus on life.

Overwork is a major culprit in unwellness. Doing anything to excess falls within this category. Obsessive, compulsive exercise, work, or study, even if it is something you love to do, will deplete the energy of the Liver and the Kidney meridians if it is not balanced with relaxation and rest. On the other hand, too much "relaxation," in the form of partying, drinking, taking recreational drugs, and indulging in excessive amounts of sex will also, at the very minimum, deplete the Liver and Kidney energy.

Lack of exercise and improper diet will dissipate your vitality as fast as the lifestyle and emotional factors listed above. Imbalanced eating habits, grabbing fast food and working through dinner, forfeiting a balanced meal for cups of espresso and a chocolate bar, or forgetting to eat at all, lead to exhaustion and a depletion of the body's resources.

Taking medication, especially over-the-counter drugs when they are not absolutely necessary, zaps vitality because drugs can cause a toxic build-up once the Liver and Kidney's filtering functions are weakened and exhausted. There isn't much information available in traditional Chinese texts on the negative effects of medication on the body, since this is largely a symptom of modern society. But Oriental medical practitioners uniformly recognize the toxic effects of drugs on the system.

Cultivating a Positive Attitude

Depression and illness can interact insidiously with one another to prevent us from switching back into a functioning state and from cultivating positive energy. You can do something about this. Use the fact that change is the basic law of the universe. Everything changes. Ask yourself if you really, truly want to get better, feel differently. Because if you really don't, if you are getting something out of being sick that you will lose if you get well, you are greatly decreasing your chances of getting well.

Assuming that you are definitely sure you want your condition to be transformed into health and balance, suspend disbelief for a minute and begin to act as if you really think your condition can and will change.

See yourself now as existing in one point in time. That time is now. See yourself healthy, functioning. That point is sometime in the future. Now mentally draw the two together. Give yourself permission to become your healthy version of yourself.

Imagine yourself healthy, happy, and balanced every day. Give this vision time and energy. Feed and nurture it. Take a small step today to move toward it. Tell people you are doing something today to change. Start small; don't try taking on the big pieces at once. Don't overwhelm yourself with this project. Commit yourself to it and feel the excitement. But remember that lasting change occurs over a longer period of time. Don't burst and burn out.

Practice looking at the positive things that happen to you on a daily basis. Along with building those positive images and repeating affirmations ("I possess unlimited health and energy, a calm, clear mind, and a supple body," "My reproductive system is functioning healthily," "I am glowing with health, warmth, and adaptability") begin to root out negativity. Try to identify one belief that sabotages your vision of health for yourself. Think about your day yesterday and recall at least one moment when you had a negative response to something or someone. Mentally take that thought and turn it into a positive thought. Put out the best to attract the best.

Working on illness is more complicated than nurturing the garden-variety positive attitude because you're dealing with a condition that your instinct tells you to fight, deny, and struggle against. Healing requires acceptance of the situation, however, with hope that things will change. Change refers to the ups as well as the downs of life. If you find yourself going "down" regularly, with the coming of winter, for example, use that time to settle into a kind of hibernation and allow your psyche to regenerate. Don't feel guilty that you can't keep up with the pace of the rest of the world, and try to do all this without getting angry or upset with yourself.

Once you accept the depression and surrender to it, you have reached your most Yin point. It follows that change will come soon. Knowing that this is not the end, that depression doesn't last forever, helps one get through the hard times. Try to have faith in your vision of health and what you and your physician are doing to make you well. And when times get rough, call a good friend you have enlisted beforehand to support you in your healing efforts. Ask this person to send you positive energy when you are down (if no one around you ordinarily does this), and open yourself to receiving that positive energy. Let it lift you. Let it renew your hope. Letting your negative thoughts run away with you keeps you focused on the "bad," and takes energy away from your healing change.

Endnotes

*1 Qigong is a type of exercise composed of slow movements combined with deep breathing that is used as a warm-up to tai'chi and kung fu. Practiced by itself it enhances concentration and relaxation, and promotes the smooth flow of Qi.

*2 Ted Kaptchuck, *The Web That Has No Weaver* (New York: Congdon & Weed, 1983), p.35.

C H A P T E R 7

Choosing a Practitioner
and a Practice

Once a person's illness has developed into severe suffering, then they are in great haste to seek a physician. Since they have not selected one before, they now entrust themselves foolishly to someone whom they may know from hearsay or whose self-advertisement they believe, and in this way they eventually destroy themselves. ...One should start one's search and become aware of who is a brilliant physician when one is healthy.[1]

The Yellow Emperor's Classic of Medicine

Who knows how to get the best medical treatment? A good doctor is hard to find. Patients want doctors with whom they can communicate and from whom they feel they receive the best care possible. But there are no guarantees. Finding a holistic practitioner or a practitioner of Oriental medicine can be even more intimidating because many of us are not even familiar with the field. For what conditions is it appropriate to consult an Oriental medicine practitioner? If you have a condition that is not life-threatening and that does not require immediate, urgent treatment, consider the possibility of acupuncture before seeing a conventional Western medicine doctor.

Those of us who have never experienced acupuncture treatment have nothing to compare a practitioner's treatment to. How do we know if the treatment was good? How do we know if our practitioner's course of therapy is going to work?

Checklist for Finding a Really Good Practitioner

1. What are the practitioner's credentials?

Has the practitioner graduated from a nationally accredited program in Oriental medicine, or attended a smaller institute for acupuncture? Licensing varies enormously from state to state. All states allow physicians to practice acupuncture, but only 14 (as of 1994) require them to have formal training in it. If the practitioner is also a doctor, ask if he or she is a member of the American Academy of Medical Acupuncture (A.A.M.A.), which requires at least 200 hours of training for membership. Licensing requirements exist and are as tough or tougher for non-physician practitioners than for physicians in Alaska, California, Colorado, Florida, Hawaii, Maine, Maryland, Massachusetts, Montana, Nevada, New Jersey, New Mexico, New York, Oregon, Pennsylvania, Rhode Island, Utah, Washington, Wisconsin, and the District of Columbia.

To find a qualified practitioner in your area, call the National Commission for the Certification of Acupuncturists (N.C.C.A.)(202-232-1404) for a listing of certified acupuncturists ($3 plus postage) or the A.A.M.A.(1-800-521-2262).

Practitioners certified by the N.C.C.A. will have a Dipl.Ac. (Diploma of Acupuncture), Dipl.T.O.M. (Diploma of Traditional Oriental Medicine), or M.T.O.M. (Master of Traditional Oriental Medicine) following their names. At the very least this means these acupuncturists have completed the standard American N.C.C.A.-approved course for acupuncture at an accredited school and passed a written and practical test before receiving a license. Some practitioners, however, have studied for many years in Asia and their schools, programs of study, and degrees may be unfamiliar to you. Ask them to describe their backgrounds and discuss their licensing. Does the practitioner seem trustworthy and professional?

2. What is the practitioner's reputation?

Word of mouth, however, is probably the best way to find a reputable practitioner. If you are thinking of visiting an acupuncturist, ask around first. Find someone who has had a positive experience at a clinic. Before you make an appointment, call the acupuncturist, explain your condition, and ask if he or she thinks acupuncture treatment can benefit your condition. Look for an understanding response. Do you get the feeling that you would be comfortable visiting the clinic and working with the practitioner? Rely on your intuition.

3. How experienced is the practitioner?

How long has the practitioner been in practice? The answer may make a difference in the type, style, and smoothness of treatment. Experience in China, Taiwan, Korea, or Japan may have helped the practitioner develop a technique, or have exposed him or her to knowledge that we have yet to integrate into studies of Oriental medicine in the United States.

4. How's the rapport?

Once you have met your practitioner it is important to make a quick preliminary evaluation of him or her. Do you feel comfortable with the practitioner? Are you on your way to establishing a good rapport? Do you feel the person listens to you and respects what you have to say? Can you speak honestly of your condition, no matter how embarrassing it may be or difficult for you to express?

5. Have you discussed the costs and estimated length of treatment?

Oriental medicine is not usually covered by health insurance. Expect to pay between $40 and $100 (¥4,000 to ¥8,000) for a first visit and slightly less for subsequent treatments. Discuss payment deferral plans if your condition requires long-term treatment and you cannot afford the regular fees all at once. And be careful. The highest prices do not correspond to the quality of care and expertise offered.

6. Does the practitioner seem healthy?

This may seem like an odd question, but no one wants to be seeing a sick health-care provider. A harried, overworked doctor should be thinking about slowing down and taking care of him- or herself rather than extending further. Also, ask yourself whether the person demonstrates a commitment to self-development, both professionally and personally. Look for a vital, healthy, and grounded practitioner who communicates clearly.

7. Have you discussed your expectations of treatment?

Ask your practitioner how long treatment will likely take. If you have a chronic condition that has been with you for a long time, don't expect to hear an answer of one or two treatments. If you do hear that, head for the door. On the other hand, if you decide to have the treatments and do not notice a change after six to eight treatments, you may want to reconsider. Discussing your expectations with your practitioner will also help. Sometimes the practitioner depends on the client's cooperation, e.g., that he stop eating sweets, which he does—except for chocolate chip cookies. He does everything else and goes regularly for treatments, but nothing changes. A talk with the practitioner could help uncover the mysterious reason that the therapy doesn't seem to be working.

8. Does the practitioner include you as part of the healing team?

Are you receiving clear explanations and answers to your questions? Does the practitioner make it clear that your understanding of your condition and your cooperation in rebalancing your body is important? Does he or she offer suggestions (exercises you can do, foods you can eliminate from or add to your diet) so that you see yourself as a partner in the healing process?

9. If the therapy seems not to be working, does your practitioner recommend an alternative type of treatment?

Acupuncturists and Oriental medicine practitioners should understand the limitations of their modality, and can usually suggest another practitioner or a different type of therapy if Oriental medicine does not seem appropriate for your condition.

10. Does this practitioner respect your personal space and maintain his or her integrity?

I know of a practitioner whose women patients complain that he makes comments about their bodies, jokingly whisks sheets off them while they lay on the treatment table so he can sneak glances at their naked bodies, and makes crass, sexually oriented remarks during treatment. This practitioner works in Japan where there are no laws protecting clients from this sort of thing. *Inappropriate behavior or sexual advances should not occur under any condition.*

Pathfinding

There is an exciting moment for a practitioner working with a new patient: the moment that an unsure, inexperienced client asks how he or she will know whether acupuncture is the right course of treatment, what diet is best, what type of exercise is appropriate, and what kind of spiritual disciplines or meditative practices might improve or influence his or her condition.

The moment the patient asks these questions, the practitioner understands the client is opening, is trusting the process, and is ready to explore. Just as important, these questions signal a major shift in the patient's outlook, from that of a passive treatment recipient to an active participant in the healing process. Joyfully and without bias, the caring practitioner suggests that the patient explore at his or her own pace. The client can be seeking in the direction of physical, emotional, or spiritual development; here again there are no absolutes and no rights and wrongs. All the major traditions of thought, movement, and medicine have value. Rest assured that experimentation is fine and is to be encouraged.

• Explore the alternatives

At the point of experimentation a synchronistic mechanism is often triggered, leading patients down innumerable roads, sometimes to delve into Eastern philosophies and spiritual schools of thought—Tibetan Buddhism, Taoism, Sufism— sometimes to explore spiritual traditions with Western roots—Celtic religions, esoteric Christianity, Jungian psychology. Patients may find themselves reading about other forms of holistic healing—Western naturopathy, homeopathy, the Bach Flower Remedies, or forms of bodywork. The patient benefits from learning as much as possible about what is available. These studies feed the healing process and reflect the loosening up of belief systems that have so far worked to keep the patient mired in negativity and/or illness.

Feel free to explore but remember to maintain a critical distance, especially in the beginning. Attending classes is a good way to meet people on the same path and perhaps a teacher you may want to work with. But beware of teachers who claim that they alone know the way or that their way is the only way; this attitude fosters unhealthy dependence, plants uneasiness in the student, and dampens the student's growing sense of trust in his or her own judgment. After lessons or lectures, privately remind yourself that you can keep what "jells" with you and leave the rest.

Another supportive boost along the pathfinding journey is to read about the lives of men and women who have contributed significantly to the world around them as a result of finding their own paths, or who have acted as illumined guides along the way for many others. Biographies of Gandhi, Paramahansa Yogananda, Krishnamurti, Mother Teresa, or Thomas Merton can uplift one and foster the will to strive for health as one begins to emulate their lives.

• Learn to nurture and energize the body and stabilize the emotions

While exploring the world of ideas and spirit, do not neglect the body and the emotions. A strong, healthy body is a pain-free body, full of vitality and energy. Physically, we begin building toward this state a step at a time, by trying a form of movement that interests us and feels comfortable, then by committing ourselves to practice on a regular basis. For example, make a commitment to attend a new type of movement class once a week for ten weeks, or to go to the gym or the pool, or to practice your Nordic Track for 10 minutes a day. The benefits of exercise are well documented and it does not take much to make a big difference in how you feel. Breathing exercises with movement—yoga and qigong, for example—increase energy without straining the body's resources, worth keeping in mind if you are trying to rebalance a Deficient condition.

Affirm your body as you move and reacquaint yourself with it in a new way. Strive to develop a relationship of acceptance with your body, treat it not as an enemy to stop, to control, or to punish, but as your vehicle, your temple, a part of you that you care for and respect.

Becoming emotionally centered is a process that takes a short time for some and a lifetime for others. Whatever state you are in emotionally, becoming aware of the relationship between the physical body and the emotions greatly contributes to the level of health you can enjoy. Begin this exploration with a goal, something you really want out of the process—clarity, peace, or stability—and hold that goal in mind. Think about it daily as you meditate, practice stress reduction, and exercise. If fears of being punished by God or religious authority hinder your explorations into other realms, perhaps talking to teachers about your fears will help allay them. In the meantime, you will know if you are on the right path when something you try leaves you feeling as if you want to continue and learn more, when you wake up the next morning and feel good about being involved with it. These are clues for you to follow.

A common trap new path-seekers fall into is to become involved in a new practice and overextend themselves. Back to balance means taking it easy and making a small but consistent effort. This usually proves to be more valuable than a great spurt of enthusiasm at the start that fizzles out in days or weeks. We practice to create a stable base and to unify body and mind; that is why finding something that suits you is so important.

• Make slow changes and build flexibility into your diet

It is incredible that food, something so basic, should have become such a problem for so many of us. Right diet challenges all of us. Whatever your practitioner tells you to do in terms of altering your diet, one helpful piece of advice is to take it slow. Major changes instituted overnight are not likely to stick. Change at your own pace, and be gentle with yourself if you are floundering. Be extra gentle if you feel agitated by today's eating mistakes and feel the internal Task Master telling you that you must eat perfectly tomorrow. "Gentle restraint," arguably the two most useful words in Buddhism, can really help when you have cravings and urges to binge or break a dietary restriction. To put gentle restraint into action, tell yourself that "just for today" you are going to pass up a tempting food or drink. Tomorrow is another day.

Being open to changes that will occur in your eating patterns is essential. A fixed diet won't work forever because your body and its needs are constantly changing and its needs are as well. We eat according to no law except that of nature. Take the lessons you learn about eating and diet with you as you move forward along your healing path.

• Practice gratitude and ask for guidance

Another tip for finding and sticking to your path is acknowledging the forces of nature and goodness that are guiding you. Gratitude is like lubricating oil in the cogs of your process; it keeps the good things coming. "My personal prayer at the end of each day is only two words," says Peter. "Thank you." It does not matter to what God or gods one subscribes, he adds; the point is to feel a thankfulness for all the blessings one receives every day and to express that gratitude regularly.

One last pathfinding tip that Peter and I both know works is to ask for guidance. Ask God, ask Kuan Yin, ask the Buddha, ask the I-Ching, ask the entire Greek pantheon, ask a shooting star, ask the universe, ask your higher self, ask your soul. Ask sincerely and the answer comes.

Endnote

*1   Paul Unschuld, ed. *Introductory Readings in Classical Chinese Medicine* (Netherlands: Kluwer Academic Publishers, 1989).

Self-Care

Adapting to Stress and Building the Immune System

Not so long ago there were people known as achieved beings who had true virtue, understood the way of life, and were able to adapt to and harmonize with the universe and the seasons.[1]

The Yellow Emperor's Classic of Medicine

While our lives are changing faster than at any other time in human history, very little has been done to help men and women deal with the gap that exists between our technological progress and our physiological/psychological capacity to deal with it. On the other hand, an emerging body of evidence is indicating that those who live longest in our culture are people who adapt well to change and handle stress positively.

The Burned-out Body Electric

In the *Shang Han Lun* (*Shō Kan Ron*), an early classic of herbal medicine from the Later Han Dynasty (25–220 A.D.), the course of illness is divided into six stages, which map the progress of disease from Yang (external) to Yin (internal). Each stage describes a pattern of symptoms that emerges from the struggle between external pathogenic agents (Wind, Cold, Heat, Dampness, and Dryness—see Chapter 2) and the body's resistance (Wei Qi and Ying Qi—see later in chapter).

In the Yang stages, the body's resistance is considered still relatively strong and the body is able to resist the progress of pathogenic attack. The symptomatic picture remains on the body's exterior—in the skin, muscles, and joints. Areas that are not considered to be part of the body's interior, such as the respiratory tract—technically considered part of the skin—or the intestines, may also manifest symptoms. Due to the relative strength of both the body and the pathogen, the severity of the symptoms is acute. We have all heard of someone who is "as strong as an ox—he never gets sick." But Oriental practitioners know that when this person does fall ill, the battle is likely to be spectacular. Only a strong pathogen could threaten this system, and the system itself will have the resources to stage a mighty defense.

Discussion of Cold-Induced Disorders

SHÀNG HÁN LÙN
SHŌ KAN RON

A symptomatic pair, chills and fever, for example, appears in the first Yang stage (called Tai Yang) and is considered a superficial condition. Superficial because at the Yang stage, fever is said to be caused by the energetic struggle between the body's surface resistance (Wei Qi, or the Protective Qi, which flows between the skin and muscles, see later in this chapter) and the attacking pathogen. The pores open in response to the fever and expose the body to cold, which produces chills.

This is very different from a pattern in which the person feels *only* chills or *only* fever. Existing by themselves, they are considered deeper internal confirmations of Heat and Cold; the surface Wei Qi is no longer involved.

People showing symptoms of the first Yang stage (Tai Yang) have a better chance of recovery than those with very weak, chronic symptoms, says the *Shang Han Lun*, which is why Oriental medical treatment—acupuncture, herbs, massage, and qigong—all aim at strengthening the body's resistance. In treating a stronger person exhibiting the Tai Yang symptoms, treatment is more vigorous because the body can handle it, and the results of treatment are more immediate.

Oriental medicine distinguishes two forms of resistance: the Wei Qi, which we have discussed, and the Ying (not Yin) Qi. Ying Qi is translated as Nutrient energy; unlike Wei Qi, it flows inside the channels or meridians. Its function is to both nourish and defend the organ structures and other components of the deeper levels of the body.

If the pathogen is stronger than the body's resistance, the pathogen continues its progress inside the body, moving gradually from surface (Yang) to interior (Yin). Yang also describes the relative *activity* of the body resistance—as the pathogen progresses more deeply, we can say that the body's Yang (function) becomes more and more depleted.

The direct encounter between the gut-borne pathogens and the Ying Qi in the Stomach and Intestines is characterized as the Yang Ming stage of resistance. It is a more internal stage of Yang (active) resistance than Tai Yang, blocking entrance to the Yin (the bloodstream). Symptoms at the Yang Ming stage of resistance include constipation, fever, and abdominal distention and pain (usually associated with bacterial infection).

The Yang Ming stage is also the deepest barrier between Yang and Yin, or between the body's active resistance to invasion and its inability to fight off disease. Once the crossover into the Yin stages is made, not only has the location of the pathogenic activity changed (gone deeper), but the resistance (Yang) has become almost exhausted. In the Yin stages, consequently, not only are the functional activities (Yang) of the body disturbed, but the actual substance of the *body tissue* (Yin) begins to undergo pathological change.

The difference between Tai Yang and Yang Ming diseases can be compared to the difference between airborne and entero infections as viewed from allopathic medicine. From the allopathic point of view, infectious disease results from a pathogenic attack on an entry point of the body, usually either the respiratory system (airborne) or the digestive system (gutborne). From here, the progress of disease according to allopathy follows a patterrn similar to that taught in Oriental medicine. The allopathic viewpoint, however, emphasizes the pathogen's progress while practically ignoring the significance of the body's relative resistance.

There is a third Yang stage, Shao Yang, associated with a pattern of symptoms that reflects the fact that the pathogen has neither been confined to the exterior, nor has it truly penetrated into the interior. It is referred to as the "half inside/half outside stage." In allopathic terms, this stage may describe accurately the activity of a so-called "dormant" pathogen, which can become active under certain conditions, usually when the immune response is lowered. Diseases such as hepatitis, herpes, and malaria fall under this stage.

If the pathogen succeeds in penetrating the second line of defense, the Ying Qi, the person will move from the Yang stage patterns to the Yin stages. This sudden transition to the Yin stage is clinically very significant. It means that the patient is no longer able to resist disease, which has now entered the bloodstream, that the body is already very much weakened, that the symptoms will be less severe because there is less struggle, and that the prognosis is not good.

In Oriental Medical terms, the move through the three Yin stages is characterized by a similar range of symptoms, all of which involve not only weakened organ function but degenerative change to the organ tissue structure itself. Classically, the final stage, Jue Yin (Absolute Yin), described a condition where Yin and Yang became depleted to such a degree that they could no longer maintain their fundamental relationship, at which point they separated, and death followed.

To a layperson, the symptoms of an illness that has reached this level may not seem severe: chronic, low-key symptoms such as chilliness, low-grade fever, diarrhea, loss of appetite, and fatigue. Certainly these symptoms don't seem as serious as the fever, aches, and other symptoms that characterize a Yang stage illness. But to an Oriental medical practitioner, this person has entered the first of the Yin stages of illness and is, in fact, quite ill. The disease has become much more difficult to treat and will take much more time to be resolved. In allopathic terms, this progression from Yang to Yin is symbolic of the shift from infectious disease toward systemic illness (one in which several systems and body tissue become involved).

The early stages of Chronic Fatigue Syndrome, for example, the causes of which are not yet fully understood, are marked by flu-like symptoms that fit one or other of the Yang stages in Oriental medicine. But due to weakened body resistance (Wei Qi/Ying Qi), the progression into the Yin stages brings with it many systemic problems—candida, central nervous symtpom (CNS) disorders, fatigue, fibromyalsia, diarrhea, and malabsorption.

Deeper, chronic, and systemic diseases involve the degenerative process of body substance rather than impaired function. Acupuncture is used to manipulate the Qi that flows through the organs, which affects function. Herbal medicine, however, is more effective in treating degenerative diseases because it involves adding substances to the body, which affect the body's substance. Yin stage illnesses are treated with both acupuncture and herbs, especially herbal tonics.

The significance of the body's Yang energy (resistance in the form of Wei/Yin Qi) is key in the Oriental understanding of the disease process. It is comparable to the immune system in Western medical terms. In Oriental medicine it is related specifically to the function of the Triple Heater (see later in the chapter).

One of the major health problems we face today is the effect of modern, stressful lifestyles on our immune systems. To an Oriental medicine practitioner, two of the most glaringly problematic characteristics of contemporary lifestyles are a conspicuous lack of exercise resulting in lowered aerobic capacity, and a poor or erratic diet. The combination of these factors causes a disruption in the two major sources of energy in the body—oxygen from the Lungs and nutrients from food—and can lead to a serious breakdown of the body's defense system as a whole. Defensive Qi can be strengthened, however, by tonifying the digestive system, which basically refers to the Spleen/Stomach channels and organ systems, and strengthening the Lung and its organ system. In China, advice concerning diet and exercise was usually given alongside acupuncture, moxibustion, and herbal treatment in cases of illness. Traditionally, *preventative* health practices have also long focused on forms of exercise and diet to keep the body strong and disease-free.

Although it is not within the scope of this book, we would like to add that there is a case to be made for the use of the Theory of the Six Stages in charting the pathology of viral activity in the body, particularly in the cases of immune-compromised patients. The theory could prove useful in the treatment of chronic hepatitis, herpes, Epstein-Barr, Chronic Fatigue Syndrome, AIDS, and AIDS-related-complex (ARC). This area could yield fruitful results with further research.

The Stress Response

Environmental irritations such as noise pollution, air conditioning, air pollution, illness and injury, tedious or demanding work, conflict, confrontation, trauma, and all other stressors cause the body to resort to a particular set of biochemical reactions called the stress response. Stress causes an increase in the adrenal gland hormones, especially in the corticosteroids and catecholamines. These hormones inhibit white blood cells and cause the thymus to shrink, leading to a suppressed immune system. Today people commonly live under a constant state of stress, continually triggering the stress response and depleting valuable reserves of defensive energy, or what Westerners call the immune function.

Stress begins to take a toll when the body is depleted of reserves. Eventually there is a reduced capacity to adapt to stress as well as a breakdown in the immune system.

Structuring Lifestyle to Better Cope with Change

There are structural or lifestyle factors that affect one's tolerance to stress and the ability to handle it. Oriental practitioners recognize these factors and can be frequently heard telling their clients to simplify their lives to reduce stress and speed recovery. Peter points out to his students that when some asceticism or simplicity is kept in life, the ability to shift and deal with periods of extreme stress comes more easily.

For some people, just the thought of simplifying life can produce stress. If you are one of them, rather than responding to the idea of simplicity with an automatic rejection, open to it slowly. Remind yourself that it is something you can take your time doing. Oriental doctors are the first to recognize that slow change produces real change. Sudden, radical shifts often result in more frustration and stress. Make one change, let it settle in, and learn to trust what is happening. Other changes will follow once the first takes root.

If you think you need to make some changes in your life, begin by asking, when a new commitment presents itself, whether you really need that experience. Steady weeding according to this measure will help cultivate balance naturally, slowly, and will carve out a Middle Way shaped to your specific needs.

Cultivating Adaptive Ability

■ *Practicing a discipline*

Practicing a discipline that incorporates deep breathing, meditation, and some physical movement increases your adaptive power enormously. Yoga, tai'chi, qigong, martial arts, or any form of prayer or contemplation will do. An active practice requires commitment and dedication; it is something you do every day, even when you don't feel like it.

Training strengthens on a physical level, increases endurance, lowers the blood pressure, and tones the parasympathetic nervous system. It strengthens and clarifies on a mental level as well. Mentally the practitioner becomes less vulnerable to external factors that can invade the body and cause illness. Some practices claim to refine energy, leading the practitioner to a calmer, more serene state of mind. Training helps ready the mind for action: when you really need to use your mind, it will be capable of clear, crisp functioning.

■ *Positive empowering*

Working on a discipline is not so different from, or goes hand in hand with, learning to change your outlook on life. Developing a positive attitude augments your ability to keep disease away, and people who have done it have no doubt that it influences the strength of the Protective Qi around the body. Eliminate sarcasm, cynicism, and negative points of view and you will free up energy that was tied to attracting negative influences to yourself. You will allow that energy to attract and invite health and positive influences to you.

■ *Adaptogens*

Ironically, the solution to the problem of maintaining one's health in a rapidly paced society, one of increasing technology and an ever-more alienating environment may have natural roots. Nature supplies us with innumerable antistress agents, and there are whole fields of herbology, Eastern and Western, devoted to discovering how to strengthen and nourish the body during periods of intense stress, the kind of stress that astronauts and athletes experience.

Adaptogen is a term originated by the renowned Canadian authority on stress, the late Hans Selye, who first defined the body's adaptive reaction to stress. Adaptogens, be they plant, animal or synthetic, are nontoxic substances that reinforce the body's ability to adapt to stress. Generally, they are something one takes to help balance the stress response. The pill-popping mentality that so often dominates health-related attitudes has made the authors of this book reluctant to recommend herbs and foods that work as adaptogens. The best way to strengthen the immune system is to live, eat, and sleep in measures that are appropriate for the needs of one's own system before one actually becomes ill. What the authors perceive as a rapid reduction in many people's physical strength and resistance against disease, however, influenced the decision to include adaptogen therapy in the main body of this book.

Oriental Medical Energetics

In Oriental medicine, the meridian system that relates to the adaptogenic response is called the Triple Heater. The Triple Heater is a Yang, or Fire, functional system that does not have a corresponding organ in Western terms. Basically, the Triple Heater integrates the functions of metabolism and elimination. Modern Chinese researchers believe that this process of integration is related to the hypothalamus, a section of the brain that controls

Triple Heater

SĀN JIĀO
SAN SHŌ

basic life functions such as appetite and body temperature.

For our purposes, the Triple Heater is important because it is responsible for the production of two types of essential energy in the body. In Oriental medicine, these are called the Ying Qi, or the nutritive type of energy that flows through meridians, and the defensive Wei Qi, or the energy that flows through the flesh, under the skin's surface, and defends the body against attacks of external forces like viruses and bacteria.

The Triple Heater is composed of three energy centers: the Upper Burner is in the thoracic cavity and is related to the Heart and Lung. It is in charge of distributing the body's essential energy.

The Middle Burner is in the abdominal cavity. It is related to the Stomach and Spleen organs and channels, and controls the extraction of energy from food and the breakdown of food into basic components.

The Lower Burner in the pelvic area is connected to the Liver, Kidney, and Bladder, and is in charge of absorption of nutrients, elimination of wastes, energy storage, and reproduction.

Establishing a harmoniously functioning Triple Heater is essential to health. An ability to effectively deal with stress and change is a sign that all is well in your Triple Heater.

When stress triggers certain problems in the body, it could be a sign that the corresponding "burner" and the Defensive Qi are weak. It is natural for something to "act up" during stressful periods. Some people get heartburn or digestive difficulties. Others break out into fiery, raw acne. Some people suffer from insomnia. Other people lose their will to fight and become depressed. Many children experience asthma attacks at the change of season. Even something as simple and natural as a change in the weather can be a stress, and there are many types of responses the body could have to it.

Internal Applications: Immune System Builders

• Avoid foods that numb the body and mind, that injure the Spleen and strain the Liver and Kidneys: alcohol, drugs, tobacco, coffee and caffeinated beverages, excessively spicy foods, heavy red meat; fatty, greasy, rich foods; also avoid food additives, preservatives, and overeating.

• Avoid sugar and fat—overconsumption of sugar and fat inhibits immune function. One hundred grams of sugar, the amount in two sodas, is enough to decrease the white cell's ability to devour harmful substances in the body. Sugar in fruit, juice, honey, maple syrup, and white and brown sugar are all simple carbohydrates that should be reduced or avoided altogether. The average American consumes 150 grams of simple sugars every day, leading researchers to the logical conclusion that "most Americans have chronically depressed immune systems."[2] A diet high in fats suppresses the immune function by hampering the production of prostaglandins, biochemicals in the body that control the activity of T-cells, important disease fighters. Fats also impede lymphocytes' ability to proliferate and produce antibodies, and the ability of neutrophils to migrate to areas of infection and engulf and destroy invading, infectious organisms.[3]

• Include more protein-rich foods in the diet; these include vegetable sources and pulses as well as meat, fish, and dairy products. Many functions of the immune system depend on an adequate protein intake. When the body fights disease it burns amino acids metabolized from protein. When you have an infection, the life span of your infection-fighting white blood cells is shortened considerably, but amino acids slow their breakdown.

• Also eat more foods that tone and fortify the Kidneys (see under Food Influences in Chapter 3). Weak, Deficient Kidneys can lead to stagnation in the Lungs, according to the Five Element Theory, resulting in shallow breathing, dryness in the mouth, nose, and throat, vulnerability to colds and coughs, frequent urination, or urinary retention. Left unchecked, the condition could degenerate into any number of Lung diseases.

>—Eating pork kidneys is a traditional and powerful method of strengthening the Kidneys. (See Preparing Organ Meats in the Appendix.)

>—Once the kidneys have been prepared, cook them in a dashi broth (see Appendix for recipe) with any combination of carrots, baby onions, bamboo shoots, burdock root, pumpkin, and lotus root. Add some precooked azuki beans if you like. Crushed Japanese peppercorns make this into an exotically aromatic dish.

>—Or slice the kidneys and serve them hot, covered with a sauce of slivered scallions, green pepper, soy sauce, sesame seed oil, ginger and vinegar in proportions to taste.

>—The sweet potato is also believed to be a Kidney strengthener. Black sesame seeds, string beans, white sword beans, and wheat have Kidney-tonifying effects as well. Wheat and wheat gluten are common allergens, however, so avoid overconsumption.

>—Add lycium berries often to soups, stews, and simmered dishes. Reconstitute with hot water, *sake*, or wine and add to dressings and sauces. Lycium berries are also tonic to the Liver.

>—Azuki and kidney beans are important source foods for Kidney support. Eat them weekly if possible. They can be purchased precooked either in vacuum-packs or canned. (See Azuki Bean Broth in the Appendix.)

• Tone the digestive system by eating warming broths and following the Spleen/Stomach-toning meal plan of fresh vegetables—especially yellow and orange squashes and root vegetables—also legumes, whole grains, small amounts of tofu and soybean products, fish, chicken, pork, beef. Cut down on dairy, caffeine, refined white flour, and sugar.

• Reishi and shiitake are two types of mushroom (the reishi is a type of shiitake) that are proven immune-system builders. They raise T-cell levels and have antibacterial, antitumor, and energizing effects. The fairly rare reishi mushroom is difficult to cultivate. It has been used in Oriental herbology for at least two thousand years. One of its active ingredients, lentinan, was authorized for clinical testing by AIDS researchers. Researchers at Kobe University have shown that shiitake contains interferon, a substance that helps cells resist viral infection.

• Change of Season Tea is an ancient prescription for precisely the problem of stress at the change of the seasons. The tea is made of four tonic herbs, all well known and often used in China by common people in their daily cooking. The herbs can be combined and decocted, and drunk twice daily whenever stress levels reach uncomfortable heights. (See recipe in the Appendix.) Drink twice a day after meals. Save the herbs and cook them again the next day.

• Wild Siberian ginseng is another herb known for its antistress properties. In more than

1,000 tests conducted over the last 30 years in China, Japan, and Russia, including among them tests on Olympic contenders, sailors making long-term voyages, and astronauts, this herb has consistently shown its value by bringing support to the body in situations of chronic and acute stress. Initial experiments with workers and athletes at the Institute of Biologically Active Substances in Vladivostok showed Siberian ginseng to have both tonic and stimulant properties. Later, it was proven not only to improve health but to protect against and speed the recovery of illness. It instills a sense of well-being in those taking it who suffer from anxiety, depression, and irritability and has a normalizing effect on the metabolism.

• People with extremely high blood pressure, those who tend to get spontaneous nosebleeds, women with excessive bleeding during menstrual periods, and people who often feel hot and dry should use Siberian ginseng with caution, under the care of a trained herbal practitioner. (See A Ginseng Aside in the section on Sexuality.)

• In cases of low energy ma huang is indicated for its energy tonic and stimulant properties. It aids in the reduction of bronchial spasms, asthma, colds, hay fever, and sinus trouble. Those with high blood pressure should not use it at all. It should be used only occasionally and is quite drying. (See the Appendix.)

• Try an herbal brew of Chinese cinnamon, ginger, dried tangerine peel, and Chinese licorice for added energy, to improve poor circulation, and to give a digestive-system boost. Add equal amounts (3–5 g) of each to $^3/_4$ of a liter or quart of water, and simmer in a fireproof, earthenware pot until the liquid is reduced by a third. Divide into two or three portions and drink two or three times a day until the condition improves.

• Make sure to eat foods that contain the following nutrients, which are particularly important to immune function:

• Vitamin A (beta-carotene)
broccoli, carrots, dandelion greens, fish liver oils, garlic, kale, mustard greens, organ meats—chicken, beef, and pork, parsley, red peppers, sweet potatoes, Swiss chard, turnip greens, yellow squashes, watercress

• Vitamin B
beef, bran, brewer's yeast, brown rice, desiccated liver, eggs, fish, green leafy vegetables, legumes, liver, milk, molasses, poultry, soy beans, whole wheat, other whole grains

• Vitamin C
Brussels sprouts, collard greens, daikon radish, green peas, kale, lemons, mustard greens, onions, oranges, parsley, persimmon, radish, spinach, strawberry, sweet bell peppers, tomato, watercress

• Vitamin E
brown rice, dark green leafy vegetables, dry beans, cold-pressed oils, cornmeal, legumes, nuts and seeds, whole grains and cereals

• Bioflavonoids*
black currants, buckwheat, citrus fruits, peppers

*Quercetin, a bioflavonoid found in blue-green algae, can be taken in supplement form with bromelin. The two work synergistically. Blue-green algae can be purchased in dried form from herb stores and suppliers.

- **Calcium**
green leafy vegetables, sardines, seafood, sesame seeds
- **Potassium**
apricots, avocados, bananas, blackstrap molasses, brown rice, dates, dried fruit, figs, garlic, nuts, potatoes, raisins, wheat bran, winter squash, yams
- **Selenium** (an antioxidant found in soil)
brewer's yeast, broccoli, brown rice, chicken, dairy products, garlic, liver, molasses, onions, salmon, seafood, tuna, most vegetables, wheat germ, whole grains
- **Zinc**
bee pollen granules, fish, legumes, meat, oysters, poultry, seafood, whole grains

"Superfoods" can fortify the immune system. To build immune strength, take supplements of one or more of the following:
- **Bee pollen** is a metabolic balancer and immune strengthener because its high protein content causes it to raise the body's gamma globulin (most antibodies are gamma globulins) levels; it stimulates the build-up of weight and energy in convalescents.
- **Chaparral** is a bitter herb that scavenges free radicals and is wellknown for its antioxidant and anticancer properties. It also relieves pain, relaxes the blood vessels, and increases ascorbic acid levels in the adrenals.
- **Chinese licorice** (contraindicated in cases of fluid retention and high blood pressure) strengthens the digestive system, treats ulcers, improves energy, detoxifies, treats sore throats, coughs, and lung dryness.
- **Echinacea** stimulates the immune system to resist infection and inflammations. In his book *Planetary Herbology*, Michael Tierra calls it "one of the most powerful and effective remedies against all kinds of bacterial and viral infections."[4]
- **Garlic** stimulates metabolism, strengthens digestion, and treats lower back and joint pains, urogenital problems, and lung and bronchial infections.
- **Ginkgo** is believed to increase memory and brain function. It also helps expel mucus from the Lungs, and has a regulating and toning influence on Kidney (and Jing)-related functions.
- **Goldenseal root** (tincture form is most stable) fights infections, colds, and flu, cleanses blood, and alleviates indigestion.
- **Lecithin** increases vital energy and enables fats to be dispersed in water and removed from the body.
- **Propolis** (the material bees use with beeswax to cement their honeycombs to the hive and to close the entrance of the hive against intruders; made from resinous juice and sap of trees and tree buds) is a Qi tonic, stimulates phagocytosis, is antibiotic, antiviral, aids infections of the mouth and throat, and promotes the healing of skin eruptions and ulcers.
- **Royal Jelly** is a Qi tonic, contains all the B vitamins, and strengthens the immune system.
- **Shiitake** and **reishi mushrooms** are excellent immune system tonics; they raise T-cell levels and are therefore used to treat immune disorders including AIDS and Chronic Fatigue Syndrome. They also have antibacterial, antiviral, antitumor, and general rejuvenative effects.
- **Spirulina** contains high concentrations of nutrients, protects the immune system, and helps reduce cholesterol.
- **Wheatgrass** is used to treat any number of disorders, increases energy and stamina, and

enhances feelings of well-being.

In the Chinese pharmacopeia, several herbs that strengthen the immune function are becoming the focus of increasing scientific attention:

• **Astragalus** is believed to boost the life expectancy of cancer patients who have undergone chemotherapy,[5] strengthens digestion, raises metabolism, strengthens the immune system, promotes the healing of wounds, and treats chronic weakness of the lungs, lack of energy, organ prolapse, sudden sweating, chronic lesions, and deficiency edema.

• **Codonopsis** has properties similar to *Panax ginseng*. It increases energy levels, facilitates the transformation of white blood cells into T-cells, and builds resistance to disease.

• **Ginseng** is an excellent energy tonic. It restores and revitalizes the entire body, is a potent sexual tonic, and is said to replace lost Qi in the organs and the meridians, increase stamina, benefit the Three Treasures (Jing, Qi and Shen), extend adaptive ability, and increase longevity. It is beneficial for men and women. (See A Ginseng Aside in the Sexuality section).

• **Schizandra berries** are used as an astringent and an energy tonic. They enhance mental function and relieve insomnia.

• **White atractylodes** root is used to expel excess moisture, settle the stomach, improve digestion and appetite, and treat fatigue, restlessness, and dizziness.

• **Ligustrum berries** are a Yin tonic used to treat consumptive wasting diseases, premature graying hair, lower back pain, blurred vision, tinnitus, and knee and joint pains.

External Applications

• Don't forget to have yourself a good laugh. Concentrations of salivary virus fighters (immunoglobulin A) increased in students at Western New England College in Springfield, Massachusetts, after they watched a videotape of Richard Pryor. And patients in the San Francisco area were able to reduce their doses of painkillers by taking part in a four-week game in which they made each other laugh.[6]

• Exercise has a positive effect on the immune response. Studies suggest that endorphins can enhance T-cell activity. Exercise also stimulates the growth of the thymus gland, the site where lymphocytes taken from the bloodstream are trained to function as T-cells. Aerobic activity warms the body, enhancing the effects of vitamins A and D. Interferon levels double in usually sedentary people who exercise steadily for half an hour.

Endnotes

[1] *The Yellow Emperor's Classic of Medicine*, Chapter 1, trans. Maoshing Ni (Boston: Shambhala Publications, 1995), p. 4.

[2] Michael Murray, and Joseph Pizzorno, *Encyclopedia of Natural Medicine*, (Rocklin, Ca.: Prima Publishing, 1991), p. 63.

[3] Ibid.

[4] Michael Tierra, *Planetary Herbology*, (Santa Fe, NM: Lotus Press, 1988), p.191.

[5] *Nutrition News*, Vol.IX, no.9, 1986.

[6] *Nutrition News*, Vol. XI, no. 1, 1988.

Allergies

Includes: allergic rhinitis (hay fever), allergic itching, and hives. For rashes and other skin reactions see the section on Skin.

Oriental Medical Energetics

In Western mèdicine, an allergy is defined as the inappropriate response to the body's immune system to a substance that is not normally harmful.

Oriental medicine, however, does not include the diagnosis "allergy." Instead, the problem is treated according to the symptoms accompanying the disorder. Further, Westerner practitioners of alternative medicine today, aware that they are treating something called "allergies" as well as "Damp Heat Poisoning," are interested in why some people are susceptible to allergies while others are not. There are causes of allergies that seem rooted in factors not directly related to the allergen itself—personal history, lifestyle, and physiognomy—that contribute to the appearance of allergic reactions. A weakened immune system is also implicated in the appearance of allergies, recent studies show. Many of the allergy sufferers Peter sees in the clinic suffer from imbalance in the Stomach/Spleen or Lung/Large Intestine organ and meridians. His experience with allergies tends to back up researchers' findings that allergies are somehow related to weakness in the immune system.

A weak Stomach/Spleen network, compounded by weakened Kidney Fire (Yang energy) in the Kidneys

The weak digestive function combined with Deficient Kidney Yang weaken the Protective Qi and make the body more vulnerable to Wind poisoning, resulting in allergic reaction. A weak Stomach/Spleen and Deficient Kidney are usually due to chronic stress or overwork. Coffee, alcohol, and chocolate exhaust the energy supply of the Kidneys and exacerbate this condition. As a result, foods are not metabolized properly, mucus is created, and fluid imbalance results. Anger and frustration at this point could lead to a Rising Liver Yang condition, when hot Liver energy invades the Lungs, chest, or head, to manifest as hay fever, watery eyes, sinus headache, or hives when the body comes into contact with a specific allergen or is under stress.

Hay fever, or allergic rhinitis, is a chronic inflammation of the nose, throat, and sinuses induced by external irritants, usually pollens carried in the air. Spring hay fever is related to tree pollen, summer to grass pollen, and autumn to weed—such as ragweed and goldenrod—pollen.

Nonseasonal allergies are usually due to household irritants such as dust, animal hair, droppings of the house dust mite, hay, straw, insect stings and bites, medicines such as aspirin and penicillin, some metals (particularly nickel), chemicals in soaps, and washing powders.

Food allergies—or food intolerance, as it is also called due to the food's triggering unpleasant or allergy-like effects in some people who do not have a scratch-test reaction to them—are another nonseasonal allergy subset. A mountain of evidence out there shows that food allergies can produce dramatic changes in mood, behavior, and physical well-being, causing symptoms such as abdominal pains, headache, insomnia, anxiety, depression, hives, and rash. Eye, ear, and throat problems are also often triggered by food intolerance. Food additives, milk, eggs, chocolate, wheat, and cheese are common problems.

Dermatitis and asthma are often related to allergies, as are migraine, irritable bowel syndrome, arthritis, ulcerative colitis, hyperactivity, skin disease, and gynecological disorders.

Allergic Rhinitis (Hay fever)

If this is your first bout of hay fever or sinusitis, it may be time to examine your lifestyle. The aggravating effects of alcohol and smoking on the respiratory system are well documented, as are those of stress, overwork, and air pollution. Chances are that if you are new to a metropolitan or surrounding area, you are coping with increases of all the problems listed above. If that is the case, you may find it beneficial to build a de-stressing program or relaxation methods into your new lifestyle as soon as possible. Eliminating cigarettes and alcohol will immeasurably increase your body's ability to reduce its hyper response to allergens.

Many studies have shown that food allergies play an important role in asthma and hay fever. Food allergy reactions are sometimes delayed, so they remain hidden and you don't realize you have one. Elimination diets have been successful in treating food allergies. Consider reading up on them if you think this may apply to you.

Self-Help Strategies

—Avoid known allergens whenever possible. You may wish to invest in an air filter to help make your home or office more comfortable during the pollen onslaught.
—Alleviate inflammation of nose, throat, sinuses, and eyes.
—Stimulate your body's antihistamine response in the nose and belly.
—Strengthen the Liver to support its filtering of toxins out of the system.
—Support the Kidneys and the adrenal glands (see the section Adapting to Stress and Building the Immune System in Part II).
—Desensitize yourself prior to hay fever season.

Internal Applications

• Foods that weaken the immune system, such as refined sugar, coffee, and white flour should be eliminated from the diet. (See the section Adapting to Stress and Building the Immune System in Part II.)

• Foods with a high fat content can clog the lymph system and increase congestion. Reduce or avoid them altogether.

• Excessively spicy foods that could irritate the Lungs/Large Intestine should also be eliminated from your diet.

• Reduce your intake of animal protein. Some tests have shown that completely vegan diets have had a high success rate in preventing recurrence of symptoms in children with asthma and allergic rhinitis. Check with a nutritionist and an Ayurvedic practitioner.

• Eat more shiitake mushrooms, which contain antiviral compounds that increase interferon production. Try cooking them with onions and garlic for a triple-whammy anti-inflammatory immuno-strengthening meal.

• Try to incorporate suggestions from the Spleen/Stomach or Middle Burner-strengthening diet in Chapter 3 and in the section Adapting the Stress and Building the Immune System in Part II.

• Eat quantities of foods rich in roughage, such as fresh vegetables, beans, and whole grains to keep the colon and Large Intestine clear.

• Ginger is tonic to the mucous membranes. Make a decoction with fresh or dried root and add a few grams of Chinese licorice to help relieve inflammation.

• Cayenne pepper helps moisten dry, hot mucous membranes, acts as a peripheral blood circulating stimulant, and relieves frontal headaches caused by dry mucous membranes. Add it to lemon juice and olive oil and drink first thing in the morning to get the intestines moving. This will help constipation and moisten overworked, dried-out nasal passages.

• Broth of onion and daikon radish strengthens the system against itchy inflammation and a tightening of the chest characteristic of asthma. The onion has an antihistamine effect while the daikon helps clear phlegm and inflammation. Drink it frequently to aid prevention of allergic reaction.

• Fenugreek seeds can be boiled into a tea to sip when you have allergic symptoms. Besides being a Yang tonic, they have restorative and demulcent properties for which they have been used traditionally to counteract catarrh and phlegm.

• Fresh coriander (cilantro) and watercress can be juiced to treat symptoms of hay fever and allergies. They are cooling to the body.

• Bee pollen is an immune system strengthener. (See the section Adapting to Stress and Building the Immune System.) It should also be taken at least a couple of months before the allergy season. Take the dose recommended on the bottle at first, or just a tiny pinch if you are taking it fresh. If no symptoms of constricted throat, itchy skin, teary eyes, or a shortness of breath develop after a few days, gradually increase to a teaspoon a day. Keep the pollen refrigerated.

• Dang gui has been shown to cause significant improvement in hay fever sufferers. It has long been used as an allergy and hay fever preventative and relief medicine in China. Start drinking as a decoction two months prior to hay fever season.

• Green tea supports hay fever treatment due to its theophylline content and antioxidant components.

• For allergies with sneezing, itchy eyes, runny nose, cough, wheezing, nasal drip, sore throat, and headache, try Bi Yan Pian (called Xanthium 12, manufactured by Seven Forests, in the United States) tablets. Dose: 6 tablets 4 times a day until symptoms are relieved. 6 tabs twice a day prevents an attack. Helps pollen-related allergies by reducing sensitivity to external irritants.

External Applications

Reflexology for allergy symptoms

Allergy sufferers can relieve their runny noses, sneezing, and itchy eyes by rubbing:

—the big toe with the thumb, in an upward movement toward the nail; the webbed area between each toe on the top of the foot (to stimulate the lymph system);

—the Large Intestine points that run in a line above the heel. Press points thoroughly with the thumb (to reduce mucus).

The Chinese recommend drinking three glasses of warm water following reflexology treatment.

Allergic Itching

• Neuralgic and allergic itching can be treated with Job's tears. Make a decoction using 9 g to 1½ cups water. Drink warm twice a day. Take a bath afterward, with hot enough water to force a sweat.

• You will need fresh loquat leaves, which contain an active ingredient that stops inflammation, for this. Ask at your local natural foods store or Korean grocery. Wash, cut slightly, slip them into a wine bottle, and add ethyl alcohol. Let soak for a week or until the leaves have turned old and discolored. Strain leaves out and massage the remaining dark liquid into affected areas after bath. Follow the nerve paths, but be careful around the face not to touch delicate membranes of the eye and mouth with the solution. Fresh loquat leaves can also be applied directly to the skin and fastened in place.

Acupressure for allergic itching and prickly rash

(See BodyMap for the location of points. Abbreviations of points are explained in the BodyMap.)

Uranaitei—On the sole of foot, a finger's width below the second toe. Moxibustion can be used very effectively here. Use 3 to 5 pieces on each foot.

GV. 14—Press here with fingernail 5 to 7 times or use 3 pieces of moxa to clear pathogens in the Yang channels and to clear Lung Heat.

BL. 13—Press, apply ginger moxa, or use a moxa stick to regulate Lung Qi, alleviate asthma and cough.

BL. 21—Press to transform and disperse Damp. Press, rub, or apply moxa.

Hives (Urticaria)

Hives are intensely itchy raised and swollen welts on the skin caused by a release of histamine within the skin. Angioedema is an eruption of the skin similar to hives but structures under the skin are affected. These conditions are basically related to allergy conditions. If an attack of hives lasts for six weeks or less it is designated acute, if it lasts longer, it is chronic.

Its causes and triggers are diverse. Excessive friction, overheating, excessive mental stress, reactions to the sun, cold or heat contact, contact with water, overexercise, and sudden changes in temperature can bring it on.

External influences such as hive-inducing drugs (particularly aspirin and penicillin), food, food colorants, flavorings, preservatives, emulsifiers, and stabilizers can cause allergic reactions resulting in hives.

Hives are a symptom of Rebellious Qi and Water Toxin in Oriental medicine terms. This condition can fall into various categories that often overlap.

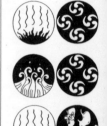

1) Wind Heat is lodged in the superficial channels below the skin.

This produces a deep red rash with severe itching.

2) Wind Damp is lodged in the superficial channels below the skin.

This produces a lighter colored rash, less itching than the above case, a heavy feeling in the body, and fluid retention.

3) Heat accumulation in the Stomach and Intestines

This syndrome produces a red rash accompanied by abdominal pain, constipation, and a strong thirst.

The basic therapeutic approach is to identify and control all the factors that are causing the outbreak of hives. This usually means working closely with a practitioner.

Internal Applications

• Avoid food allergens: the most common triggers are milk, fish, poultry, meat, eggs, beans, and nuts.
• Eliminate all food additives. Additives appear to be a major factor in many cases of chronic hives in children. Azo dyes, flavorings (salicylates, aspartame), preservatives (benzoates, nitrates, sorbic acid), antioxidants (hydroxytoluene, sulfite, gallate), and emulsifiers/stabilizers (polysorbates, vegetable gums) have all been found to trigger hives. Allergy to the food colorant tartrazine, commonly found in packaged foods, is common in people allergic to aspirin. It increases cells related to inflammatory reactions.[1]
• Foods that produce Damp and Phlegm should also be avoided if possible (see Chapter 3).
• Avoid foods that irritate the Stomach/Spleen (see Chapter 3).
• Avoid foods that weaken the Kidneys (see Chapter 3).
• Foods that nourish the Kidneys are recommended (see Chapter 3).
• Include more foods that nourish the Stomach/Spleen (see recommendations in Chapter 3 and the section Adapting to Stress and Building the Immune System in Part II).
• Infections are a major cause of hives in children. Strep throat, a bacterial infection, can also lead to an acute case of hives. In adults, bacterial, viral, and yeast infections can lead to hives. So can chronic trichomoniasis and hepatitis-B. See a practitioner if you think you may be suffering from any of these.
• If you suspect infection, get plenty of rest, limit sugar consumption, and take echinacea,

goldenseal, or Chinese Chinese licorice, proven blood cleansers, two to three times a day. Follow the dosage on the bottle. Note: if taking Chinese licorice for a prolonged period, eat more calcium-rich foods.

• Drinking a skin nutritive and tonic made of lightly toasted sesame seeds and a few drops of honey in 3 tsp. of *sake* twice a day is said to help clear up hives. Water instead of the *sake* is fine.

External Applications

• For itchy skin, slice a Japanese radish or daikon radish into rounds and apply the cut end directly to skin. The enzymes in the daikon radish help relieve itching and Heat under the skin.

• Infuse chrysanthemum leaves (one ounce per two cups water) in a covered ceramic pot for 15 minutes; add a few drops of vinegar, cool the mixture to skin temperature, and apply over affected area to relieve itching.

• Cucumber juice can help relieve swelling and inflammation. Peel and grate a cucumber and squeeze in a cotton cloth or cheese cloth to extract juice. Add a small amount of herbal borax powder and apply over affected area.

• Garlic's powerful antibacterial properties can be taken advantage of when hives are due to bacterial infection. Bathe the area in a broth made from chopped and boiled garlic.

• Fresh perilla leaves can be placed over affected areas. Eat them raw also, particularly if oily fish such as sardines or mackerel has triggered hives.

Recipe: Chicken Liver, Scallions, and Ginkgo Nuts

This recipe applies the theory of the Doctrine of Signatures (the theory of like-cures-like[2]) through the use of chicken liver. It is said to strengthen the Liver and fortify its filtering function. Chinese Chinese licorice is indicated to relieve inflammation. It is also a detoxification agent.

Serves 2

    200 g chicken livers
    1-inch piece fresh ginger
    $1/3$ c sliced leeks, or
    $1/2$ a round cooking onion
    1–2 cloves garlic

    1 tbsp. soy sauce
    $1 1/2$ tsp. mirin
    3 g Chinese Chinese licorice
    12 ginkgo nuts
    1 sweet red pepper
    1 or 2 bunches green or yellow Chinese chives or scallions
    canola oil

To prepare:

    1. Wash and cut liver into bite-sized pieces.
    2. Slice ginger and crush roughly with the heel of a knife,

chop onion or leek.

3. Add liver, half the amount of garlic and ginger, soy sauce, mirin, $1^1/_2$ tbsp. water, and Chinese licorice to pot. Braise until the juice has evaporated.

4. Prepare ginkgo nuts. Hull and boil until soft.

5. Cut pepper into very thin julienne strips and cut the chives or scallions into 4 cm lengths.

6. Add oil and remaining ginger and garlic to wok. When hot, add peppers, ginkgo, nuts and leek or onion. Once softened, add liver and finish cooking over a high flame. Place in the center of the serving dish.

7. In an empty wok, add a touch of oil, chives, a dash of salt and pepper, and cook over high heat until the color comes out. Spread in a ring around the liver and peppers, or mix together.

Endnotes

*1 For a brief, concise introduction to food allergies, see Michael Murray and Joseph Pizzorno, *Encyclopedia of Natural Medicine* (Rocklin, Ca.: Prima Publishing, 1991), pp.305–321.

*2 The Doctrine of Signatures is regarded by many today as an old wives' tale, yet in our experience it has proven effective in many cases. The truth lies in the testing.

Anemia

Oriental Medical Energetics

Anemia, according to Western medicine a condition of not having enough red blood cells, is called Blood Deficiency in Oriental medicine. But remember that from the Eastern point of view, Blood refers to more than the red liquid that flows through veins and arteries. It is the means by which the nutrients that flow through the blood are produced; it is the function of nourishing the body's tissues and then storing the nutrients.

A diagnosis of Blood Deficiency means, essentially, either that the Blood does not contain enough nutrients to adequately nourish the tissues or that there is not enough blood, or red blood cells, circulating in a particular area at any one time.

Weak, deficient Blood occurs as a result of weakness in related organs and their meridian systems.

1) Deficient Spleen

The Spleen is a primary player in the production of Blood. It converts nutrients from broken-down food into Blood. If one's diet does not contain ample nutrition, or if the Spleen is already weakened by irregular eating habits, stress, or long-term illness, it will be unable to produce Blood to feed the body. The Spleen also holds the blood vessels in place, and if the Qi in the Spleen is weak, Blood will be easily lost, as in the case of a woman who loses excessive blood during menstruation. Excessive loss of blood will create a shortage or lack of healthy Blood, which could eventually lead to irregular periods or amenorrhea.

Accompanying symptoms could include a sallow complexion, anorexia, fullness and distention in the epigastrium and abdomen, abdominal pain relieved by pressure, fatigue and weakness in the arms and legs, nausea, and a loose stool.

2) Deficient Jing energy

The Kidney may also be involved in Blood Deficiency. In this case, the Jing energy, the body's generative and sexual energy, is housed in the Kidney and creates a substance called Marrow, not to be confused with the fatty, vascular tissue that fills the cavities of most bones. Think of this Marrow as a matrix out of which the spinal column, brain, and bone marrow are formed. Bone marrow produces Blood. If the Jing is weak, it follows that the Blood will be weak, as will the brain function and bones.

Symptoms of a lack of Jing include premature aging, graying hair, hair loss, loss of teeth, poor memory, senility, gradual worsening of sight and hearing, weakening of bones, and sexual dysfunction. In males it can manifest as impotence; in females as a lack of interest in sex or insufficient vaginal secretions; in children as mental or physical retardation, bed-wetting, poor bone development, and retarded sexual development.

3) Liver Blood Deficiency

A Liver involvement could also play a significant part in Blood Deficiency. The Liver stores Blood when the body is at rest and releases it to the control of the Heart when the body goes into motion. Dizziness and fainting that occur when the body is moved could be the result of the Liver not releasing Blood when it is needed. This could be due to hemorrhage, chronic disease, worry, fatigue, and eyestrain, all of which deplete stores of Blood in the Liver.

Symptoms include a sallow complexion, dry skin, dizziness, dry eyes, blurred or failing vision, spots in front of the eyes, insomnia, dream-disturbed sleep, irritability, becoming easily startled, pale lips, tinnitus, pale finger and toe nails, tremors, spasms, involuntary movements, light menstrual flow, amenorrhea, and late menses.

Symptoms of these imbalances hardly ever manifest in pure form; instead, they are often mixed and show up in any number of combinations. Generally, a Spleen imbalance can be identified through the presence of abdominal bloating, diarrhea with undigested food, a tendency to bruise or hemorrhage, and anorexia. In women, weak Jing in the Kidney usually shows up as lower back pain, especially prior to menstruation in women, impaired menstruation, a lack of vaginal secretion; men might suffer from lower back pain, a weakened libido, impotence, and premature ejaculation. Other symptoms are fuzzy thinking and an inability to concentrate. A weak Liver can be identified through dry skin in the face, brittle nails, dizziness, and blurred vision.

There is a simple test for anemia in the book *Healing Ourselves* by Naboru Muramoto. Stretch your hand out and make it slightly tense. The fingers should stretch in a convex manner upward. If the fingernails stay white, you are anemic. If you don't have to stretch your hand to get the whiteness, the condition is severe, he says. Double-check by pulling down the lower eyelid to see if it is pale underneath. It should be red.

Internal Applications
• Avoid toxic substances. The tannins in tea and coffee inhibit iron absorption. So do additives found in dairy products, beer, candy bars, and soft drinks. Cigarettes contain cadmium, which also interferes with iron absorption.
• Avoid raw foods and cold or iced foods and drinks.
• Foods that strengthen the digestive function and the Stomach/Spleen organs and meridians nurture the Qi and tone the Blood: chicken and vegetable broths with lightly cooked vegetables, rice porridge with Chinese red dates, leeks, or scallions, yellow and orange vegetables, root vegetable stews and simmered dishes, lightly steamed greens, whole grains.
• The Anti-hypoglycemic Stew, listed under Recipes in the Heart Problems section, is good for people with anemia, as well.

• Try to include foods that tone and cleanse the Blood (see Chapter 3).

• Kidney organ and meridian tonics strengthen the Kidney Yang and Jing and can be helpful for anemia (see Chapter 3).

• Include foods that detoxify and tone the Liver (see Chapter 3). Liver organ meats are toning; dandelion greens are particularly good.

• Dang gui is one of the major Blood builders and cleansers in the Oriental medical pharmacopeia. It can be used by both men and women to strengthen the Blood. It has a warm energy that tonifies the Heart, Liver, Spleen, and Kidney. Cooked dang gui works to warm the inner organs, strengthen the Blood, and enhance skin quality and Blood circulation. It regulates the female endocrine system. It also harmonizes the Blood, making sure its consistency and nutritive balance is appropriate to the body's needs. It has mild sedative effects and contains vitamin B_{12}, which is necessary to prevent anemia.

You don't need to use dang gui as a medicine. It can be used regularly in cooking, about three times a week, without a problem, but do not take dang gui while menstruating. It will increase the blood flow. I add dang gui to codonopsis, dioscorea, Chinese red dates, and sometimes peony root. To make this broth, see the recipe in the Appendix. Add a few slices of dang gui to chicken—a naturally delicious pair; cooked with garlic, onion, ginger, Japanese kabocha pumpkin, rutabaga, turnips, or carrots, they make a fortifying soup or stew for body and Blood.

• Cooked di huang (*Rehmannia glutinosa*) is one of the most effective Blood and Kidney tonics. (There is a raw version that has other medicinal effects.) It tones up the Marrow, strengthens bones and tendons, eyes and ears. Rehmannia aids blood circulation in the legs and is also used after childbirth to strengthen the female reproductive system and relieve abdominal pain. It can be decocted and drunk in a tea with dang gui, peony root, and the Chinese herb ligusticum as a woman's tonic. Or add 1 to 3 grams to stews, soups, and other simmered dishes. Or see a practitioner for a diagnosis and prescription. Try it and see how you like it; it can be too oily for some people's stomachs.

• Di huang is also the main component of a patent medicine called Shou Wu Chih, manufactured by The United Pharmaceutical Manufactory of Kwangchow in the People's Republic of China. Although it is available in the United States as a dietary supplement, it has not been approved for sale in Canada and its sale is in contravention of the Canadian Food and Drug Act for containing unspecified amounts of digitalis, a powerful heart stimulant.

The tonic is supposed to be a version of a very common woman's tonic called Four Things Soup, which strengthens the Blood, warms and strengthens the body, builds immune function, strengthens women's sexual organs, and regulates menstruation. See the recipe for Four Things Vegetable Soup in the Appendix.

• Longan, dried litchi fruit, is another herb recommended for anemia. It strengthens the Heart and helps the body cope with stress. It is also a Spleen, Blood, and energy tonic. It combines well with simmered meat dishes and soups. It is fairly sweet, so use it sparingly unless you like a sweet, glazed meat type of dish. Try it with chicken gizzards, lamb, or beef. For breakfast, boil longan meats with slivered ginger. Longan can also be added to green leafy vegetable dishes simmered with baby onion, garlic, and ginger, for example, in a light oyster or dark miso sauce. To prepare this, lightly brown garlic and ginger in a wok or frying pan with a small amount of oil, add 6 to 8 shelled longan fruits with or without the seed, $^1/_2$ cup of water, and 6 to 8 baby onions, and simmer for 5 minutes. Add spinach, bok choy, or other green leafy vegetables, turn up the heat, and stir-fry quickly to preserve the fresh green color of the vegetable.

• Organ meats strengthen organs, at least according to the theory of like-heals-like, which holds that a weak Liver or Kidney will benefit from liver and kidney organ meats. Liver cooked with Chinese cinnamon and soaked Chinese black dates with a bunch of greens and red pepper thrown in at the end is a delicious way to eat it. Lamb, by the way, is very Warming and is called "woman's meat" in China. (See the Appendix for directions on the proper preparation of organ meats.)

• Wheatgrass is a highly nutritious food that has a chlorophyll molecular structure similar to hemoglobin's, the blood's protein in charge of transporting oxygen. The similarity of the two might explain why experiments with anemic animals have shown that their blood counts return to normal after four or five days of receiving chlorophyll in wheatgrass. Alfalfa is also high in chlorophyll and detoxifies the system, especially the liver. Dandelion cleanses the Blood, and nettle is an overall body tonic, recommended in cases of anemia.

• Blackstrap molasses contains iron and essential B vitamins. Take a tablespoon a day to strengthen the Blood.

• Dokudami, found in several Japanese health teas available in the United States and in pharmacies and natural food stores in Japan (see the back of the book for ordering information), is traditionally drunk in Japan to help cleanse and build healthy Blood and aid digestion.

• Saffron is indicated in Oriental medicine in cases of weak Blood.

• **Saffron Wine**
>   1 tsp. saffron
>   1 liter of 45° alcohol
>   optional: $^1/_2$ cup honey or granulated sugar

Let this sit for a week and drink a *sake* cupful nightly.

• Iron is necessary to make hemoglobin. To increase amounts of iron in the Blood, for a while eat fewer almonds, less asparagus, beets, cashews, chocolate, kale, rhubarb, sorrel, spinach, Swiss chard, and most nuts and beans. They contain oxalic acid, which cuts down on iron absorption.

• Egg oil can be taken daily for anemia, Kidney and Liver trouble, a weak constitution, low blood pressure, hemorrhoids, and vaginal problems. The liquid is extremely bitter. Dilute with 5 drops to 15 drops of water. (See the recipe for The Essential Egg in the Appendix.)

External Applications

Moxibustion for the Spleen and digestive function
(See BodyMap for the location of points. Meanings of abbreviations are also included in the BodyMap.)

>   SP. 6—Tones the digestive function and harmonizes with ST. 36.
>   ST. 36—Tones the Qi of the entire body, strengthens and regulates the digestive function. Use 4 to 5 balls of moxa once or twice a day.
>   C.V. 12—An old Korean remedy works to warm and stimulate the point with 50 tiny balls of moxa burned there daily. Alternatively, warm with a moxa stick.

Arthritis (rheumatoid)

Two common forms of arthritis are osteoarthritis and rheumatoid arthritis. Osteoarthritis affects the cartilage covering the bones in a joint. The cartilage erodes, creating friction, while the tendons, ligaments, and muscles holding the joint together weaken and the joint itself becomes deformed, painful, and stiff. Osteoarthritis is a natural process of aging, although it tends to run in families and is more common in women.

Rheumatoid arthritis is characterized by a swelling, thickening, and folding of the synovial membranes, the membranes in joint cavities that secrete lubricating fluids. This swelling and thickening spreads over the cartilage and, together with the enzymes in the synovial fluid, eats away at the bone underneath. The joints become unstable, painful, swollen, and in advanced stages, greatly deformed. The body as a whole also suffers, leaving the person feeling weak, tired, feverish, and generally ill with a loss of appetite. The remedies included in this section deal primarily with arthritic pain of the rheumatoid type, bursitis, and tendonitis.

Oriental Medical Energetics

Obstruction

BI
HI

These pathologies are referred to as *Bi*, a word used in Oriental medicine to mean pain or obstruction. Bi is caused by an obstruction of Qi energy and Blood circulation due to an invasion of Wind, Cold, and Damp in the body. Spending too much time in damp environments, working in wet clothes, wearing wet, sweaty clothes during sports for too long—all these can play a significant role in the development of Bi, of which there are four common patterns:

1) A change in the weather, cold, or rain triggers pain that moves from place to place.

Wind Bi, also called Wandering Bi, manifests as pain moving to different areas in the body. It typically manifests as lower back pain that disappears following a visit to the doctor, but is soon replaced by a dreadful shoulder or knee pain. The pain is often accompanied by chills and a fever, and suggests Liver involvement to the practitioner. Wind Bi can be effectively treated through acupuncture.

2) Pain is worse when it is cold.

Cold Bi, or Painful Bi, is characterized by severe fixed pain that feels worse when it is cold and is relieved by warmth. Cold Bi is treated with moxibustion.

3) The joints feel sore and heavy when it rains.

Damp Bi, or Obvious Bi, manifests as skin and muscle numbness or a sore, heavy sensation around the joints. Walking and any type of movement is worse in damp, wet weather and the sufferer often has a problem with edema and fluid build-up. This is treated with a combination of moxibustion and acupuncture.

4) Heat causes the joints to swell with an achy burn.

The fourth type is called Febrile Bi, characterized by painful, swollen joints, inflammation, and a feeling of heat in the body or around the joints. This form is treated with acupuncture.

All forms of Bi or arthritis will also be treated by the practitioner with herbal formulas based on each individual case. Treatment focuses on increasing circulation and ridding the body of Damp or Heat. In advanced cases, Oriental medicine cannot help the sufferer regain what has already been lost, but it can stop the pain and slow down the degenerative process. Inflammatory diseases of the joints, soft tissue, neuralgia, sciatic nerve pain, facial nerve problems, intercostal pain, and intercostal hernia are all related to the syndrome.

Years of unhealthy living, poor nutrition, an unhealthy environment, overeating, emotional and physical stress, a sedentary lifestyle, and the lack of a positive outlook contribute to metabolic imbalance and the breakdown of body functions. This results in damage to the normal channels of elimination: Kidneys, bladder and bowels, Liver, Lungs, and skin, resulting in a large build-up of toxins in the joints.

Self-Help Strategies

—Cleanse the body of toxins (Damp, Cold, Wind) and tone the organs of elimination and the vital organs. Clear constipation.

—Cleanse and tone the Blood and Qi.

—Strengthen the immune system (see the section, Adapting to Stress and Building the Immune System).

Internal Applications

• Avoid foods that create Damp (see Chapter 3).

• Reduce intake of cooling foods such as asparagus, celery, cucumbers, seaweed, soybean products, spinach; cold or iced beverages, and cold, raw, and iced foods.

• Avoid refined, processed foods, including white rice and white flour. Limit your intake of starchy foods, particularly at night.

• Eliminate or reduce sugar—it drains vitamin B, which is necessary for general muscle flexibility and organ muscle tone of the heart, stomach, and intestines.

• Niacin, or vitamin B_3, is needed for healthy nerve function. Some natural sources are beef, broccoli, carrots, corn flour, and fish.

• Add foods that clear and strengthen the Liver (see Chapter 3).

• Make a pot of mugwort tea in the morning and keep it on hand during the day to sip instead of coffee and caffeinated tea; it cleanses the Liver and the Blood.

• Ginger warms the entire system. Eat it often in stir-fries, simmered dishes, or slivered on fish or rice porridge. Drink ginger tea decocted with Chinese licorice to warm, nourish, and cleanse the system.

• Job's tears can be eaten with brown rice in soups. It clears the Large Intestine.

• Sesame seeds are rich in calcium, reduce the nerves' sensitivity to pain, and help relieve inflammation in the nerves.

• Clear the Large Intestine by eating konnyaku, okara, burdock root, celery and the sea vegetable wakame. Eat them in large quantities at first; once the intestines clear, gradually add more vegetables and brown rice.

• Safflower cleanses the Blood and warms the body. Decoct a tablespoon with 2 tbsp. Job's tears (the grain, not the roasted tea) purchased from a herb shop or Chinese pharmacy and 2 tbsp. red lycium berries. The Job's tears are Sweet and Cooling, have diuretic and sedative properties, and relieve nerve pain, along with stomach inflammation, edema, and warts. The lycium berries are Sweet and Neutral, are tonic to the Liver, aid exhaustion, dizziness, headache, and diabetes. You can use this mixture to cook with as an antidote to pain due to Damp Bi. Try it in a stew with chicken, shiitake, long green onion, bamboo shoots, and carrots. Add a dash of soy sauce, *sake*, and ginger, and simmer until the vegetables are cooked through.

• Rice porridge with walnuts, topped with slivered ginger and chopped scallions, benefits Cold Bi, is tonic to the Kidneys, warms and strengthens the Stomach/Spleen, and helps clear the Large Intestine. Cooked with dang gui (10 g), the porridge will also help relieve inflammation. (See the Appendix for directions for porridge.)

External Applications

• Relax, so much so that you allow yourself to feel dimwitted, or even really out of it for a while. Take a week off, visit a hot spring retreat, stay in a country bed and breakfast inn, or develop an intimate relationship with a beach—whatever it takes—complete relaxation is crucial. It will allow your system to let go of stress and begin to release the toxins that perpetuate disease.

• Sunlight—get some everyday (unless you have sensitive skin or another skin condition that is exacerbated by sunlight), but avoid *over*exposure. Ten minutes a day is enough. Try to stay out of the sun between 10 A.M. and 3 P.M., when the sun's rays are strongest.

• A ginger compress directly on the points of pain, or soaking hands in ginger juice, helps warm the body and gets the blood circulating. More blood in circulation means blocked energy will become unblocked more quickly, and the Chinese always say that where there is pain, there is blockage.

• Ginger and red pepper poultice is a variation on this theme, touted as a "miracle cure" for rheumatic pain. Grate 3 to 4 nubs of ginger. Then boil 5 finely chopped dried hot red peppers in 100 ml of water until reduced by about a quarter. Mix the ginger and water together, add a small amount of rice or barley flour until you have formed a smooth cream, spread onto half a cotton cloth and fold the other half over the spread cream, and apply to the painful area. Cover this with gauze and plastic wrap, and tape into place with surgical tape. If you have sensitive skin use less pepper. Remove immediately if skin irritation beyond a little redness results.

• Foot and hip ginger baths are recommended for painful rheumatism. Grate $1/4$ to $1/2$ cup of ginger root and boil in 2 quarts of water until it turns quite dark and emits a strong ginger smell. Add this to bath water or your foot-soaking bucket.

• Mugwort baths are recommended for nerve pain and rheumatism. Boil 2 handfuls of the dried leaves in 2 quarts of water, strain, and add to your bath water. This also improves the circulation.

Back Pain

Includes: chronic back pain, lumbago, and sciatica.

Chronic back pain is one of the most frequent complaints in an acupuncture clinic and rivals only arthritis as being the cause of the most missed days of work. The causes of chronic back pain are many, but the pain can usually be attributed to incorrect posture, improper lifting, pushing and pulling during daily activities, or to internal disorders, such as overwork and stress that weaken the Kidney and Liver organs and meridian systems with possible involvement of the Heart or Spleen. Four common syndromes are included below.

Oriental Medical Energetics

1) Imbalance or weakness in the Kidney

The most common causes of lower back pain are external, such as the ones listed above. When an internal imbalance is involved, the Kidney is the organ network most affected. Excessively practicing detoxifying diets, a diet high in salt or in raw foods, or constant purging, for example, can weaken the Kidney Qi and the Blood. This condition can be accompanied by Blood Stagnation, which could manifest, for example, as sciatica or clots in the menstrual blood. Lumbar pain would be only one of a whole set of symptoms. If you fall into any of these patterns, see a practitioner. The Kidney organ is crucial to a long life full of vigor and vitality, so you don't want to put it in jeopardy.

Weakness in the Kidney organ and meridian system can manifest as cold extremities, hearing loss or ringing in the ears, fatigue, an increased need to sleep, a loss of stamina, sore throats, frequent or difficult urination, puffiness around the eyes, impotence or diminished libido, forgetfulness, and a fearful, depressed, or grumpy disposition, in addition to lower back pain.

Self-Help Strategy

—In this case, the primary treatment principle is to protect and tone the Kidney.

2) Heart imbalance

If the Heart is involved, the lumbar pain and weakness along the spine may be accompanied by mood swings and extremes, disturbed sleeping patterns, lack of muscle tone and joint flexibility, anxiety, restlessness, an easily excitable nature that burns out quickly, nausea, diarrhea or frequent urination related to mood shifts, phobias, manic-depressive behavior, a craving for salty, spicy, stimulating foods, and thyroid imbalance.

Self-Help Strategy

—Harmonize the Kidney and the Heart.

3) Spleen Deficiency

To identify Spleen Deficiency look for signs of sluggish digestion, bloating, distention, constipation and water retention after overeating, dry skin and mouth, sore or swollen face, hands, feet, muscles, or joints, chills or cold extremities, diarrhea or loose stools with bloating, urination irregularities—too little, too much, or too frequent—gingivitis, cystitis, or urethritis, prostate trouble, a craving for sweet or salty food, and an apathetic or insecure personality.

Self-Help Strategy

—In this case, the practitioner would harmonize the Spleen and Kidney.

4) Excess Liver Yang

The Liver imbalance usually associated with lumbar pain is the Excess of Liver Yang Energy. This imbalance is often seen in middle-aged men who also suffer headaches, neck and shoulder pain, red eyes and face, insomnia, palpitation, vertigo, irritability, and weakness in the lower part of the body.

Self-Help Strategies

—Lower the Yang.
—Build the Kidney Yin, which nourishes the Liver Yin.

Internal Applications

• Avoid coffee, tea, alcohol.

• For Kidney imbalance, stay away from excessively salty foods, raw food, and cold drinks.

• For Spleen involvement, eliminate foods that weaken the Stomach/Spleen: greasy oily foods and cold or iced foods and beverages.

• For Heart involvement, try not to eat foods that overstimulate the body: chili pepper, wasabi, horseradish, caffeine, alcohol.

• For Liver involvement, eliminate foods that aggravate the Liver (see Chapter 3).

• Eat more foods that tone Qi and Blood: fresh and lightly steamed vegetables, whole grains, and legumes (see Chapter 3).

• For Kidney involvement, include foods that tone the Kidney and build Kidney fire. Azuki beans, kidney beans, fish, and kidney organ meats are recommended (see Chapter 3. For directions for preparing kidney organ meat, see the Appendix). Also try the Azuki Bean Broth (see Recipes in the Appendix).

• For Spleen involvement, include foods that tone the Spleen and Middle Burner (see Chapter 3).

• For Heart involvement, eat foods that tone the Heart. (See Chapter 3.)

• For Liver Yang, foods that cool and lower the rising Qi and tone the Liver Yin are helpful (see Chapter 3). See a practitioner for help in getting the balance right. It may be that the Yin is so depleted that too many Cooling foods could stop the Liver's ability to keep its fire under control.

• Cooked di huang (rehmannia) is indicated for a weak Kidney. Add 3 to 5 g to soup with dioscorea, peony root, and dang gui to make Four Things Soup. (See the Appendix for Four Things Vegetable Soup.) Also, see a practitioner for a proper diagnosis and an herbal formula containing di huang appropriate for your condition.

External Applications

• Massage by a qualified therapist should help relieve symptoms. Practitioners worth their salt should work on educating the clients in ways to prevent back pain from returning. The therapist teaches exercises to improve posture and strengthen the related muscles, and helps integrate the therapy into the client's everyday life. Simply relieving the pain is not adequate treatment. Before beginning therapy, mention any injuries you may have incurred so that the therapist can take them into consideration and proceed more slowly during the treatment, in response to possible scarring of tissue. This way the pain can be gradually released without the therapy itself causing more trauma.

• Postural realignment is indicated if your back problems are chronic and due to poor posture. Try Iyengar yoga to realign posture, or see a specialist, such as a Rolfer or Alexander Technique practitioner, for realignment and backup sessions to follow up on the realignment.

• Simple exercises can help alleviate back pain, but please note before doing than that the spine is very delicate. Exercises affecting it should always be performed carefully and slowly. Never force movements, and stop at the first signs of discomfort. Increase repetitions and the length of time the positions are held gradually, paying attention to any muscle or spinal soreness that might occur in the next few days after exercising.

—Stand up with the feet hip-width apart and revolve the hips in small then larger circles in both directions, then rock the pelvis gently forward and backward to get more movement in the spine.

—Stretch the hamstrings by bending forward while standing with the legs together. If you have trouble keeping this position separate your legs until you can hold the position comfortably. The stretch should move into the spine. Breathe deeply and hold this for as long as is comfortable.

—Traditional neck rolls, which normally help stretch the neck and shoulder area, could cause muscle spasms or changes in an arthritic condition. Instead, gently rock the head backward and forward, then turn it to the left and the right, four times each.

—A common yoga stretch that helps with mid—and upper back pain is to lift the right arm over the head, bend at the elbow, and grasp the elbow with the left hand. Rotate the elbow inward and upward so that you stretch the inner arm and the armpit muscles. Hold this for 10 seconds. Then take the left hand behind and grasp the right hand in the back. Hold this for as long as possible. Repeat both stretches on the opposite side.

—Try sitting sideways on a straight-backed chair with the feet forward and flat on the floor. Exhale, then twist and grasp the back of the chair firmly with both hands. Breathe deeply, allowing the breath to fill the lower back area. Hold for a minute and switch to the other side.

—To stretch the entire back and shoulders, sit in your chair, hold a towel in both hands and extend the arms up over your head. Let the shoulders ride up toward the ears. Hold this for 10 seconds and release quickly down. Repeat several times, letting all the tightness out with a big sigh on the release.

—To invigorate the upper back and shoulders, stand up and swing the arms in big circles around toward the front as fast as you can for a count of 10. Then swing toward the back for ten. The energy in your arms should race down to your fingertips.

Sciatica

The sciatic nerve starts at the base of the spine and travels down through the buttock, the thigh, and the lower leg to the foot. Sciatica is a swelling or pain that could be the result of an injury to the nerve, causing pain, soreness, or tingling. Another cause could be misalignment of the body. If you suffer from back pain that travels down the leg, please see a qualified practitioner.

Oriental Medical Energetics

1) Wind Cold or Wind Damp invade the body and block Qi.

In Oriental medicine, pain that occurs on one side of the body is interpreted as an obstruction of Qi or energy flow resulting from an injury or an invasion of an environmental factor, either Wind Cold or Wind Damp, that block the energy flow. Pain that shifts location is said to be influenced by Wind. Cold contracts, freezes, and blocks normal movement, producing sharp and intense pain. Damp sciatic pain in the lumbar and legs is heavy and turbid, worsening on wet days.

These energy imbalances can occur in the Gallbladder channel down the outside of the leg, in the Bladder channel down the back of the leg, or along the Stomach channel, which runs down the outer front of the leg.

Self-Help Strategies

—Disperse blocked Qi with warmth.
—See a practitioner for a proper diagnosis.

2) Blood Stagnation

Sciatic pain can be caused by Blood Stagnation from injury or menstrual problems. It can be produced by overexposure to the natural elements of cold and wind.

Self-Help Strategies

—Reduce or eliminate exposure to wind and cold.
—Get the Blood circulating. This may require professional treatment.

Internal Applications

• Avoid Damp-producing foods, such as ice cream, cold, raw foods, and oily or deep-fried foods, which can worsen sciatica.

• Cut down on coffee. Instant coffee has been shown to block the opiate receptors in rat brains, making the body more receptive to pain.

External Applications

• Ginger compresses are helpful. Make a broth from grated ginger decocted in a cup of water until it turns a dark golden color, then soak a clean white cloth in the broth; or boil grated ginger in water and add the solution to bath water for a ginger bath. Also try a massage oil with the juice from grated ginger (or essential oil of ginger) and sesame oil. Apply directly onto painful areas. In cases where sciatica is related to Stagnant Blood and menstrual problems, apply poultices to the lower abdomen as well.

• Strong acupressure or moxibustion applied to a particular point along the Bladder meridian may help. To find the point, press in the hollow behind the outer ankle bone, then come up 3 to 5 inches until you find a sore or sensitive spot. Press strongly or burn moxibustion balls or warm the point with a moxa stick for 5 to 10 minutes on both sides. You can also press the inside crease of the leg to relieve obstruction along the Bladder meridian, but do not use moxa here. (See the BodyMap for an illustration of points along the Urinary Bladder meridian.)

• If you have back trouble, avoid sports such as baseball, basketball, football, golf, tennis, and weight lifting. The movements involved in these sports are potentially very damaging to the back. Swimming and light yoga are more appropriate choices.

Body Odor and Bad Breath

The body has three ways to eliminate toxins and wastes. The primary system is through digestion. Foods are broken down and processed out through the intestines. When this system becomes blocked, however, as sometimes happens, other systems are called in to help with the work. Those systems are the skin and the respiratory system.

Oriental Medical Energetics

Traditionally, smell was an important indicator of illness or imbalance in Oriental medicine. Chinese doctors regularly checked a patient's breath, stool, and urine to determine where imbalance lay. On a simpler level, we, too, are aware of these smells. Think of going to a bedridden person's bedroom or to a hospital room; the distinctive odor is instantly recognizable. Each smell is different for each person, but there are commonalities among these odors that hold valuable information for a doctor of Oriental medicine.

According to the Five Element Theory, each element is associated with an organ and meridian system; each element also has a corresponding smell. It is not easy for an untrained nose to discern the odor at all, and to place it within an olfactory spectrum might seem an impossible task. But with training it can be done.

For example, people with trouble in the Lung meridian or the lung itself might give off a fishy, rotting smell when they sweat profusely. The smell is often manifested in combination with a white color in the cheeks or a pale complexion with pink or red spots on the cheeks, and a tendency to have a weak, forceless, or weepy voice. This condition might be accompanied by a sunken chest or a large, expanded chest while the person breathes only superficially, from the upper lung cavity. Emotionally this person may whine, complain, need to grieve, or may be overindulging in grief.

Kidney disorders give off a putrid, metallic, sulfurous smell. The skin color associated with a Kidney disorder is brownish to dark gray or bluish black, especially around the eyes. It could be accompanied by urinary problems, such as excessive urination or difficulty in urinating. The voice may sound fearful or hesitant, and the person might seem afraid of commitment and lack clarity.

Liver disorders are characterized by their rancid, sour, or sharp odors, like rancid butter or sour milk. This could be accompanied by a greenish hue in the face, sore and reddish, dry, itchy eyes, abdominal bloating, and tightness in the lower ribs. Emotionally, this person may exhibit irritability and could be easily aroused to anger. Inversely, the person might never feel angry and instead feel depressed all the time—in psychological terms, depression is anger turned inward. The voice could sound domineering or depressed.

The smell of an imbalanced Heart meridian is slightly scorched, dry, or burned. The smell and imbalance are accompanied by symptoms of insomnia, anxiety, or heart palpitation. This person might be unable to express emotions or may feel overexuberant, tending toward restlessness or endless searching for gratification, without ever feeling satiated or satisfied. The voice tends to be jumpy and breathless and the speech may race. This person sometimes squeaks and laughs inappropriately.

The Spleen odor is sweet, a cloying and overpowering smell, like too many flowers in one room. Spleen disorders may be accompanied by a yellowish tinge in the skin that ranges in hue from a barely noticeable golden tone to a deep ocher. In Oriental medicine jaundice is related to Stomach/Spleen problems rather than to Liver problems. This person may also have digestion problems, a sweet, sticky taste in the mouth, a loose stool with undigested food in it, and a craving for sweets or salty junk food.

Self-Help Strategies

—Clear the Large Intestine.
—Rebalance other organ systems.

All these smells and disorders point to an accumulation of toxins in the body that have to be eliminated somehow. When the odors are strong and easily discernible, the main channel of elimination, the Large Intestine, is generally blocked. Constipation forces the toxins to make their way out of the body through the breath and the pores.

Menstrual smells are an exception. Regularly changing body odors naturally accompany a woman's cycle, reflecting healthy hormonal shifts. The odors have an aphrodisiac effect, some people say, and they indicate a woman's body is doing its job well. Leukorrhea, a thick yellow, greenish, or clear discharge, is not normal and indicates a build-up of Damp Heat or Damp Cold. In these cases, see a practitioner.

Internal Applications
• Avoid foods that clog the intestines: dairy products, refined and processed foods, particularly white flour and sugar, greasy, oily, deep-fried foods, heavy red meats, and red, oily fish.
• Eliminate alcohol, caffeinated beverages, and tobacco.
• A whole foods diet, consisting of fresh, fiber-rich, lightly steamed vegetables, legumes, soy beans and soy products, small amounts of chicken and fish, and whole grains is conducive to smooth and efficient elimination. (See Constipation in the Digestion Disorders section in Part II.)

External Applications
• Exercise is a must. It encourages intestinal action, which helps move the stool, promotes

sweat and the elimination of toxins through the skin, and encourages the deep intake of oxygen, cleansing the Lungs and increasing the amount of oxygen or Air Qi that comes into the body, leaving you nourished and invigorated.

• A skin brush can be used to regularly dry-brush the skin. A natural bristle brush helps clear the pores and promotes the release of toxins through the skin.

• Some women in Japan swear by finely powdered sea salt for washing in the bath and shower as a deep cleanser and purifier. Rub it directly onto wet skin or sprinkle it onto a washcloth and scrub with it. The salt stings a little but leaves a fresh afterglow and really does seem to counter body odor.

Bad Breath

Halitosis is understood to be stagnation and congestion in the digestive system, particularly the Large Intestine, Stomach or Lungs. Again, an overconsumption of fats, refined sugar, alcohol, and heavy red meat are believed to lie at the root of the problem.

• See Constipation in the Digestive Disorders section of Part II.

• Jasmine tea is appreciated for the sweetness and clearness it gives the breath after a meal. It is especially good after a garlicky or oily meal.

Colds, Coughs, and Sore Throat

Includes: the common cold, coughs, sore throats, fevers, and mucus.

When a person receives pernicious influences on his body, there must be a place where they are granted entrance. These influences have gone there because they responded to a summons. As long as a person's essence and spirits are complete and strong, no external evil will dare to offend that person.[1]

The Yellow Emperor's Classic of Medicine

There are so many components to colds that we will look at each symptom separately as well as discuss self-help strategies and remedies for the two basic types of colds: the Cold type and the Hot type, which are determined by the type of mucus given off and by the presence of a fever or chills.

The Common Cold

Stomach/Spleen Deficiency

It is a rule of thumb in Oriental medicine that people with digestive problems frequently catch colds. Unmetabolized fluids generated by a weak Spleen Yang build up, and invade the Lungs and their Yang partner under the element metal, the Large Intestine. The fluid then combines with Hot, Cold, and sometimes Wind, and—looking for a route toward elimination—rises to create congestion in the head, build-up in the nose and sinus passages, aches and soreness in the neck and shoulders, a sore throat, and congested Lungs. The fluid can eventually settle deep down in the Lungs, resulting in serious problems: pneumonia, whooping cough, and tuberculosis. Alternatively, the fluid can invade the digestion system itself, leaving the body run-down, affecting the Liver, causing chronic diarrhea, constipation, and pleurisy, and leaving the body vulnerable to attacking pathogens. There is no set pattern to the direction of this fluid as it settles further into the system.

Self-Help Strategies

—Strengthen the Stomach/Spleen function.
—Reduce excess internal fluid.

Internal Applications

• Avoid caffeine, white refined flour and sugar, tobacco, alcohol, dairy products, iced foods and drinks, and excessive intake of spicy foods, which disrupt the smooth functioning of the Stomach, Spleen, Liver, and Kidney.

• Strengthen the immune system (see the section Adapting to Stress and Building the Immune System in Part II).

• Tone and fortify the Kidneys. Weak, Deficient Kidneys can drain the Lungs, according to the Five Element Theory, resulting in shallow breathing, dryness in the mouth, nose, and throat, vulnerability to colds and coughs, frequent urination or urinary retention. Left unchecked, the condition could degenerate into any number of Lung diseases.

• Eating pork kidneys is a traditional and powerful method of strengthening the Kidneys. (See the section on Preparing Organ Meats in the Appendix.)

• The sweet potato is also believed to be a Kidney strengthener. (See Chapter 3 for more Kidney Yang tonifying foods.)

• Add lycium berries often to soups, stews, and simmered dishes. Reconstitute them with hot water, *sake*, mirin, or wine and add to dressings and sauces. Lycium berries are tonic to the Kidney and the Liver.

• Azuki and kidney beans are important source foods for Kidney support. Eat them weekly if you can. Also, if you have enough time to cook them yourself, make the Azuki Bean Broth (see under Recipes in the Appendix).

• Prepare and keep Garlic Liquor on hand and drink when you feel rundown to prevent colds.

• Garlic Cold Concoction

Warming and Pungent, garlic affects the Lungs, Stomach, and Spleen. It expels Cold, counteracts toxins, and warms the digestive system. Honey has Neutral energy, a Sweet flavor, and is often used to alleviate Dry coughs, constipation, sinusitis, and to counteract toxins.

5 cloves garlic
500 g honey

Steam the garlic until it is very soft. Crush it, place in a thick saucepan, add the honey, and simmer on lowest heat setting. Do not add water but stir regularly, if not constantly, until the garlic is thoroughly cooked and gives off its characteristic fragrance. Take a teaspoon in hot water three times a day whenever you feel a cold coming on or take a teaspoon or two before bed to quell a painful throat or cough. This is good for children, too. Keeps well in the refrigerator.

• Long Green Onion (Leek) Broth

Long green onions are Spicy in flavor and Warm/Neutral in energy. The white inner parts are Spicy and Neutral. They strengthen digestion, have sudorific and diuretic properties, promote appetite and digestion, break down toxins, help prevent hardening of the arteries, and bring cold relief.

> 3 cloves garlic, crushed or pressed
> 1-inch piece ginger, finely sliced
> 2 long green onions (leeks)
> 2 cups chicken stock or water
> 1–2 dried shiitake mushrooms
> 3–4 tbsp. white or red miso (optional)

Chop the garlic and ginger and add with shiitake mushrooms to broth, heat on medium, and cook until the mushrooms are soft. Remove shiitake, cool until you can cut them, remove the stems, slice the caps, and add to the broth. Slice off the tops of the leeks and discard. Then remove the outer green leaves of the lower end of the leeks and save in the refrigerator for another dish; it is the white inside parts of the leek that contain the active healing ingredient. Add the leeks and cook until soft. Turn down the heat and add miso, if desired. Serve hot. Follow this with a very warm bath and go to bed immediately.

• Grilled tangerine skin tea is a traditional remedy for a cold accompanied by a scratchy throat, coarse voice, and achy back. Peel a tangerine after grilling or broiling it so the skin is well-browned, and boil the dried skin with $1\frac{1}{2}$ cups water. The tangerine skin's active ingredients promote sweating. Scrub the skin well with a scratchy brush before grilling to thoroughly clean off any insecticides or better yet, use organically grown fruit.

• A cup of peach leaf tea contains about 20 times more vitamin C than a whole lemon. It's great for colds and cold prevention, promotes resistance to disease and bleeding of gums, high blood pressure, and hardening of the arteries. Slightly diuretic. Use two spoonfuls per cup, let steep about 7 minutes. If you pick the leaves yourself, the young leaves of June are best.

External Applications

• For relief of sinus infection and nasal congestion, make a poultice using a regular round onion or the white part of a long green leek by grating it, dipping absorbent cotton pads in the juice, and lightly pressing the depressions under each nostril. If it's too powerful, then soak the pads in a tiny amount of salad oil and reapply. Some people find relief by putting rounds of onion over their upper sinus tract above the bridge of the nose and above the eyes, but this is quite strong. Some people put the onion over a cotton pad and then hold it over the sinuses.

• If you are prone to colds with a stuffy nose and slight fever yearly when the weather changes, try washing the nostrils with lukewarm water by simply holding the water in the palm of your hand in front of the nostrils, tipping your head slightly to one side, and quickly inhaling and breathing the water out again.

Acupressure for stuffy noses

First, stop smoking and drinking alcohol if this applies to you. Smoking stimulates the mucous membranes in the nose, resulting in an increase of phlegm. Alcohol dilates the blood vessels of the nose, causing further swelling and irritation. (See the BodyMap for location of points and the meanings of the abbreviations.)

Indō—Press the Third Eye point, in the middle of the eyebrows, with as intense a pressure as you can stand. Use the knuckle of your thumb. Notice the irritation begin to decrease after several minutes.

L.I. 20—Find the slight depressions at the outside corners of the nostrils; press and rub. Unblocks the nose and clears Heat.

BL. 2—Press the points on the bone of the inner corners of the eyes.

L.I. 4—This is a major point for facial problems, especially those involving the nose. Press with medium pressure, 5–10 times.

Coughs

In Chinese medicine a cough is seen as a symptom of a Deficiency or an Excess Cold, Heat, or Dry condition, determined by the amount and quality of mucus produced by the body. Learning to recognize your cough is your first step in self-help treatment. This may be confusing. See a practitioner at first to discuss and confirm your findings. Five common cough patterns are included here.

1) Excess Heat causes thick, sticky, green mucus.

The cough is wraking and expectoration may be difficult. There is thick, sticky, green phlegm. The cough may be accompanied by a fever, thirst, sweating, and difficulty in sleeping. This is a Heat type cough. Thick green phlegm and high fever point to an Excess condition, which means the body can tolerate strong treatment.

Self-Help Strategies

—Clear Heat.
—Relieve thirst.
—Calm the cough.
—Loosen phlegm.

Internal Applications

• Avoid mucus-generating foods: bananas, dairy products, starches (except for barley and rice), deep-fried, greasy foods, roasted peanuts, iced foods and drinks, refined sugar.

• Eat cooling foods. (See Chapter 3.) Try barley soup with mung bean sprouts and watercress with some freshly ground or prepared horseradish, wasabi, or hot mustard as a condiment. These three roots help expel mucus.

• Chinese green tea and chrysanthemum tea are cooling and indicated for this condition.

• For coughs, colds, and asthma, make your own garlic syrup by adding a teaspoon of garlic juice to honey. From 20 to 30 drops of garlic juice help to remove mucus from the throat and lungs.

• A garlic poultice on the foot overnight helps clear up catarrhal coughs with thick, white phlegm or even gray phlegm from the nose. Crush a small piece of garlic into a paste with a little cooking oil. Wrap the garlic clove in a thin layer of cotton, place this on the sole of the foot, wrap with a gauze bandage, and put a sock over it to keep it in place. (Garlic kept directly on the skin for a long period of time may burn.)

• Cayenne pepper also helps restore moisture to hot, dry mucous membranes. Add it to foods or to a dressing of olive oil and lemon for steamed vegetables.

• A nasty cough will be relieved by taking honey-soaked daikon radish. Cut an inch-long round and dice, then add enough honey to completely cover the pieces. Leave for 2 to 3 days so that the daikon releases water. Mix well and take a spoonful as needed. Or add a spoonful to a cup of warm water and drink.

When you don't have time, grate the daikon and mix with $^1/_3$ the amount of honey. Use the same way as above. These preparations are especially good for children.

External Applications

• To treat the cough, soothe the throat and bronchi, and loosen any excessive mucus try a steam inhalation of freshly crushed garlic or garlic tincture. Add a little thyme oil to this: one of the most powerful bacterial oils, it is useful in combating a cough due to bacterial infection.

• Gentle massage of the throat and chest either alone or with the inhalant is also effective.

2) Excess Cold causes cough with quantities of clear mucus.

A cough that easily expectorates large quantities of clear, colorless phlegm, and is accompanied by cold, clammy hands and feet, chills, a desire for warm drinks, listlessness, and a pale complexion, points to a Cold condition in the body. The cougher's listlessness is a sign of a Deficiency.

Self-Help Strategies

—Stimulate circulation, perspiration, and expectoration.

—Avoid overstimulation.

—Tone and replenish Qi.

Internal Applications

• Avoid sugar, refined flour, caffeine, and raw fruits and vegetables. Take it easy on the oranges and the orange juice. Raw fruit increases the moisture in the body, which is exactly what caused this condition. Aspirin, alcohol, analgesics, antidepressants, anticoagulants, oral contraceptives, and steroids may reduce levels of vitamin C in the body.

• Warming vegetables and broths made from them are best. Add chives, scallions, onion, yam, carrot, string beans, winter squash, turnips, okra, and shiitake to the stock. They also help decongest moisture. Spices such as ginger, coriander, and cinnamon can be added for warmth, to increase circulation, and to regulate perspiration. Rice, Job's tears, black beans, kidney beans, broad beans, pork and beef kidney, carp, mackerel, shrimp, eel, and mussels are warming and decongesting.

• For vitamin C, eat more asparagus, beet greens, broccoli, mustard and turnip greens, brussel sprouts, green peas, radishes, Swiss chard, and parsley.

• Of the Chinese herbs, ma huang has been a trusty remedy to reduce bronchial spasms, asthma, colds, hay fever, and sinus trouble. It is very drying and has stimulant properties. It should not be used by people with high blood pressure. Stop taking it after 10 days, or once the condition has cleared up if that happens before 10 days have passed. (The Food and Drug Administration issued a warning on an herbal formula containing ma huang. See the Appendix for more information.)

3) Dehydration has set in after a fever, setting the stage for a Dry/Heat type hacking cough with little phlegm.

A third type of cough is the post-fever hack. It is accompanied by a dry, scratchy throat, difficulty in sleeping, red and parched lips but no particular thirst. This cough can be tinged with blood. It is of the Deficient type. The Heat is no longer due to fever but dehydration, or, diagnostically speaking, to Deficiency of Moisture and Dispersion of Qi. The lack of thirst indicates that the body has been weakened and does not have the energy to recover by itself.

Self-Help Strategies

—Consult a practitioner.
—Clear Heat.
—Moisten the Lungs.
—Clear phlegm.
—Tone and build Qi.

This combination of symptoms is a deep condition for which it is advised to see a practitioner. Herbal formulas work very well for this type of cough, says Peter, but they should be prescribed. In the meantime, warming foods, no cold drinks, and staying away from raw fruit and vegetables will help tremendously. Follow the dietary suggestions under Cough type one.

4) Cold has invaded the body, the illness has penetrated more deeply, producing a chronic, rattling cough.

Another type of cough is the rattling type in the chest following a cold. This cough produces large amounts of frothy sputnum in the morning and may be accompanied by loose bowel movements, chills, and a loss of appetite. This cough may indicate that the body has not recovered from the cold. More likely, the illness has penetrated deeper.

Self-Help Strategies

—Consult a practitioner.
—Warm the body.
—Stimulate the metabolism.
—Restore Qi.

Internal Applications
• Avoid Cold and Cool foods (see Chapter 3).
• Try to stay away from mucus-producing and fluid-producing foods (see Chapter 3).
• Reduce or eliminate your intake of caffeine, refined flour and sugar, alcohol, and tobacco.
• Follow other dietary suggestions under Cough type 2.
• To supplement Qi, sweet potato, mustard greens, yam, potato, celery, carrots, string beans, winter squash, turnips, okra, shiitake, and chestnuts are also good. Combine them with your usual diet or add a couple to rice porridge as an ideal way to warm and nourish the body.

• Moxibustion for deeply penetrating Cold

(See Chapter 4 for instructions on the use of moxibustion. See the BodyMap for the location of points and the meanings of abbreviations.) Warm the following:

> L.I. 4—Activates Qi and Blood in the entire body, disperses Wind Heat and Wind Cold.
> ST. 36—Tonifies the entire body, readjusts functions of Stomach/Spleen.

The sternum area and the upper back between the shoulder blades are directly related to the Lungs and will also benefit from moxa's warmth.

5) Weather influences affect the Lungs to produce a cough.

A dry late autumn, a time when Peter sees a definite rise in respiratory and bronchial problems, can affect the Lungs. Cold weather can affect the Kidneys, weakening a stressed-out body further to bring about a cough and dry mouth, accompanied by lower back pain, frequent urination or urinary problems. Damp, humid weather affects the Spleen/Stomach. The results are digestion difficulties and a cough with thick, yellow phlegm or lots of white, frothy phlegm, depending on whether one has a Heat or a Cold condition.

Self-Help Strategies

—Take proper weather precautions.
—Strengthen the entire body and the immune system.

Sore Throats

According to Chinese medicinal theory, the throat and nose are governed by the Lung meridian network, which is involved whenever you have a cold, cough, or throat infection. Additionally, many meridians pass through the throat, and any imbalance of energy in the Heart, Spleen, Kidney, or Stomach systems could result in a sore throat. The accompanying symptoms (stomach ache, nausea, fever, and chills) are determined by the channel(s) the disharmony exists in. Visit a qualified practitioner for a proper diagnosis and treatment if the sore throat persists.

Internal Applications

• Chinese licorice is used in a commercially prepared powdered drink for throat pain, sold in Japan as *Kanzōtō*.

• The old honey and lemon in hot water standby for symptomatic treatment of sore throats is still his favorite, Peter says.

• Eat some fresh pineapple which contains the meat-digesting enzyme bromelin. The enzyme aids in healing the throat by digesting the dead tissues left by infection. Some people add a teaspoon of cream of tartar to $^1/_2$ cup of pineapple juice for a similar effect.

• The odor of garlic has always been unpopular in Japan. In response, one traditional garlic remedy for a sore throat calls for steaming the garlic cloves before smashing, then simmering them on low heat with honey (no water) until well cooked to produce a thick syrup, and taking a teaspoon whenever the throat hurts.

• Traditionally in Japan, plums are credited with having great sore-throat-relieving qualities. One folk remedy still in use today calls for crushed plum extract, which you can find at most natural foods stores, and a grated clove of garlic. Put them both together in a teacup, add hot water, stir, and drink. To make this more effective, one of my favorite home remedy collectors, Yuriko Tojo, suggests mixing the plum extract with salted bancha tea and a pinch of brown sugar, then gargling, spitting it out, and swallowing a mouthful, repeating until the cupful is finished.

• This mixture includes lotus root, daikon radish, and goldenseal. Grate $1/4$ cup of daikon, $1/4$ cup of lotus root, and boil them for 10 to 15 minutes with 2 cups of water and 3–5 g goldenseal for an anti-bacterial, blood cleansing, throat soothing drink. Drink three times a day. Grating a daikon radish creates much more volume than one would expect, so use a large pot. For children, add honey to sweeten.

• Burdock root is good for red, inflamed throats with slight fever. Grate the burdock root and strain through a cotton cloth. Adults should take two tbsp. three times a day, children one tbsp. three times a day. Burdock root juice also makes a good gargle.

• Mugwort has antibiotic effects and can be used to help heal a red, inflamed throat. Boil a handful of dried leaves in 2 cups of water, turn down the heat, and cook over a low flame for 10 minutes. Use this to gargle with several times a day.

External Applications

• Gargle with quite warm salt water every two or three hours. The heat increases blood flow to the affected area and the tissues are bathed in a restorative solution. You can add gold-enseal powder, an antibacterial herb, to the salt water, or goldenseal and red pepper to taste. The Japanese add rice vinegar, although white vinegar acts just as well.

• Another vinegar remedy for a sore throat is to inhale the steam of hot vinegar. Take care when you do this—you don't have to get too close for it to work.

• Strong black tea, cooled until it is just warm, makes an excellent gargle. Use it every hour until the throat is eased.

• A ginger compress can be made by grating about a half-inch-thick piece of ginger into 45° alcohol and heating the mixture until it is hot and the ginger gives off an odor. Dip a clean cotton fabric into the mixture and wrap or hold in place until it cools. Repeat several times. It's important that the alcohol is hot during application.

Acupressure for a sore throat

(See BodyMap for the exact location of points and the meanings of abbreviations.)

C.V. 22—Press the bottom of the Adam's apple, down into the depression, with quite a bit of pressure three to five times. Clears phlegm, throat blockages, and calms cough.

LU. 11—Press three to five times, for 15 seconds with quite heavy pressure. This is good to eliminate Heat in the throat, and alleviates loss of voice with a sore throat.

L.I. 4—Lies on the outside of the hand in the fleshy area between the thumb and the index finger. This point activates Qi in the entire body. Pressure or moxa is recom-mended. This is also good for headaches.

G.B. 20—Clears cold symptoms and dispels sore throat.

BL. 12—Is for moxibustion, but if you don't have a partner to help you, use a blow-dryer to warm this area. According to Oriental medicine, Cold and Wind enter the body through this point and linger at Fū Chi (G.B. 20), the previous point.

Lump in the Throat

The lump-in-the-throat sensation may worry those who suffer from it. Many people with this condition think they have throat cancer and rush to the doctor, who is often unable to find anything wrong with them. It gets written off as a neurosis, *globus hystericus*, and is virtually untreatable by Western medicine, comments Peter (see Liver Problems, under Liver Imbalance in Oriental Medical Terms). In Oriental medicine, this condition is diagnosed as disharmony of the Liver energy, which rises and becomes blocked in the throat. It is frequently caused by worry and emotional trouble. Don't worry about it, but do consult a practitioner to restore balance to the Liver organ and meridian system.

Fevers

• Grated fresh ginger boiled in water with a little honey warms the body and promotes urination and sweating. Make a ginger broth with sliced long green onion (leek) or round cooking onion, and daikon radish, with bonito flakes sprinkled on top.

• Daikon radish is Spicy/Sweet, Cool/Neutral. When cooked, it moistens the Lungs, stops coughs, lowers fever, aids digestion, relieves colds, and restores voice. is rich in vitamin C and contains enzymes that promote digestion. The spicy quality of the raw, cool vegetable promotes sweating and moves Heat/Phlegm blocks.

• To bring down a fever, make a quick watercress soup by finely dicing the watercress and grating a slice of fresh ginger and a slice of fresh daikon radish if it is on hand. Place the pile of vegetables in a bowl of hot water and add a dash of soy sauce. The watercress is cooling and has diuretic properties.

• Make and take the Green Onion Broth listed under General Colds in this Section.

Mucus

• For mucus, grill a piece of ginger root over an open flame until it is thoroughly charred, wrap in aluminum foil and then steam, pour hot water over, and gargle with the liquid when it has cooled.

• **Kumquat Anti-mucus Syrup**

The fruit is bittersweet but wonderfully fragrant, lending this wine a full-bodied flavor. The fruit has been used traditionally in Japan and China as a cough medicine. Also drives away mucus, aids the Stomach, and alleviates exhaustion.

$^1/_2$ kilo kumquats
200 g crystallized sugar
3 tbsp. honey

Place the bittersweet mini-oranges in a wide-mouth jar and cover with the crystallized sugar. Let sit until the sugar becomes gooey. Then add the honey, mix well, and let sit until the entire mixture becomes thick and orange-honey-colored. Take a cupful every 3 hours or so for a cough or to expectorate a dry, hacking cough.

• Try lotus root when mucus is a problem. Grate a large, unpeeled lotus root, wrap in cotton, and squeeze out the juice. Drink this slightly warm with honey once or twice a day for two to three days. Lotus root has antiseptic qualities and is also said to benefit mucus problems.

• **Perilla Leaf Anti-mucus Brew**

    100–200 g green perilla leaves
    $^1/_4$ c crystallized sugar
    720 ml 45° alcohol

Wash and slice the perilla leaves and place them in a wide-mouth jar with the alcohol and crystallized sugar. Let sit for three months, strain, and take one *sake* cupful for irritating coughs. Dilute with water if the alcohol is too strong. Also makes a good gargle.

Cold Prevention Measures

Cold Prevention Herbal Wine I

This clear brown pleasant-tasting elixir aids a run-down feeling and poor appetite; it increases metabolism, improves blood circulation at the surface of the skin, regulates urinary function, clears the head, and is beneficial as an overall body tonic. Take when you feel vulnerable to catching a cold but not *after catching one.*

    30 g ginseng root
    40 g astragalus
    15 g Chinese licorice
    15 g Chinese cinnamon
    1 liter 45° alcohol
    50 g fructose
    100 g granulated sugar

Place all ingredients in a glass container and let the mixture mature for at least a month before drinking. Dose: 20 ml, about a *sake* cupful, 2–3 times a day before meals on an empty stomach.

Cold Prevention Wine II

This fragrant, light brown, round-tasting liquor strengthens a weak constitution, improves digestion, helps the body to ward off colds. Its gentle action makes it safe to drink continuously through the cold months. It can be drunk by young and old alike. The peony builds Blood and vitality, while the dates and licorice warm and reinforce the action of the peony, bring relief to aches and pains, and soothe cramps.

    30 g peony
    20 g Chinese cinnamon
    20 g red dates
    15 g Chinese licorice
    10 g dried ginger
    1 liter 45° alcohol
    250 g honey

Mix ingredients together, place in a glass container, and let mixture mature for a month before drinking. Drink 20 ml, a *sake* cupful, 3 times a day before meals.

• Cough Relief Wine

Make this in the summer and keep it on hand all year long. The apricot is slightly Cool, Sweet/Sour, clears Heat, detoxifies, and quenches thirst. Overconsumption reverses the cough-alleviating properties.

1 kilo apricots, half ripe, half unripe
400 g crystallized sugar
1 liter 45° alcohol

Cut the apricots in half and remove pits. Add ice sugar and a liter of alcohol. Remove fruit after three months and let the wine mature for two to three more months. Take 20 ml when needed, not to exceed 3 doses a day.

• Quince Cough Wine

This is another one to make well in advance—it needs a year to age properly.

5–6 yellow quince
150 g crystallized sugar
3 lemons
1 liter 45° alcohol

Cover quince with a towel and let sit for several days so that the nectar accumulates on the skin. Then add to alcohol with three peeled lemons and the sugar in a wide-mouth jar. Remove the lemons after three months; let the brew mature for a year. It's good for cough due to colds and asthma. Take 20 ml as needed, not to exceed 3 doses per day.

Endnote

*1 Paul Unschuld, ed., *Introductory Readings in Classical Chinese Medicine* (Netherlands: Kluwer Academic Publishers, 1988).

Compulsive/Addictive Disorders

Oriental Medical Energetics

Compulsive disorders such as addiction are diagnosed as Disturbed Shen by Oriental medicine practitioners. The Shen, the spiritual energy of the body, is out of balance, affecting the Heart meridian and other energy systems, depending on the nature of the disorder. This translates into a serious emotional disorder that is throwing things off balance.

Course of Treatment

Typically, a practitioner might initially respond with the following:

• Acupuncture to rebalance the Heart meridian and other systems that are affected. Acupuncture is a front-line, simple, nonintrusive way to treat Shen imbalance. Acupuncture allows a person to experience his or her own energy quietly and in safe surroundings. There is no intermediary between the person and the person's feelings. This intimacy with the self allows one to connect with the path to one's highest good. It helps one become activated to work for one's own recovery and encourages a building-up of trust in the therapy at one's own pace.

• Acupressure, massage, herbal treatment: serious addicts and emotionally distraught people often respond well to therapeutic touch and the calming effects of herbs.

Once some progress has been made, in addition to the somatic therapy the practitioner might begin a second level of treatment in the form of encouragement in these terms:

• Too much of any behavior throws the whole system off balance. Moderation in exercise, eating, drinking, and sex is best.

• Reinforcing attempts to break self-destructive behaviors, from nail-biting to drug and alcohol addiction, requires commitment and perseverance on the part of the individual, support from others, and the inculcation of discipline in oneself through constructive new habits.

• Fostering habits that meet the needs that the destructive behavior is now meeting can help break the habit more easily.

After a while, the acupuncturist might move to the third line—encouragement meant to help empower the patient:

• **You have a choice.**

It's important to realize you have a choice in your behaviors. Before you pick up that first drink or piece of cake, stop and ask yourself if you *have* to have it now. Sometimes if you can stop and think, you can switch gears and practice a little gentle restraint with yourself. Rather than eating or drinking something immediately, tell yourself you can have it in an hour if you still crave it then. Chances are you will have forgotten about it, particularly if you physically remove yourself from the premises or involve yourself in an engrossing project.

Many addicts complain they cannot stop and think before they act. Meditation develops the mind's ability to identify and elongate the "Stop!" moment. We consider meditation one of the most effective addiction-breaking tools.

• **You have power, the substance doesn't have power.**

Addictive substances—alcohol, drugs, food—and behaviors—gambling, compulsive sex—are not intrinsically bad in themselves. Our attitudes toward them become the problem. Alcohol is a problem because a person is unable to handle it; he abuses it because it satisfies a need to numb or cover up pain, i.e., the disturbance in the Shen. When the underlying causes of addiction are identified and dealt with, the dependence on the substance loosens and can eventually disappear completely.

Try visualizing yourself in a life without your primary addiction. Imagine an entire day, from waking up in the morning to going to bed at night. Imagine yourself going through the motions of the day, confronting problems that ordinarily give you difficulty, but this time, in your mind, you are able to deal with a troublesome person or situation by practicing a new coping skill—deep-breathing, repeating to yourself that you are safe and being taken care of, or making a telephone call when the stress becomes intense. Seeing yourself acting in a healthy, powerful manner taps into the health and power that already exists inside.

• **Become conscious.**

A practice of meditation of any kind, and disciplines such as yoga, qigong, tai'chi, and karate slowly begin to chip away at the desire to overindulge in anything, be it food, alcohol, or drugs. Maintaining a practice of this sort also helps us become more conscious of what we do.

• **Focus on the positive: what you can have or do.**

To break any kind of habit, instead of dwelling on breaking the habit, which is essentially dwelling on and feeding what you can't have with energy and attention, concentrate on behaviors that serve you better.

This is a strategy that has far-reaching benefits if you practice it. For example, rather than feeling deprived of addictive substances and the network of friends you had surrounding that activity, you can use the time you would have spent in your past activities to go out and take a class, connect with people who are interested in what you are, and slowly begin to build a new social circle for yourself. Or better yet, you could support your efforts to break your addiction by joining a group of people who are actively working on their emotional or spiritual development. Their energy could help buoy your recovery efforts and the new connections could lead to new possibilities and directions that you had never thought of.

• **Find effective methods to release stress, anger, and fear.**

Sometimes addictive habits serve to release stress, tension, and other emotions that build up but are not effectively channeled out. Creating releases that nourish the body such as dancing, running, punching a punching bag, practicing a martial art, singing loudly, or a combination of any or all of these are good substitutes. Be creative. Be spontaneous, be outrageous, and have fun with this part of recovery. One Tokyo woman's favorite method of releasing anger was to throw eggs at the back of her house! It also helps to be prepared for difficult times by making a list of five things you can do to relieve stress and keeping this list on hand for emergencies.

Battling keeps the energy stuck there. An argument is a good example of this dynamic. When we are embroiled in the heat of an argument, perpetuating the argument means that nothing changes. Listening, discussing, and working with the feelings and opinions of both parties, however, leads to breakthroughs. Letting others and yourself be as they are allows the energy of irritation to taper away. Let go of irritation. To do this, when you feel really piqued, try repeating to yourself that nothing is more important than your peace of mind.

• **Develop new coping tools.**

We are now broaching the area of acceptance, specifically self-acceptance. Breaking an addictive-compulsive habit is accomplished with less resistance when the addicted person acknowledges that the behavior served an important function for a while because it helped him or her survive an otherwise intolerable situation. What is needed now are some tools for handling the situation or changing it completely to eliminate the need for a self-destructive response. Conventional counseling and nontraditional counseling methods such as hypnotherapy or Neurolinguistic Programming (NLP) can help us do this.

• **Nurture 100% resolve.**

People who have successfully broken their habits have all had one thing in common: they all desperately wanted to break their habits. They accepted backsliding as a battle lost but not the war, as a lesson taking them one step closer to freedom. They were willing to make choices and sacrifices to feel the benefits of life without the monkey on their backs. Are you?

External Applications

• Practice deep breathing whenever you have a food or alcohol craving.

• See an Oriental medicine practitioner, someone who can help you work out an eating program that is suitable for your body, that meets your nutritional needs, that strengthens and balances. This will eventually remove the need to binge on a physical level and can help rectify the imbalances—which can be quite serious—you have caused your body through the addiction.

• To treat sugar cravings:

1. In Oriental medicine the taste of Bitter is said to remove sugar cravings. Almonds, endive, radish sprouts, romaine lettuce, rye, and turnips are some foods in the Bitter category. The bitter flavor stimulates the pancreas, which is directly related to the Spleen function.

2. Protein also helps: nuts, beans and legumes, soybeans and soybean products such as tofu, soy milk, and miso. Some people who experience sugar cravings do not take in adequate

protein: for thin, protein-lacking bodies that are gaseous and have severe cravings, a diet low in carbohydrates and rich in milk and dairy products is good.

To illustrate, Peter had a friend who put himself on a fairly rigid diet—mainly brown rice, soba noodles, some tofu, and cooked vegetables—not because he was ill, but because he thought it was good for him. He developed strong sweet cravings, however, and started to binge on sugar. He also suffered from a lot of gas, abdominal bloating, a loose stool, and weight loss. After incorporating more protein into his diet, along with some fats, a wider variety of vegetables—including bitters such as dandelion greens and endive—the sweet cravings, diarrhea, bloating, and gas diappeared, while his energy level improved. Evidently what we think is good for us and what actually *is* good for us often prove to be two different things.

3. In Japan, the salty, sour taste of an umeboshi is recommended for putting an end to a sugar craving.

Acupressure to treat food or alcohol cravings
(See the BodyMap for the exact location of points and the meanings of abbreviations.)

G.B. 2—In the depression by the protuberance of the flesh in front of the ear at the notch at the top of the tragus.

S.I. 19—Between the tragus of the ear and the mandible joint, where a depression is formed when the mouth is opened wide.

Depression

Oriental Medical Energetics

Oriental medicine views depression as a symptom of imbalance related to the Liver and/or the Heart organs and channels. Peter believes that acupuncture can be an effective method of treating chronic emotional disorders: it treats the symptom at the root of the imbalance. Acupuncture also releases endorphins, the body's natural painkillers and anti-depressants, which elevate the mood and increase one's sense of hopefulness. "Once the depressive cycle is broken through the release of the endorphins, and by giving hope, the client is more open to other forms of helpful therapy," says Peter.

1) Stagnant Liver Qi

Eating large quantities of greasy and heavy foods, drinking iced drinks or alcohol, and repressing intense emotions such as anger and frustration can lead to Stagnating energy in the Liver meridian and the lower abdomen, leading to depression. Conversely, prolonged depression can also cause Stagnant Qi in the Liver channel.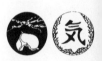

2) Depleted Heart and Shen

Our emotional nature, the Shen, is believed to reside in the Heart, according to Oriental medicine. When the soundness of this organ and meridian system are undermined by over-work, suppressed emotions, stress, and high levels of anxiety, the "Shen withdraws" and feelings of loneliness, despair, and a lack of desire to do anything—classic Yin symptoms—result.

3) Deficient Spleen

When the energy of the Spleen is imbalanced, the body becomes unable to transform and transport nutrients. The Earth loses its grounding, balancing influence on the system. Excessive worry, obsession with detail, or excessively thinking about the past, in combination with an improper diet, result in the stagnation of body fluids, which causes digestive difficulty accompanied by depression, Blood and menstrual disorders, sluggishness, and foggy thinking.

Internal Applications

• Avoid foods that aggravate the Liver and congest Qi (See Chapter 3).

• Excessively spicy foods aggravate the Heart and are best avoided.

• Foods that help disperse Liver Qi congestion and rebalance the Spleen include warming foods that dispel Cold—chicken cooked with Chinese red dates and dang gui, onions, garlic, ginger, pork kidney, beef and chicken livers, yellow and orange vegetables, whole grains and cereals. Eat them frequently.

• Foods to calm the mind—longan, rice, rosemary, wheat, wheat germ, mushrooms—should also be incorporated into the diet.

External Applications

• Bodywork can be helpful in getting over that no-energy, hopeless feeling. "The depressed client's breathing is depressed," says Rolfer Ashuan Seow, a Chinese-Australian Rolfer and founder of Body Link, a bodywork institute in Australia. "One of the first issues that Rolfing deals with is to increase the breathing capacity so more energy can be generated." Rolfing and deep tissue massage "open and release all that is suppressed and compressed via the physical form to create the potential to treat the whole being in stages."

• For depression relief, commit yourself to regular daily exercise. This does not necessarily mean you must join a health club. You could go out for a run with the dogs for half an hour a day or jump up and down to danceable music for half an hour first thing in the morning. Take a long walk practicing deep abdominal breathing as you go, and try not to think of anything but how grateful you are to be alive on such a beautiful day. (This can be considered a mental exercise at first. Move the body and mind, and the heart follows.) Break a sweat and get the breath going. Results should be noticeable within a few weeks. You may not want to exercise, but force yourself to do it.

• When one is depressed many elements of one's life are out of order. Treating depression at the symptomatic level is a temporary measure, but simple steps, such as enlisting the help of another person, can help break the feeling of isolation. Counseling or simply talking frequently to a confidant are valuable methods of releasing the suppressed anger.

• Replace worrying, obsessive, and angry tapes in your head with positive messages, a prayer, or a mantra when you notice yourself slipping into this habit.

• Many plants produce antidepressant essential oils. Oils such as camomile are also sedative, while others, such as bergamot and rose, can help lift the mood without sedating. Consult an aromatherapist who is skilled in blending oils appropriate for specific conditions.

• For hundreds of years Japanese women have taken baths with fresh fruit or flowers to alleviate depression. Try slicing a fresh lemon, orange, or *yuzu*, scatter the rings across the bath water, and slide in for a while to uplift the spirits. Plum and cherry blossoms in season permeate the body with the energy and fragrance of spring. Sprinkle fresh rose petals on a bath of cool water and go for a soothing, sensual dip during the balmy days of summer. In winter make a strong infusion of dang gui and add it to the bath water for its warming and mildly sedating properties. Freshly cut evergreen branches can be sliced, packed into a cloth bag, and added to the bath for some revitalizing energy.

Depression in Women

Irritability, low spirits, moodiness, and difficulty in concentrating, socializing, and being active are familiar to those suffering from hormonal fluctuations characteristic of Premenstrual Syndrome and postnatal depression. In addition, women with a history of depression can be seriously affected by menopause-related stress.

According to the Pacific Post-Partum Society, 80% of women experience the postnatal "fourth day blues," caused by a dramatic reduction of estrogen and progesterone in the bloodstream. Extreme emotional sensitivity, anger, depression, feeling overwhelmed and out of control ensue. This phase lasts about 24 hours, when the milk for nursing mothers comes in and hormone levels start building again.

Postpartum blues is a euphemism for an often devastating depression that can appear anywhere from three to six months after the birth. This occurs in about 20% of women. Symptoms include anorexia or overeating, insomnia or prolonged and extreme fatigue, migraine headaches, uncontrollable anger, having violent thoughts about the baby, isolating oneself from the outside world, feeling unable to cope, and hallucinations.

The causes are several, says Maya Shah, a former instructor of postpartum depression workshops for new parents in Tokyo. A new mother is at risk if any or all of the following factors are present: she does not feel good or positive about the pregnancy and birth, does not communicate well with her partner, has strong PMS, is in a mixed marriage lacking the cultural support for validating her beliefs on child-rearing.

Postpartum Depression Prevention

• Prepare for a change in lifestyle while pregnant. Meet other pregnant women and set up a support network to counter isolation. Educate the father on ways to support you through this major change.

• Make necessary dietary changes: increase intake of vitamins B and E.

• Exercise gently and avoid sudden weight loss.

• Treat yourself to massages and essential oil treatments to counter negative feelings, and to relax and uplift you. Try oils of bergamot, camomile, geranium, lavender, lemon, neroli, orange, and especially tangerine.

• Women on the pill should know that it depletes at least four essential brain nutrients: vitamins B_6, B_{12}, and C, and folic acid. Consider using an alternative method of birth control or taking multivitamin and mineral supplements, including trace minerals. The authors believe, however, that essential nutrients are ideally ingested through food sources. Foods rich in vitamin B_6 are brewer's yeast, carrots, chicken, eggs, fish, meat, peas, spinach, sunflower seeds, walnuts, and wheat germ. For B_{12} try blue cheese, clams, eggs, herring, kidney and liver organ meat, mackerel, milk, seafood, and tofu. Vitamin C is found in high amounts in green vegetables, citrus fruits, and berries. Folic acid is found in barley, beans, beef, bran, brewer's yeast, brown rice, cheese, chicken, dates, green leafy vegetables, split peas, pork, liver organ meat, oranges, root vegetables, salmon, tuna, whole grains, and yeast.

Digestive Disorders

Includes: constipation, diarrhea, flatulence, indigestion, stomachache, stomatitis, nausea, vomiting, food poisoning, gastric and duodenal ulcers, heartburn/ acid reflux, cold sores, loss of appetite, and overeating.

Chronic digestion problems are certainly some of the most common problems that walk through an acupuncturist's door. Peter estimates half his patients suffer from digestive disorders or related problems. The most common three complaints are constipation, diarrhea, and flatulence. These can be accompanied by abdominal distention and bloating, pain before and after eating, and acid reflux, or heartburn. The causes of these problems are many, but they can be effectively treated through a combination of a change in diet, Chinese herbs, acupuncture, and other self-help measures.

According to the Chinese model, malfunctioning in the digestive system is usually symptomatic of either Deficient or Excessive energy in the Stomach/Spleen and Liver systems; we will explore this more in depth momentarily.

Diet and the conditions under which we eat are major factors in digestion. The most common mistakes we make in relation to the digestive system is to eat when we are upset, to overeat, to eat heavy meals late at night, and to imbibe large quantities of iced liquid with meals. The Liver organ and meridian system are already under stress when you are upset. Eating on top of that strains the Liver Qi and prevents the smooth flow of Qi to the Stomach and Spleen to break down and transport essential nutrients to the rest of the body. Overeating further stresses the Liver. Eating large meals late at night withholds a period of rest from the digestive system during sleep and interrupts the 11 P.M. to 3 A.M. active period for the Liver, when it revitalizes itself.

Try to keep twelve hours between the last meal of the day and breakfast the next morning. Do not eat anything once you have finished dinner or supper. The word breakfast denotes the idea that there should be this period of no food, or a "fast," following dinner. The first meal of the day should "break" that fast. Regularity is an ancient pattern with thousands of years of common sense holding it up.

Ice-cold drinks put the Stomach and Spleen under stress, particularly during the winter, when people thoughtlessly consume them out of habit rather than from the need or desire for them. Those large ice waters, teas, and sodas consumed with meals fill the stomach with cold liquid, which lowers the temperature of the food contents, dilutes the hydrochloric acid in the stomach, forces the Stomach and Pancreas to work harder to heat the food so it can be broken down, and hinders the rate and efficiency of the body's digestion process. Eventually, in an already Deficient type, this can put the fire of the Spleen and Stomach out, causing pain, indigestion, and stomach acid reflux.

Instead of drinking cold beverages with meals, try a little oolong tea with a Chinese or a vegetarian meal or steamed or stir-fried vegetables. A small amount of wine, too, can stimulate the gastric juices.

General Topics

• Taking antacids after meals makes the discomfort worse.

Do not keep taking antacids for chronic digestion problems. They tend to compound the problem, Peter says. Older people, for example, produce less hydrochloric acid in their stomachs. Then they reach for the antacids when their stomachs bother them, when the problem is not excessive stomach acids but too little acid.

• Poor elimination prompted the use of laxatives, but now the bowels won't move without them.

Laxatives have a deleterious effect on energy-deficient constitutions, especially. In this case the body does not have enough energy to move the feces. Taking laxatives further weakens the muscles in the intestines, creating a vicious cycle of dependence on the drugs, preventing recovery. The elimination system can be regulated; the body will need to be nourished and strengthened to provide the elimination system with enough energy to perform its job, however. Be prepared for some discomfort in the beginning of treatment. A dietary change to add more fiber will help immensely.

Constipation

1) Damp and Heat injury to the Spleen

Damp accumulating in the Spleen transforms to Heat due to prolonged ingestion of quantities of alcohol, fatty, rich foods, and sweets. The continued consumption of these foods injures the Stomach/Spleen, leading to an accumulation of Damp and Heat that will probably involve the Liver and Gallbladder. Other symptoms include a tendency toward anorexia, nausea, vomiting, fever, thirst (or conversely, no desire for drinks), a bitter taste in the mouth (Gallbladder), sweet sticky taste (Spleen), abdominal distention, epigastric discomfort, jaundice or pale complexion, constipation or foul-smelling diarrhea, dark and scanty urine. Left unchecked these conditions can develop into the Western pathologies of acute pancreatitis, acute hepatitis, acute cholestasis (sluggish liver), and cirrhosis of the Liver.

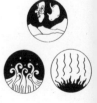

Self-Help Strategies

—Dispel Heat and Damp, best done under a practitioner's care.
—Nourish the Spleen/Stomach.
—Cleanse and tone the Liver/Gallbladder.

2) Fire in the Liver system

Excessive drinking, smoking, eating fatty foods, chronic depression, or extreme emotions generate Fire in the Liver channel. Symptoms may include constipation appearing with a migraine headache with dizziness, vertigo, redness in the face, red painful eyes, conjunctivitis, a buzzing in the ears that sounds like waves, irritability with outbursts of anger, thirst, dry mouth with a bitter taste, vomiting sour or bitter fluid, insomnia, restlessness, hypertension, and, if severe, the blood vessels may be affected, manifesting as frequent bloody noses.

Self-Help Strategies

—See a practitioner.
—Treatment should clear the Fire.
—Calm the Liver.

3) Deficient Kidney Qi

Long-term illness, excessive sexual activity, early childbirth or too many births, miscarriage or abortion, or overwork/ too much studying with insufficient rest result in Deficient Kidney Yin. This, in combination with an over-reliance on stimulants and relaxants such as coffee and alcohol, creates a symptomatic picture that combines constipation with chronic hearing or ear problems, poor memory, lumbago, aching in the lower legs or heels, thirst, dry throat, night sweats, heightened libido, afternoon flush, hypertension, diabetes mellitus, chronic nephritis. This can be combined with anxiety and disturbed sleep (Heart energy complication), dry eyes, blurry vision, headache and menstrual irregularities (Liver complications), or a dry cough, sore throat, and coughing of blood (Lung channel).

Self-Help Strategies

—See a practitioner to clear the Deficient Fire (thirst, dry eyes, irritability, flush or fever)
    and nourish the crucial Kidney Yin.
—Tone the Kidneys.
—Nourish the Yin.

4) Qi Stagnation in the Large Intestine

This results from food stagnation, parasites, or Blood Stagnation, which clog the Intestine. In this case, abdominal distention and bloating are painful when pressure is applied. The Qi can back up and affect the Stomach Qi, causing it to rise, resulting in nausea and vomiting. Also, a Stagnation of Qi and Blood as the result of overeating or of an inability to adapt to weather changes can cause the Qi to become blocked. This creates severe pain in the lower abdomen, constipation or diarrhea, fever, and vomiting.

Self-Help Strategies

—Disperse Qi and blockages of Blood or food.
—Avoid overeating.

—Calm the Stomach Qi.

Internal Applications

• Avoid foods that aggravate the Liver, dampen the Stomach/Spleen function, and stress the Kidney: (See Chapter 3.)

• Before eating anything in the morning, drink a glass of warm water with a spoonful of honey upon waking to lubricate the intestines and get things moving. Wait an hour before eating breakfast.

• Again, first thing in the morning, drink a cup of warm water with a spoonful of blackstrap molasses. Drink a cup of this before bed, too.

• One more wake-up drink: a cup of warm water with sea salt. The sea salt is full of magnesium and stimulates peristalsis. This is contraindicated for anyone with a heart condition and should not be drunk regularly. Eat calcium-rich vegetables such as broccoli, asparagus, collards, kale, and parsley later during the day if you do drink this.

• An effective tonic is the juice of half a squeezed lemon, 2 tbsp. olive oil, and a pinch of cayenne pepper. This drink is especially good for stimulating bile production.

• Try cooking and eating azuki beans and kombu together. Azuki beans are very nearly considered constipation miracle drugs in the Oriental folk remedy annals. According to Japanese tradition, the best foods to clear out the intestinal lining are brown rice, azuki beans, burdock root, hijiki, soybeans, the insoluble residue from tofu production (okara), and devil's tongue (or yam cake, as it is sometimes translated when sold in Western markets—konnyaku). Garlic, Chinese chives (nira), and scallions should be eaten daily, along with small amounts of fermented foods such as miso, soy sauce, nattō and umeboshi.

External Applications

• A bath of dried daikon radish leaves is recommended to increase circulation in the lower abdomen, stimulate the Liver and Kidneys, and relieve constipation and diarrhea.

• Regular exercise and stretching are extraordinarily helpful in helping the bowels to move along.

• Try these yoga stretches, taking special care to perform all exercises involving the spine very splowly and carefully. Never strain or force the muscles.

Forward bend

    —Stand up looking straight ahead.

    —Raise the arms straight over the head and bend down from the hips, bringing the arms down to touch the floor.

    —Touch the palms to the floor at the sides of the feet if you can. Breathe deeply, using the breath to expand the lower abdomen.

    —Imagine you have two balloons inside the lower abdomen that start at the bottom of the rib cage and run down into the kidney area all the way to the pelvic bone (iliac bone).

    —Half close the eyes and inhale and exhale into your balloons 20 times.

Twist

    —Sit on the floor with the legs straight out. Keep the hands on the floor behind you, palms down.

—Now cross right leg over left and place the right foot down on the outside of the left knee.

—Turn the torso to the right.

—Place the left elbow on the outside of the right knee to keep it from flopping to the right.

—Readjust the right hand on the floor if you need to.

—Using all your lower back strength, work the spine into a straight position. Imagine lifting the head toward the heavens from the lower back. Try to eliminate any hunching forward.

—Open the chest.

—Breathe into your lower back balloons. Imagine wringing and squeezing out the area on the exhale. Do 10 full cycles of breaths.

—Change sides.

Diarrhea

Diarrhea's causes are many, although the problem usually involves a Deficiency in the Stomach and Spleen. Trouble here can be triggered by emotional anxiety, overeating foods with laxative properties, drinking large quantities of beer, a minor bacterial or viral infection, and sometimes extreme fatigue. Food intolerance can cause diarrhea in babies, and is often indicative of an allergy to dairy products. Antibiotics can also cause diarrhea.

Even a quick bout of diarrhea depletes the body's potassium and magnesium levels and dehydrates the body. It is important to drink plenty of clear liquids to avoid depletion and dehydration: boiled water drunk warm, noncaffeinated teas, and broths.

"Holiday tummy" often occurs when we travel to foreign countries and ingest organisms we lack antibodies for. This is usually no cause for worry. A 24-hour attack is definitely normal. Eat less or fast the next day, drinking noncaffeinated teas and broths to help balance.

A chronic case of diarrhea should be treated by a practitioner, who can do some fine-tuning with the diet and add the correct herbs as well.

1) Sinking Stomach/Spleen Qi

An overindulgence in cold foods and drinks, irregular eating habits, excessive worry or mental strain, or long-term illness lead to diarrhea and Stomach weakness. Spleen Qi Sinking is marked by a sallow complexion, a tendency toward anorexia, fullness and distention in the stomach and abdominal area after eating that is relieved by pressure, a heavy, "bearing down" sensation, and diarrhea. Uterine, rectal, and visceral prolapse may already exist. The body and limbs may feel tired. And there may be hemorrhoids.

2) Spleen Yang Deficiency

This condition may be a progression of the first, it may be due to ingesting excessive quantities of cold or raw foods, or it may stem from a Kidney Yang Deficiency where the Kidney Fire is unable to warm the Spleen. The symptoms are similar to the above. There is pain and coldness in the abdomen that can be relieved by applying a hot-water bottle or moxibustion. The stool is loose with undigested food. Mental and physical fatigue, edema, gastric or duodenal ulcer, chronic gastritis, gastric neurosis, anorexia, chronic enteritis, and chronic diarrhea may result from a lack of Spleen Fire.

3) Damaged Spleen Fire

Again, the overconsumption of Cold damages the Spleen Fire, preventing efficient food metabolism. Fluids accumulate, mix with Cold from the lack of Spleen Fire, and chronic diarrhea results. Other symptoms include distention in the abdomen and epigastric area. Nausea, vomiting, cold limbs, a fear of cold, chills, leukorrhea, lassitude, and a heavy feeling in the lower body accompany the diarrhea.

Self-Help Strategies

—See a practitioner.
—Nurture the Stomach/Spleen.
—Clear Cold and Damp.
—Control obsessive thoughts and reduce workload.

Internal Applications

• Foods that injure the Stomach/Spleen, the Liver, and the Kidney organs and meridian systems should be avoided or significantly reduced (see under Food Influences in Chapter 3). Coffee and sugar have a dilating effect on the intestines. Avoid tropical fruit and foods, dilators that dispel Heat from the body so that it is more comfortable in a tropical environment. Particularly in winter choose long-cooking (burdock root, carrots, turnips), mineral-rich (hijiki and kombu) foods that help the body retain Heat and contract the intestinal muscles.
• Reduce intake of iced drinks, frozen or chilled food and foods that produce fluid (see Food Influences in Chapter 3). Sea vegetables and tofu fall into this category. It's okay to include a little seaweed for the minerals or cooked tofu in a hot soup in your diet, but don't eat them to excess. The suggestions here are guidelines, not hard-and-fast rules.
• Foods that have a contracting effect on the intestinal tract and absorb excess fluid are recommended (see Food Influences in Chapter 3).
• Eat foods rich in magnesium and potassium. Foods rich in both include fish, meat, avocados, bananas, blackstrap molasses, and brown rice. (There are many others.)
• Sei Ro Gan pills, a Japanese herbal medicine, can be purchased all over Asia. They are an effective preventative against the siege.
• A medicinal drink made with kuzu, a powdered mountain root found in the macrobiotic section of natural foods stores, used to be a Japanese mother's equivalent of aspirin—doled out for everything. It is helpful in restoring intestinal balance. Add a heaping teaspoon of the white powder to 2 to 3 tbsp. cold water in a saucepan, mash and stir until the kuzu has dissolved. Add 1 cup of water, turn the flame to low and stir constantly for 2 to 3 minutes until the liquid turns thick and clear. Add the flesh from a small umeboshi plum.

External Applications

• Exercise aids the body's efforts to expel excess fluid through sweating, and massage can help absorption of nutrients and get the Qi moving. But continue to cut back on fluid intake until the balance is corrected.
• Warm the stomach in the morning and evening with a ginger compress covered with a hot pack for 15 to 20 minutes. (See Chapter 4 for instructions for preparing a ginger compress.)
• Yoga to tone the abdomen and inverted postures (headstands) help the digestive function

and correct prolapse. Headstands can be dangerous unless they are done with the proper guidance of a qualified yoga teacher.

• Take hip baths to stimulate the energy in the abdomen.

Moxibustion for diarrhea

(See the BodyMap for the exact location of points and the meanings of abbreviations.)

ST. 36 and SP. 6—Use three cones on all 4 points to alleviate diarrhea.

C.V. 12 and ST. 25—Use ginger moxa or a salt ring on these points.

Uranaitei—Use moxibustion for diarrhea.

Flatulence

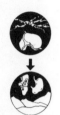

1) Overbearing Liver Attacks the Spleen

Abusing your digestive tract leads to a weak Spleen and an overbearing Liver, which together produce gas.

Flatulence, or gas, is disharmony between the Liver and the Spleen meridians and organ systems. The diagnostic name for the condition is Wood (Liver) Attacking the Earth (Spleen). Normally, Wood restrains Earth in the Control Cycle, but in this case, the Liver is overbearing. A lack of circulation between the Spleen Qi and the Liver Qi develops when the Spleen Qi is weakened by mixing too many types of foods, eating the wrong types of food, imbibing quantities of liquid with meals, or eating foods that are difficult to digest. Liver imbalance is caused by stress, improper diet, or anger, causing the Yang to rise and attack the Stomach to produce flatulence and burping.

Also, incompletely digested food doesn't become absorbed into the bloodstream in the small intestine; instead, it may sit there and ferment to result in noxious flatulence.

Self-Help Strategies

—Calm the Liver Qi.

—Tone the Spleen Qi.

—Reduce sugar intake.

—Keep the intestines clear.

Internal Applications

• Reduce intake of foods that weaken the Stomach/Spleen, and instead eat to nourish and strengthen it (see Food Influences in Chapter 3).

• Difficult-to-digest foods increase one's susceptibility to developing gas, but these foods differ for everyone. One person may be able to eat pork 'n' beans, burritos, black bean soup and hummus in a single week. That combination might send another to the moon on a self-generated cloud. Someone might not be able to tolerate the outer skin of bell peppers; another cannot eat nuts. These diet idiosyncracies are worth figuring out if you suffer from chronic gas.

• Unequivocally, the best treatment for flatulence is a simplified diet that is mostly composed of fresh, whole foods. Cook thoroughly foods that need to be cooked a long time. Brown rice and eggplants are two examples of foods that tend to be served undercooked. Cook beans after soaking in water and a teaspoon of bicarbonate of soda over night, skim-

ming the foam off when cooking, until they are completely soft. Or try adding kombu while cooking; ingesting the added minerals will stimulate intestinal activity.
• Chewing foods completely and allowing 2 to 3 hours to pass from the end of supper to bedtime also helps prevent gas.
• An infusion of powdered ginger (1 tbsp. ginger to 1 cup water) drunk warm may also help relieve intestinal spasms.

External Applications
• Taking a moment to calm the mind and body before meals can reduce episodes of flatulence. Practice some deep breathing by loosening your belt, sitting with your back straight, breathing in deeply through the nose, and letting the abdomen expand. Exhale, letting the abdomen fall in naturally. Practice deep breathing 10 minutes before eating. It strengthens the abdominal muscles and improves digestion.
• Try a ginger and mustard poultice for a painful abdomen, distention, gas, sore and stiff shoulders, and heaviness in the head. To make it, grate an inch-long chunk of unpeeled ginger. Add the same amount of Japanese yellow mustard (*karashi*, sold powdered and canned in Oriental foods markets) to the ginger and mix well. Spoon the mixture onto a handkerchief and fasten with a string or tie in the middle to make a small sack. Throw this into a pot with 2 cups of water and bring to a boil, turn the heat down, and simmer 10 minutes. Soak small hand towels in the decoction and place on abdomen, cover with a dry towel and a hot-water bottle. Change once or twice. Leave on for 30 minutes total.

Indigestion, Stomachache, and Stomatitis

Most stomachaches are due to imbalance in the Spleen channel; see the problems above for descriptions.

Internal Applications
• Stomach and abdominal pain can also be relieved by the regular ingestion of garlic, according to Japanese folk tradition. Grill 2 to 3 cloves with the skin on until they are well browned and eat these with dinner. The taste is pleasantly nutty and is good for chronic digestive problems in general.
• A cup of Japanese bancha tea or a cup of ginger infusion with 1 tsp. ume (plum) extract is recommended for stomachache.
• Stomachaches due to stress can be alleviated by eating more sticky foods; the mucilage coats the stomach lining, helping prevent the development of an ulcer. Konnyaku, nattō, taro root, and yamaimo are typical Japanese foods that fall into this category.
• Take a teaspoon of honey with warm water and do not eat for an hour after to relieve stomach inflammation and Heat in the Stomach.

External Applications
• A hot salt "stone" is recommended for indigestion, stomachache, and blood in the urine. Heat a cup of salt and wrap it in a handkerchief with the ends tied to make a sack. Set this over the painful areas to warm them, and lightly massage the internal organs.

• Give yourself a break after meals by lying down on your right side with your head in your right hand. This aids digestion and the movement of food into the duodenum.

• A ginger compress is recommended for stomachaches. Make this by grating about an inch-long chunk of peeled ginger and cooking it in 2 to 3 cups of water until the ginger tea turns dark. Steep a clean cotton towel in the mixture once the liquid cools enough to wring out, and apply over the painful area. Cover with a dry towel and a hot-water bottle.

• Try massage for intestinal pain due to gas, constipation, and food lodged in the organ of the Large and Small Intestines. Place the left hand over the right and rotate the hands in a circular motion over the lower belly while deep-breathing. Begin at the navel, move the hands to the left, then down, around over the lower abdomen, and up to the level of the bellybutton again. Repeat this 50 times. Visualize energy clearing the digestive tract as you do this.

Acupressure for Stomach Cramps
(See the BodyMap for the exact location of points and the meanings of point abbreviations.)

> BL. 17—Stimulate both sides of the 7th cervical vertebra with the thumbs, then above it and below it, 2 to 3 times, to harmonize Stomach Qi.
>
> Uranaitei—Use moxa for stomach cramps, upset and indigestion.

Nausea and Vomiting

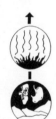

Rising Stomach Fire

Eating too fast; eating excessive quantities of rich, fatty food; or just plain overeating can cause the Stomach Fire to rise, resulting in foul belching, vomiting of sour fluid, and burning pain in the epigastrium.

Nausea can also be caused by a flu or cold virus, bacteria, rotten food, and by an internal disorder such as Cold Damp in the Spleen, which was described in the Diarrhea section, above.

Self-Help Strategies

—Pay attention to what and how you eat. Slow down, and reduce quantities where applicable.

—Cool the Stomach Qi.

Internal Applications

• If you have vomited already, drink a few cups of ginger tea with a teaspoon of ume (plum) extract.

• Drink a cup of bancha tea with $1/2$ tsp. soy sauce. Add the meat of an umeboshi pickled plum to the tea if nausea is accompanied by pain. Or drink $1/2$ tsp. ume (plum) vinegar with the juice from grated ginger in a cupful of warm bancha tea. Drink immediately.

• Follow an episode of nausea and vomiting with brown rice cream (see recipe in the Appendix) and umeboshi meats, which are full of digestion-promoting enzymes. Miso soup with scallions and a little brown rice on the side contains enzymes that aid digestion. A couple of slices of takuan pickle (see Glossary) are also recommended.

Acupressure for vomiting
(See the BodyMap for the exact location of points and the meaning of point abbreviations.)

ST. 36—Readjusts function of Spleen/Stomach.

C.V. 12—Readjusts the Stomach and subdues the ascending Qi.

Food Poisoning

• If the food poisoning was cause by fish or shellfish (it often is), cut up some raw perilla leaves and pour hot water over to make an infusion, then drink the tea. Or eat the raw leaves.

• Grate some raw lotus root, add to 3 cups of water, boil and then turn down to simmer, cook for 10 minutes, and drink hot.

• Daikon radish is indicated for food poisoning as well. Grate $^1/_3$ cup of daikon radish and 2 tbsp. fresh ginger. Add these with a dash of soy sauce to a cup of hot bancha tea or hot water and drink 3 times a day.

Gastric and Duodenal Ulcers

Unchecked Deficient Spleen Qi and Kidney Yang Deficiency

As the lack of Spleen Qi progresses (which causes indigestion, included earlier in this section), Cold signs increase; pain is relieved by warmth. Left untreated, ulcer, chronic gastritis, gastric neurosis, chronic enteritis, and dysentery may result.

The combination of Spleen Qi Deficiency, overindulgence in cold food and drinks, stress, and Kidney Yang Deficiency can develop into quite an unpleasant syndrome. Besides the pain in the abdomen, the stool is loose and includes undigested food, there is Cold and fatigue in the arms and legs, mental and physical fatigue, edema with little urination, and possibly organ prolapse.

An ulcer is a stress-related injury. If you are unsure how or why your ulcer developed, go back over what you were doing when stomach problems first developed. What new stress entered your life at that time? Has that stress continued? Has it gotten worse? Has your stomach problem continued? Gotten worse? As stress worsens, the stomach becomes unable to absorb nutrients, the cells of the lining of the stomach become unable to secrete hydrochloric acid, food cannot be digested, and weight loss occurs.

Sulfur drugs or antibiotics taken for a prolonged period of time can destroy the intestinal bacteria, upsetting the natural internal balance and facilitating the development of an ulcer.

Self-Help Strategies

—See a practitioner. This is a serious condition that needs personal treatment. Herbal treatment can be very effective.

—Tonify the Spleen.

—Warm the Middle Burner.

Internal Applications

• Avoid overeating, refined and simple sugars, animal fats, food additives and preservatives.

• Begin a stress reduction technique immediately. With regular and consistent practice, this could significantly contribute to the healing of an ulcer.

• Include more water-soluble fiber such as oats, brown rice, and beans.

• Shiitake mushrooms are ulcer-soothing contributions to any meal. Eat them frequently.

• Sesame oil contains vitamin E and aids in the healing of wounds. Add to lightly steamed vegetables and cooked salads.

• Bee propolis is also recommended for ulcers. Take according to the directions on the bottle (see the section Adapting to Stress and Building the Immune System in Part II).

Heartburn, Acid Reflux, and Cold Sores

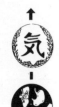

1) Ascending Stomach Qi

Overeating, especially rich food, or eating too quickly lead to undigested food in the Stomach, causing the Stomach Qi to rebel and ascend, with belching and sour regurgitation.

Self-Help Strategies

—Eat less at meals, and eat more slowly.

—Reduce intake of fats.

—Cool the Stomach Heat.

2) Stagnant Liver Qi (Wood) invades the Spleen (Earth)

Belching with acid reflux can occur when the Liver Qi Stagnates and Rises to invade the Stomach, causing nausea and epigastric pain. Ulcerations in the mouth indicate Heat in the Stomach.

Self-Help Strategies

—Tonify and free the Liver Qi.

—Eliminate rich foods from the diet.

—Cool the Stomach.

—Tonify the Spleen.

Internal Applications

• Add 1 tsp. of ume (plum) extract to a cup of bancha tea. Drink warm.

• Grated daikon radish with a small amount of soy sauce helps cool the acidic, hot stomach.

• Eat a piece of soaked, toasted kombu and chew it well.

• Eat sesame seeds with brown rice regularly.

• Well-aged takuan pickles (see Glossary) are recommended for heartburn. Find them at Japanese and sometimes Chinese markets.

• Drink a cup of gentian infusion after each meal for a month and notice that it makes a huge difference in weak constitution types with weak digestion. Do not drink this on an empty stomach.

Loss of Appetite

• Eat only when you feel hungry, not when the clock tells you it is time to eat. When the digestive system is clogged and over-stuffed, the body will not absorb nutrients in food and the additional food will make the body feel worse. Put your mind somewhere else at meal time. If you can, go to a movie or watch a video while others are eating. Try to not be in food's vicinity if you "can't help" eating.

• Drink bancha tea with toasted grains of brown rice, a teaspoon of ume (plum) extract in warm water, and decoction of *ketsumeishi*, available at Chinese pharmacies.

• Try the brown rice cream (see the Appendix for recipe). It is light, very nurturing to the Spleen/Stomach, and is full of nutrition.

• Another appetite-stimulating therapeutic meal is brown rice soup. See the end of the chapter.

External Applications
• Garlic moxibustion

"Lighting the wick" garlic moxibustion for weak constitutions with appetite loss:

—Using the largest garlic clove you can find, peel and slice a 3 ml thick round.

—Place this on the bellybutton.

—Tear and roll a small piece of moxa and place this exactly in the middle of the garlic round. It should be small enough so that it does not spill off the round. No moxa should touch the skin.

—With a lit incense stick, light the moxa ball, and allow it to burn down.

—The garlic should become quite hot. Remove it whenever the heat becomes uncomfortable. Repeat 5 to 10 times until there is a ringing sensation in the abdomen and the area is well stimulated.

—This treatment is said to rekindle the digestive fire. The belly button is actually the point Conception Vessel 8.

—This treatment is also fine for children.

—Garlic moxibustion can be applied directly over painful muscles, such as those in the back and the hips, as well.

—Dried moxa sold in rough form, in bags, works better than stick or rolled form.

Overeating

• Drink hot tea and broths to be gentle to the system and help digestion but do not imbibe too much. Too much liquid can also put undue stress on the system and harm the Spleen/Stomach.

• The bitter herb gentian aids the Stomach/Spleen and Liver after a spell of overeating. The herb was introduced into Japan during the second half of the nineteenth century as an example of a Western digestive bitter.

• Eat lightly steamed or juiced greens—kale, clover greens, dandelion, chrysanthemum leaves—as often as you can. Rich in chlorophyll, they clean and supplement the Blood. Dandelion is a bitter leaf, also good for the Liver.

• Light meals for a few days, such as boiled fish soup with coriander, or freshly slivered ginger and grated daikon radish served with a small amount of brown rice leave your body in fine shape quickly. Do not eat between meals.

Recipe: Brown Rice Soup

This is brown rice cooked in vegetable broth; it is very easy to digest and is particularly recommended for ulcers and stomach reflux. Add barley for diarrhea. Rolled oats are helpful in cases of constipation.

Vegetable broth made with any of the following: burdock root, carrots, celery, daikon radish, winter squash, eggplant, dark leafy greens, and parsley

    1 tbsp. brown rice for every cup of broth

To prepare:
1. Strain the vegetables out through a cheesecloth before cooking.
2. Add the rice to the broth and cook until the rice is soft.
3. For those with stronger digestion, add the vegetables in the same proportions of rice to liquid at the beginning of cooking.

Ear problems

Oriental Medical Energetics

Both the ears and the hearing are under the control of the Kidney system, particularly the Kidney Jing, the regenerative energy of the body. Hearing often declines during old age, when the Jing begins to suffer from depletion as well. In the Far East, interestingly, large fleshy ears with long or wide lobes are regarded as a sign of vitality and longevity, which indicates a person well endowed with Jing. Hearing problems could indicate a weakness in the Kidney organ and channel, an imbalance in the Gallbladder channel, the Triple Heater, and/or the Small Intestine channel.

1) Jing Deficiency

Gradual hearing loss points to a gradual decrease in the Kidney regenerative energy, the Jing. There may be blocked ears, ringing or buzzing sounds, ticking or gradual loss of hearing but no pain. Other symptoms might include poor memory, lumbago, dizziness, night sweats, dry throat, constipation, concentrated urine, and aching in the lower legs. Tinnitus may indicate other meridian involvement that only a practitioner can diagnose.

Self-Help Strategies

—See a practitioner. Toning and supplementing the Jing retards the aging process. There are many herbs that supplement the Jing.

—Reduce stress and overwork.

Internal Applications

• Foods that weaken the Kidneys: alcohol, coffee and caffeinated beverages, chocolate, citrus fruits and juice, and excessively spicy foods should be avoided.

• Steer the diet toward strengthening the Spleen/Stomach system (See Chapter 3).

• Foods that tone the Kidneys should also be eaten (See Chapter 3).

2) Internal Heat and Phlegm

An acute earache with discharge is present but no hearing loss is involved. This indicates a situation of internal Heat and Phlegm. This situation could occur in conjunction with a cold, or it may be more serious. If the pain is not gone in a day or two consult a practitioner.

External Applications
• For earaches, grate a small piece of daikon radish, squeeze the juice from the gratings, soak a cotton swab or a small cotton ball in the juice, wipe the ear with it, and keep it in the ear for an hour. Reapply if necessary.
• A burdock leaf infusion is indicated for inflammations of the outer ear. Use a handful of the dried (or shade-dried fresh) leaves to 1 cup of boiling water. Steep and wipe the ear once the solution is cool. Soak gauze and keep it in the ear. Burdock has antiphlogistic properties.

Acupressure for ringing in the ears
• These are local points for ear imbalance and tinnitus. An acupressure therapist will be able to administer individualized and more effective treatment, depending on the involvement of other meridian systems.
(See the BodyMap for the location of points and the meaning of the abbreviations.)

G.B. 2—Opens the ears, dispels Wind, and moves the Qi in the head.

G.B. 3—Boosts the hearing; indicated for tinnitus.

T.H. 21—Boosts hearing; indicated for tinnitus and discharges from the ears.

T.H. 17—Massage the entire back of the ear, as if trying to rub out the lumps for deafness and tinnitus. Also treats clenched jaw and poor eyesight.

Eyes

Oriental Medical Energetics

The eyes reflect the general balance of the body, according to Oriental medicine theory. Specifically, many eye problems reflect imbalance in the Liver organ and meridian system. In traditional Oriental medicine, the Liver controls the eyesight and the function of producing tears. This seems likely when we stop to consider that vitamin A, the vitamin most related to proper eye functioning, is manufactured in the liver.

1) Liver Qi Rising or Heart Fire Flaming

Red and sore eyes may indicate stagnating Liver Qi Rising up to attack the eyes or Heart Fire Flaring. Both imbalances are due in great part to stress and overwork. If the hot Liver Yang energy flares up while the Liver Yin is depleted, a vacuum will occur, called Wind Heat, which will also affect the eyes. Dry, itchy eyes signify Blood or Yin Deficiency.

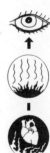

Self-Help Strategies

—Calm the Liver.
—Reduce work, study, and the use of the eyes.
—Reduce stress levels and anxiety.
—If the redness persists, see a practitioner.

2) Excess Heat in the Kidneys

Failing eyesight, on the other hand, may also be related to failing Kidneys. Chronic red, sore eyes that are not caused by eyestrain, improper lighting, or contact lenses, could reflect Excess Heat in the Kidneys, a condition best treated by a practitioner with acupuncture and herbs.

Internal Applications

• Avoid substances that strain the Liver or Kidneys (see Food Influences in Chapter 3).
• Eat some Liver-toning and -relaxing foods such as liver organ meat (see Food Influences

in Chapter 3 for more food recommendations and the section, Preparation of Organ Meats, in the Appendix).

• Also include foods that tone the Yin (see Food Influences in Chapter 3).

• For pinkeye and pains in the eye, a traditional Chinese food cure is the ingestion of bitter gourd (which can be purchased at typical Oriental markets; it looks like a wrinkled zucchini or cucumber). The regular ingestion of bitter gourd is said to improve eyesight. It is regarded as the king of bitter food and is good for those with a hot physical constitution because it cools down the internal region and improves the condition of the Liver.

• Habu-cha (*ketsumeishi*), which can be purchased from Chinese pharmacies, is indicated for all sorts of eye problems, from tired, sore eyes to nearsightedness. Decoct 3 to 9 g of the seeds in $1^1/_2$ cups of water, bring to a boil, then turn the heat down and simmer, and reduce by $^1/_3$. Drink throughout the day.

External Applications

• Tired eyes have lost a good deal of their water component. Rehydrate the eyes modestly with saline solution (commercially prepared is okay), take care to look into the distance regularly, be careful about aggravating the Liver, and keep the intestines clean.

• A traditional Sicilian remedy for red, swollen eyes is to cover them for 10 to 20 minutes with slices of tomato.

• Effective eyewashes for mild infections include an infusion of chamomile (strong chamomile tea) cooled to skin temperature, a cooled infusion of eyebright (*Euphrasia officinalis*), and rosewater.

• For irritated, sore eyelids, place cool compresses soaked in an infusion of marigold flowers (*Calendula officinalis*) over the eyes.

• Traditionally in Japan conjunctivitis was treated with a sea salt and warm water eyewash and then covered with a potato plaster. To make a potato plaster, grate 2 tbsp. regular potato or taro root, add an equal amount of flour, spread onto a piece of gauze, cover with another layer of gauze, and tape over the eye.

• For a sty, try warming garlic cloves until they are toasted and soft. Spread over gauze, cover with another layer of gauze, affix to the eye with tape, and cover with an eye bandage. The plaster takes advantage of the garlic's antibacterial properties. Cool the Heat of the sty by applying a potato plaster to the eye and taping into place at night. A sty also signifies overwork, or overextension. Take a rest for a couple of days, eat regularly, and incorporate Stomach/Spleen-toning foods into the diet. Sesame, bran, green leafy vegetables, sea vegetables, vitamin B complex, and calcium are recommended.

Acupressure and massage for eyestrain

Massage is the form of self-help treatment the Chinese and Japanese practice most for eye pain. Acupressure around the eye can relieve the muscular tension and the aches and pains that accompany eyestrain.

• Massage both sides of the top of the nose with the thumbs. Keep the other fingers slightly curved against the forehead.

• Massage the sides of the bridge of the nose using the thumb and the index finger of one hand. Press down, then up.

• Now place the index and middle fingers of both hands on either side of the nose. Remove the middle fingers and massage under the cheekbones using the index fingers.

• Press on the inner and outer corners of the eye and around the eye socket with the index finger.

• Press the Third Eye point between the eyebrows and press the outer edge of the eyebrow.

• Press the temples lightly and rub gently.

• First thing in the morning, raise the eyes up and down, to the left and right, and to the diagonal corners of the room to strengthen and alleviate tension in the muscles.

Fatigue and Chronic Fatigue Syndrome

Assuming you are not anemic or suffering from influenza, fatigue is usually associated with poor nutrition, insomnia, stress, depression, or an underlying psychological problem. Fatigue is also a side effect of narcotic painkillers, some anticonvulsants, antidepressants, antihistamines, antihypertensives, birth-control pills, cough and cold preparations with codeine, sleeping pills, muscle relaxants, and tranquilizers.

Excess fat in the diet can cause fatigue by impairing the blood's ability to deliver oxygen to body cells and hardening the arteries. Carbohydrate deficiency, alcohol, smoking, constant dieting consisting of purging and fasting can all cause fatigue. Lack of exercise is another culprit.

Feeling tired is different from Chronic Fatigue Syndrome, called Myalgic Encephelomylitis in Europe. We include the European name because it provides a descriptive term for other common symptoms that make up the Chronic Fatigue group symptoms. Myalgic refers to pain, usually in the muscles; enchephelo- has to do with the brain, and -mylitis refers to an inflammation of the brain's lining. Besides the overwhelming lack of energy and motivation that the illness is notorious for, relentless aches and pains, especially in the muscles, and disturbed brain function—including confusion, poor or lack of concentration, poor memory, and fuzzy thinking—are common among its sufferers.

The syndrome was first noticed in young, overworked, and highly stressed individuals in the 1980s who caught colds characterized by aching joints and flu-like symptoms that lingered interminably, for which it was dubbed "yuppie flu." With the passing of time, however, doctors have identified the syndrome in people from a wide range of ages and backgrounds.

Chronic Fatigue Syndrome was defined by medical and health experts at a meeting sponsored by the Centers for Disease Control in 1988,[1] as a specific set of symptoms that the patient experiences for a minimum of six months. These symptoms include energy loss—more than just fatigue, the lack of energy is devastating. The patient feels incapable of continuing the activity at hand and there is often a physical need to stop and lie down. The sufferer does not feel refreshed after sleep, experiences narrow bands of productive waking hours, and is active only during these times of day. Often the early morning (active time for the Stomach/Spleen systems) and late afternoon (the most active time of day for the Kidney) are difficult times, while midday is better.

Mental symptoms include the Central Nervous System disorders mentioned above—poor concentration, memory loss, forgetfulness, headaches, heaviness in the head, and feeling a need to put the head down. Recent studies have shown that this may be related to a lack of oxygen in certain areas of the brain or neurally mediated hypotension.[2] Emotionally, the patient is often depressed. In Oriental medicine it is said that when the Qi is blocked or depleted a person will feel depressed, but a person with Chronic Fatigue may not have felt depressed when he or she came down with the illness. As the illness progresses, however, he or she may become depressed by the inability to function normally as well as by the mechanism of the disease process itself. The depression could actually have a negative impact on the illness, whereas keeping one's spirits up can actually help the prognosis a little.

Digestive system symptoms include repeated bacterial or yeast infections in the gut, pain and distention in the abdomen, food allergies, bloating, lack of appetite, weight loss, diarrhea, undigested food in the stool, and other symptoms comprising a Tai Yin pattern of illness (the first Yin stage of illness—see the section Adapting to Stress and Building the Immune System in Part II). In allopathic medical terms, these symptoms would suggest *Candida albicans*, irritable bowel syndrome, and food allergies. They could also be associated with cholitis, Crohn's disease, and diverticulitis.

The onset of the syndrome is often caused by an acute viral attack with fever, chills, and other flu-like symptoms. The patient should be very careful to prevent a recurrence of these flu-like symptoms during the course of the disease, which can significantly weaken the body and result in a regression. Careful attention to keeping warm in winter by wrapping the areas of the back of the neck and kidney area is particularly important.

Recovery from Chronic Fatigue Syndrome can take anywhere from six months to one year for a light case, to several years for a more serious case. Oriental medicine can be used to treat the syndrome with very positive effects.

Preventative measures can be very helpful. Watch for a virulent viral attack, typically of meningitis, glandular fever, or some other ordinary flu-like virus that lingers for several weeks. Once this occurs, the body is balancing precariously on the edge of the syndrome. See a practitioner for advice immediately, and begin herbal and acupuncture treatment, a light but consistent exercise routine to increase the body's intake of oxygen, and make appropriate dietary, work, and lifestyle changes to reduce stress, frustration, and irritation. The sooner treatment begins, the better the prognosis. Currently there is no definitive test for the virus, which itself has yet to be clearly identified.

Oriental Medical Energetics

Deficiencies in the Spleen, Kidney, and/or Lung affect Blood, reduce Warmth, and create fatigue.

Chinese medicine considers air and food to be the main ways to increase energy in the body. The Lungs, of course, are the organs involved in the process of taking in Air Qi (oxy-

Air Qi

KŌNG QI
KŪ KI

Grain Qi

GŪ QI
KOKKI

Original Qi

原
気

YUÁN QI
GEN KI

gen). The Stomach/Spleen systems are most directly involved with the digestive process—including the pancreatic function of the secretion of digestive enzymes. Nutritive essence from food broken down by the Stomach/Spleen and Air Qi are thought to combine in the chest and spread throughout the body via the meridians to warm and nourish the entire system. A Deficiency in either the Lung Qi or Spleen/Stomach Qi could reduce the amount of Qi entering the body and result in fatigue.

Besides the intake of oxygen and food, the body has a second line of energy production that takes place in the Kidneys. This energy is called Hereditary Qi (or Yuan Qi). Yuan Qi is an active form of energy formed from Jing. It is stored by the Kidney and released to supplement the Nutritive Qi in times of inadequate exercise or nutrition. This mechanism acts as a system of checks and balances, providing the body with a back-up energy system during difficult or stressful periods. But overwork, excessive sexual stimulation, prolonged illness, and experiencing extreme emotions for a long period of time can drain the Kidney of these energy stores, resulting in Kidney-related fatigue.

Liver Involvement

The Liver does not produce energy, but stores and distributes it. If the Liver energy becomes stuck, usually due to frustration and anger, the Liver Qi could become excessive and stagnate, Blood will not be released when the body is in motion (an important Liver function according to Oriental medicine), and the person could feel fatigued as a result.

Characteristics of Fatigue

The nature of fatigue depends on the organ involved.

The lack of Qi in cases of Lung Deficiency results in physical tiredness, shortness of breath, lowered resistance to colds, nasal congestion or a constantly running nose, fear of wind or cold, a lack of motivation, not wanting to do things, feeling isolated and introspective. Oriental medical treatment and the gradual incorporation of a gentle exercise program will help the patient in this case.

Fatigue in cases of Stomach/Spleen Deficiency is characterized by a more physical feeling, since the Spleen and Stomach are responsible for the flesh, the substance of the body. In this case, the arms and legs feel heavy, tired, and the entire system feels sluggish. There is also mental fatigue characterized by the inability to think clearly. Oriental medical treatment and dietary measures can help this condition.

Kidney fatigue produces exhaustion—not only a heavy body or a lack of motivation, but a total lack of energy, will power, and the ability to push on. The candle has really been burned at both ends, and reserves have been completely eaten up. The patient may also experience lower back pain. In this case, the sufferer can only supplement treatment with rest.

The Lungs, Spleen, and Kidney organs are all involved in the process of creating Blood. The Kidneys add essence to the system, the Lungs add Air Qi, and the Stomach/Spleen provides nourishment so the bone marrow can produce nourishing, high quality Blood. Deficiencies in any of these systems will produce Blood of a poor quality and poor chemistry, lacking in oxygen and nutrients. Symptoms of dry skin, dizziness, pallor, fatigue, and insomnia suggest a Blood Deficiency in which Blood is unable to reach the Heart.

Chronic Fatigue

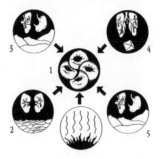

1. Blood Deficiency
2. Kidney Deficiency
3. Spleen Deficiency
4. Lung Qi Deficiency
5. Liver Qi Stagnation

Fatigue associated with Liver imbalance is a different dynamic, since the imbalance is not a deficiency problem but an excess where Qi becomes blocked. The fatigue resulting from this dynamic comes in bursts and starts; the organism's energy is not sustained. The body feels tired at times, and stuck, rigid, and blocked emotionally and physically at others. The person could demonstrate variable, manic behavior. In this case, Oriental medical treatment in addition to dynamic motion—exercise—will help activate the Qi and improve the condition. This type of fatigue is easier to treat and is not usually associated with chronic, persistant fatigue.

In terms of Yin and Yang, fatigue, caused by deficiency, understood as Damaged Yang. In the body, Yang symbolizes Qi; Yin is related to the body's substances (Blood, fluids, nutrients). When the Yang and Qi decline, the Blood and fluids are also weakened, and the body becomes fatigued. In addition, with the decline of Yang and Qi, the body's fluids accumulate and the body loses its warmth. The four limbs grow cold, the skin and lips become pale, diarrhea and cramping may appear. Oriental medicine clinicians have found that acknowledging the presence of Cold and treating it with warming herbs (such as aconite) before using tonic herbs (ginseng, astragalus) to tone the body has proven to be a pivotal point in reversing the condition.

Internal Applications

• Fatigue sufferers must realize that they have completely depleted their resources. The treatment principle is to begin to build up the body again, beginning with the digestive system. Strengthen and rebuild before considering a detoxification program or you could become even more deeply fatigued. Chronic fatigue sufferers should be working with a practitioner.

• Take measures to strengthen the immune system by following recommendations included in the section Adapting to Stress and Building the Immune System.

• Foods that weaken the Kidneys should be avoided (see Chapter 3).

• Reduce foods in the diet that are energetically Cold and Cooling. Avoid iced foods and drinks, fruit juice, raw fruits and vegetables, and greasy or deep-fried foods that weaken the Stomach/Spleen (see Chapter 3).

• Avoid tobacco, over-the-counter drugs, food additives and preservatives.

• Eat more foods that detoxify and tone the Blood—liver organ meat, mochi, and mugwort tea.

• Include foods that supplement Blood (see Chapter 3).

• Warming, Qi-toning foods tone the Spleen and the Middle Burner and are indicated for this condition (see Chapter 3).

• Try a vinegar tonic for fatigue every morning: blend 1 cup warm water with 2 tablespoons apple cider vinegar and 1 teaspoon honey. Rice vinegar is also indicated for fatigue in Oriental medicine.

• To strengthen and supplement Blood make a decoction of cooked di huang (rhemannia) (3 to 9 g) in 2 cups of water. Boil and reduce water by $1/3$. Divide into two portions and drink in the morning and evening after meals.

• Decoctions of longan berry meats strengthen the Spleen and Heart, tonify Blood and Qi, and are used to treat anemia, dizziness, and fainting. Cook 5 to 10 g with 2 cups of water, bring to a boil, then turn down heat to medium and continue cooking for 5 minutes. Drink the liquid and eat the fruit in the morning and evening with or after meals.

External Applications

• The idea of exercise may seem unbearable, but very gentle movement and breathing will aid the body's struggle to recover from fatigue. Try some slow walking, gradually picking up the pace as you feel yourself growing stronger. Qigong and deep breathing are highly recommended.

• Take sensible precautions against catching colds and flus, especially in winter. The Chinese believe Cold enters the body through the back of the neck and the kidney area—make a special effort to keep these areas covered. Catching a cold or flu could set recovery back a long way.

• Practice relaxation techniques, and try counseling to counter psychologically related fatigue.

Endnotes

*1 Department of Health and Human Services, *The Facts About Chronic Fatigue Syndrome* (Atlanta: Public Health Service Centers for Disease Control and Prevention, 1995), pp.11–12.
   The 1988 CFS working case definition was revised in 1993 because it did not effectively distinguish CFS from other types of unexplained fatigue. As such, Chronic Fatigue Syndrome is now treated as a subset of *chronic fatigue* (a broader category of unexplained fatigue of 6 months or longer), which in turn was made a subset of *prolonged fatigue* (fatigue lasting 1 month or longer). Clinically evaluated, unexplained chronic fatigue can be classified as CFS if the patient meets both the following criteria:
      1. The fatigue is not the result of ongoing exertion, is not substantially alleviated by rest, and results in substantial reduction in previous levels of occupational, educational, social, or personal activities.
      2. The concurrent occurrence of four or more of the following symptoms: substantial impairment in short-term memory or concentration; sore throat; tender lymph nodes; muscle pain; multijoint pain without swelling or redness; headaches of a new type, pattern, or severity; unrefreshing sleep; and postexertional malaise lasting more than 24 hours. These symptoms must have persisted or recurred during 6 or more consecutive months of illness and must not have predated the fatigue.
*2 Peter C. Rowe, Issam Bou-Holaigah, Jean S. Kan, and Hugh Calkins, "Is Neurally Mediated Hypotension an Unrecognised Cause of Chronic Fatigue?" *The Lancet*, March 1995, p.623.

Feet

Feet carry more than the day. They walk, run, skip, jump, hop, and climb us to our destinations. They dance us till dawn, yet they are two of the most dismally undercared-for parts of our bodies. The feet, which are said to contain a map of the entire body on the soles, are actually valuable tools for healing. Reflexology is the modality of therapy used to treat the body through a massage of the feet. Acupuncture meridians also end in the feet. One of the most common treatments for releasing blockages in the lower half of the body employs two major points on the feet. Please try to take care of your feet by keeping them clean, dry, and the toenails trimmed. Wearing sensible shoes (high heels are the worst—not only for feet but for the back and posture as well) is essential for well-being of feet and mind. But feet love exposure to air, grass, sand, and water—go barefoot whenever possible.

Athlete's Foot

This fungal infection of the skin flourishes in wet, moist environments. The best treatment is to keep the feet clean and dry.

• Try tea tree oil for skin fungal infections. It can also be used for toe- and fingernail fungal infections. Paint the oil on twice or three times a day. It is nontoxic and nonirritating. Apply full strength to infections, or dilute it with water (10% solution or $1^1/_2$ tbsp. per cup of water) to rinse and clean infected wounds. Find it in most health food stores or see the Appendix for ordering information.

• Garlic can also be applied directly to athlete's foot. Crush a clove of garlic, wrap it in gauze, and fasten it to the foot with medical tape. Cover with a sock and keep on overnight. If the garlic feels as if it is burning the skin after a couple of days, make a garlic decoction by crushing a few cloves, boiling in a cup of water, and painting on the infection.

• Chrysanthemum leaves also have antibacterial properties and were traditionally used on skin abrasions and cuts to fight infection. Use the leaves in a foot bath for athlete's foot.

• One ounce of the Chinese herb da huang (*Rhizoma Rhei*, rhubarb root) to 3 cups of water and boiled down to one cup makes a strong decoction to paint on areas affected by athlete's foot. Apply 2 or 3 times a day.

Sore, Itchy, Tired Feet

• For itchy, burning feet massage with cooling Tiger Balm, or a massage cream that contains camphor, or a small amount of White Flower Oil (see Glossary) in almond oil.
• Soak dried, cracked skin in a hot foot bath with sesame seed oil and a decoction of Job's tears(see Glossary).
• Add 2 to 3 g Sichuan peppers (*sanshō*, *Zanthoxylum bungeanum* Maxim) to the Job's tears when you decoct it. The peppers are available in the West at most shops carrying Chinese and Japanese foods and spices. This solution is also recommended for skin cracks and dry skin.
• Pomegranate is said to alleviate itching. Itchy, tired feet can soak in a pomegranate foot bath. Cut the fruit, crush the seeds, and infuse in hot water for 15 minutes. Add this solution to hot water and soak the feet for 15 minutes. Rinse with warm water and massage with Tiger Balm.
• Before you go to sleep, if you're feeling tired and irritated and your feet hurt, try soaking them in hot ginger water for 15 to 20 minutes. Follow up with a fresh lemon-juice massage. Rinse with cool water, dry completely, and practice some deep abdominal breathing to move the energy down into your belly and completely relax you before bed.
• A 15-minute foot massage feels so good that after you try it, you will want to do it for yourself at least weekly. It will put you into a deep, revitalizing sleep.

Reflexology

Reflexology is an ancient Chinese therapy designed to bring the body into balance and maintain general health. The therapy is based on the idea that the organs of the body have corresponding reflex points on other parts of the body, some of the most sensitive points being on the feet. Reflexologists have divided the body into zones in order to find the corresponding areas. Organs of one zone can be stimulated by pressing various points in a corresponding zone. All the organs of the body are represented on the feet, making them a virtual map of the body. The zones can also be interpreted as energy lines upon which the flow of Qi moves, starting from the head and ending in the hands and feet. There are lateral lines as well.

Initial palpation of the foot reveals the condition of the entire body. Tender points correspond to organs that are out of balance. Stimulating the reflex point stimulates a circulation of Qi in the corresponding organ and promotes the body's move toward balance. Imbalances can be caused by an unhealthy lifestyle, overwork, stress, diet, poor environment, illness, and pain.

The emotions are also tied in with the blockages. For example, swelling, tightness, and contraction often reflect the emotions of fear and guilt. Fear and guilt are the emotions most associated with lower back pain, reflexologists say. When fearful, the body constricts to protect itself, cutting off the flow of energy to the back. Some reflexologists think guilt manifests as an unconscious desire for self-punishment, resulting in pain in the body. It can be helpful to combine counseling while receiving reflexology treatment.

Try some basic reflexology on your own:
• **Allergy sufferers** can relieve their sneezing, runny nose, and watery eyes by rubbing the top of the first segment of the big toe with the thumb, in an upward movement toward the nail.
• For **abdominal bloating and digestive difficulties**, rub and press under the metatarso-phalangeal joint of the big toe (ball of the foot) and the entire digestive zone area—the middle part of the foot where the digestive reflexes lie. Blocks in the digestive tract will manifest on this area of the feet as bumps or deposits. To locate the bumps, first stretch back the toes. Then with the thumb, firmly stretch the instep of the foot, and use the thumb of the the other hand (starting from the innermost part of the instep) to run up the sole on a diagonal. Sensitive spots become apparent after a few deep explorations. Rub these sore spots well.
• For **digestive problems** due to acidity in the stomach or overeating try rubbing just under the ball of the foot, that is, immediately behind the metatarso-phalangeal joint of the big toe.
• Stimulate the **lymph system** by pressing the points between each toe on the top of the foot.
• Women with **menstrual pain or irregularity**, other pelvic area difficulties, or lower back pain, should rub and press the area between the ankle bone and the heel of the inner foot. Doing this regularly can significantly reduce the intensity and duration of menstrual cramping.
• There are many fine books on reflexology; it is an excellent self-help tool (see Recommended Reading in the Appendix).

Gynecological problems

Includes: dysmenorrhea (pain and cramps), dark clots in menstrual blood, lingering cycles, excessive bleeding, mood swings (irritability, sudden bursts of anger, depression), female infertility, exhaustion after periods, endometriosis, leukorrhea, yeast and vaginal infection (*Candida albicans*), fibroids and cysts, and problems in menopause.

Dysmenorrhea

This is a common gynecological problem with symptoms of lower back pain and abdominal cramping during or after menstruation. The pain is often accompanied by a pale complexion, profuse sweating, cold extremities, nausea, and vomiting.

In Oriental medicine there are several possible energetic scenarios resulting in period pain. Due to the number of related syndromes, self-help guidelines (including internal and external applications) come at the end of the section Mood Swings.

Oriental Medical Energetics

1) Stagnant Qi and Blood

Blood and Qi Stagnation do not allow for the smooth flow of Blood, causing blockage and pain. Blood and Qi Stagnation is a common diagnosis for this problem. The cramps usually stretch through the lower abdomen in this case, radiating to the sides. If the problem is mainly Qi Stagnation, the pain isn't terribly severe. You may also notice distended pain in the chest and breasts, scanty blood with dark purple clots, and an irregular cycle. Blood and Qi Stagnation is often due to nervous stress or emotional depression. Poor hygiene during menstruation or after childbirth can also lead to infection, which leads, in turn, to cramping.

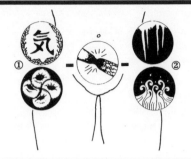

Self-Help Strategies

—Activate the Qi and Blood to remove Stagnation.

—Relieve pain.

2) Stagnant Cold and Damp

Stagnation of Cold and Damp inhibits the smooth flow of Qi and Blood, causing blockage and pain.

This second type of imbalance causes pain before or during menstruation. The pain is located in the center of the abdomen and may also radiate to the back. It is relieved by warmth and pressure. Accompanying symptoms are a pale complexion, cold hands and feet, scanty flow with purple clots, and a delayed cycle.

Caused by external influences, usually poor diet, excessive ingestion of cold drinks and foods, raw fruits and vegetables. This condition could also result from catching a chill when you are cold and wet during menstruation. Oriental practitioners are taught that resistance is weaker around the time of menstruation, when Cold can easily invade the body and be retained in the "House of Blood" (the uterus), impeding menstrual flow and causing Blood Stagnation, and consequently, pain.

Self-Help Strategies

—Warm the body and dispel Cold.

—Activate Qi.

—Relieve pain.

3) Blood and Qi Deficiency

A Deficiency of Qi and Blood prevent the body from becoming strong enough to generate a healthy, freely flowing cycle. Pain can also be caused by a Deficiency of Qi and Blood. In these cases the pain is dull and generally occurs at the end or following the cessation of the period. It feels like a "pulling down" sensation in the center of the abdomen. This pain, too, is often relieved by warmth and pressure. It may be accompanied by a pale complexion, palpitation, lack of energy, shortness of breath, a scanty, light-colored flow, and perhaps a late cycle. Other symptoms are related to poor Blood circulation, including headaches, dizziness, mood swings, irritability, neck/shoulder/lower back pain, and cold extremities.

A Deficiency of Qi and Blood as the result of a weak constitution and/or the aftereffects of a severe or chronic disease is compounded by menstruation, which is a type of stress for the body. Menstruation drains the body's supply of Blood and deprives the uterus (House of Blood) of nourishment.

Self-Help Strategies

—Strengthen the body and restore its vital energy.
—Nourish the Blood and improve circulation.
—Relieve pain.

4) Yang or Jing Deficiency

Yang deficiency will also lead to period pain because, according to Oriental medicine theory, the Blood is moved by yang energy. A lack of yang will lead to poor circulation of Qi, which in turn leads to poor blood circulation, retarded menses, and pain.

Too many births, abortions, and miscarriages can lead to generative Kidney Jing and Blood deficiencies and an undernourished uterus, causing pain in the lower abdomen.

Self-Help Strategies

—In the first scenario, tone and build the yang energy.
—Nurture the Jing in the latter case.
—Relieve pain.

Dark Clots in Menstrual Blood

Ordinarily, women don't worry about dark clots in their menstrual blood, but in Oriental medicine, the clots are a sign that all is not well with the Liver Qi. Take it as a warning and visit a practitioner. Clearing clots early on can prevent serious problems later, from endometriosis to cysts, fibroids, and even uterine and breast cancer.[1]

Oriental Medical Energetics

1) Stagnant Liver Qi and Blood

Liver Qi and Blood Stagnation cause the Blood to sit and congeal rather than flow out freely and smoothly. Dark clots are a result of Stagnant Liver Qi that lead to Liver Blood Stagnation. Ordinarily, fresh blood is a light, vivid red. Old blood that has been blocked and lying stagnant in the body will appear dark purple, or sometimes blackish, with thick clots.

Stagnant food in the Intestines due to overeating, stagnant Blood due to trauma, long-term Blood Deficiency, and Dampness can all impede Qi's flow. If you have had abdominal surgery, used an IUD, had an abortion, or are using birth control pills, you may develop a problem with Stagnant Liver Qi.

Signs of Qi Congestion and Liver Stagnation are a feeling of fullness or discomfort in the chest, belly, or head, agitation, anger, frustration, depression (anger turned inward), blood clots with the period discharge, premenstrual breast distention, irregular periods, and cramps at the beginning of the menstrual cycle.

Blood Stagnation pains are localized, stabbing, and sharp, and cramps are alleviated after the blood flows. Other signs are clots in the menstrual blood, varicose veins on the abdomen, hemorrhoids, lumps or masses, and painful intercourse with poking pain.

2) Stagnant Liver Blood combines with Cold

Stagnant Liver Blood can sometimes combine with Cold, when it then takes on a more purplish color and the body exhibits other Cold signs—a purplish or bluish tongue (which a practitioner is capable of distinguishing), and cramps that are relieved by warmth. A woman with this condition will have trouble conceiving because her uterus is also Cold.

Self-Help Strategies (for 1 and 2)

—Warm the body with warming and nourishing foods.
—Disperse Stagnant Liver Qi and Blood.
—Tone and relax the Liver.
—Activate the Qi.

Lingering Cycles

Oriental Medical Energetics

1) Kidney Yang or Jing Deficiency

Lack of Kidney Yang means the Kidney cannot regulate the reproductive function properly. Lingering cycles are the result of a Deficiency and can point to general weakness in the Kidneys. When Kidney Yang energy is Deficient, the lingering cycles may appear with lower back pain, often with a feeling of weakness or cold at the waist, a general feeling of cold, a lack of energy, withdrawal, dizziness, ringing in the ears, pallor, loose teeth, hair loss, anorexia, cold and aching knees, frequent or uncontrollable urination, urinary blockage, edema, diminished sex drive, amenorrhea, female infertility, or leukorrhea.

Self-Help Strategy

—Tone and nourish the Kidney Yang and the regenerative Jing energy.

2) Weak Spleen

Another possibility is that the Spleen is weak and unable to keep the Blood flowing in the vessels, resulting in excessive menstrual bleeding or spotting. If you suffer from digestive discomfort and are also an easy bruiser, this could be you.

Self-Help Strategy

—Concentrate on strengthening the Spleen.

Excessive Bleeding

Oriental Medical Energetics

Excessive bleeding during menstruation can be caused by an Excess or a Deficient condition.

1) Excess Heat in the Liver

An Excess Heat condition in the Liver, affecting the Blood, essentially works to push the Blood out of the body. This can be caused by overeating rich, greasy, oily, deep-fried foods or drinking too much alcohol. (Not everyone who eats a lot of deep-fried food or drinks alcohol will get this condition; it could become a problem if you are prone to this type of imbalance.)

Self-Help Strategies

—Subdue the Liver Fire.
—Tone the Liver, nurture Yin.

2) Spleen Deficiency

The other possibility, again, is Spleen Weakness, which renders the body unable to hold the Blood in the vessels. The imbalance results in excessive bleeding at first, followed by a lack of menstruation.

Self-Help Strategy

—Tone the Spleen.

Mood Swings: Irritability, Sudden Bursts of Anger, or Depression

Susan Lark, M.D., in the widely praised *PMS: Self-Help Book*, (see Recommended Reading in the Appendix) says that the most common type of PMS is characterized by anxiety, irritability, and mood swings. Symptoms worsen in the days prior to menstruation and are relieved only by its onset.

1) Stagnant Liver Qi

The syndrome is a classic case of Liver Qi Stagnation caused most often by excessive, prolonged stress. The stress causes blocks and obstructions in the Liver Qi, which then blocks the smooth flow of Blood. The blocked Blood flow further congests the Liver Qi. This vicious cycle affects the Liver organ and meridian in two ways. First, the Liver, being the organ most easily disturbed by excessive emotions, is the first to react when the body becomes overstressed. Second, functionally, the Liver is in charge of the smooth flow of Qi and Blood. When the Liver becomes imbalanced, the flow of Qi and Blood does so too. Anger is the emotion associated with the Liver. When the Liver Qi and Blood are blocked, this creates anger and irritability.

According to a leading Oriental medical gynecologist, Bob Flaws, "Their emotions come in fits and starts as the Qi first backs up behind the congestion and then vents when it accumulates sufficient pressure. Therefore, people with Liver Qi are by turns both irritable and morose."[2]

Self-Help Strategies

—Cleanse and tone the Liver.
—Activate the Liver Qi and Blood.
—Reduce stress.

Self-Help Guidelines

Primarily, women with PMS and period difficulties need to strengthen their digestive function, warm the body, tone the energy of the Stomach and Spleen, detoxify and tone the Liver, and activate Qi and Blood.

Internal Applications

• Reduce intake of iced or chilled foods or drinks, especially just prior to and during the menstrual cycle.

- Cut down on raw fruits and vegetables, salads, quantities of citrus fruits, soybeans and soybean products such as tofu (particularly served cold), millet, buckwheat, dairy products, sea vegetables, large intakes of liquid with meals, salt, and simple, refined sugars.
- Eat whole grains, but be careful that they are not undercooked.
- Eliminate excessively spicy foods and heavy red meat.
- Ice cream is particularly bad because of its high sugar content and cold, which weaken the digestive system. Dairy products in general increase the body's production of mucus and Phlegm. Many women report that eating ice cream before a menstrual cycle brings on more severe cramping than they would ordinarily experience.
- Try to avoid taxing the Liver with over-the-counter drugs, preservatives and food additives.
- Don't overeat.
- Do eat more warming foods that are easy to digest. Foods that tone the Spleen/Stomach are recommended (see Chapter 3 and the section Adapting to Stress and Building the Immune System).
- Typically, vegetarian diets don't include enough protein. Oriental medicine encourages the intake of small amounts of animal protein to strengthen the Blood and Qi. Organ meats are highly recommended dietary supplements but please see the Appendix for instructions for their proper preparation.
- Eat more foods to activate Qi in cases of Qi Stagnation (see Chapter 3).
- To activate Blood in cases of Blood Stagnation, eat well-cooked eggplant, amazake, saffron, basil, and chestnuts (whole or use the flour in cooking) along with the warming, Spleen-strengthening foods.
- To further nourish, clean, and build the Blood, incorporate wheatgrass, spirulina, chlorophyll, blackstrap molasses, di huang (rhemannia), dried and decocted longan fruit meats, dandelion, mugwort, and safflower into your daily diet. Sweet rice cakes (mochi), liver and kidney organ meat, congealed pork or cow's blood, and oyster are also recommended.
- To relax the Liver in cases of high stress to the organ or in one's life, try black sesame seed, cooked celery, kelp, liver organ meat, mulberry, mussel, nori, and plum.
- Dang gui is used to tonify the Blood, regulate menstruation, treat dysmenorrhea, and promote blood circulation, relieving pain caused by Stagnant Blood. It can be added to cooked foods or drunk as a tea with red dates, Chinese licorice, and peony root. Add about 3 grams of each to 3 cups distilled water in an earthenware pot. Bring to a boil, then simmer gently until the water is reduced by a third. Drink twice a day. Avoid taking dang gui during menstruation, the early stages of pregnancy, and if there is bloating and abdominal congestion.
- A dang gui broth can be used regularly in cooking. (See the Appendix for recipe.)
- Chicken is definitely indicated for its warming properties. Once, after several months of no period again, I went to China during the winter. There was no heat where I was staying and I woke up half frozen in the mornings. Besides a regular program of kung fu and qigong practice, my teacher had me eat chicken everyday, in soups, stews, and sometimes cooked in a medicinal herb cooker with dang gui, red dates, or an egg. Interestingly, my teacher, who ate everything I ate, broke out with acne after a week or so. When I asked him why, he explained that the chicken was creating too much heat in his body. I, on the other hand, had no other response but a cheerfully bright red, healthy menstrual cycle at the end of that month despite the cold weather.

• Black Chicken Pills, White Phoenix Pills, and Chicken Broth supplements are patent supplements indicated for Stagnant Liver Qi, period cramps, Yang and Blood Deficiency, and poor Blood circulation. They are sold at Oriental medicine pharmacies and can also be purchased by mail-order. See the Shopping information at the back of the book.

• Jasmine tea steeped with a teaspoon of thyme is believed to help calm jangled hormonally out-of-balance nerves. The smell is wonderfully delicate and soothing.

• Evening primrose, black currant seed, and borage oils are rich in GLA (gamma linoleic acid) and can help alleviate cramps. They can be taken as supplements (500 mg twice a day). But better than supplements, try to build these GLA-rich foods and oils into your diet: sunflower seed oil, corn oil, kidneys, brains, sweetbreads, lean meats, legumes, green vegetables, fish (especially oily fish such as herring and mackerel), fish liver and flaxseed oils. Choose cold-pressed oils—they haven't had their natural anti-oxidants removed in processing.

• **Drink Mood Swing Wine** (see recipe in the Appendix).

External Applications

• Freshly grated ginger compress is a commonly used and dependable pain reliever. Leave in place for 20 minutes. It also helps if you place a heating pad on your lower back. (See Chapter 4 for instructions on making a compress.)

Acupressure for cramps, moods swings
(See BodyMap for the exact location of points and explanations of abbreviations.)

SP. 6—Balances the Liver and Kidney energies, tones the lower Yin channels, invigorates the circulation of Qi and Blood, and is frequently used for female reproductive system difficulties. Use ginger and moxibustion or hard finger pressure.

G.V. 20—For irritability, press this point that lies at the very top of your head. Also "pulls up" the center, alleviates the "pulling down" sensation.

C.V. 12—Corrects the central Qi, warms and strengthens the Stomach/Spleen, tonifies the entire body. Press here upon exhalation.

SP. 9—Balances the Kidney and Liver energy. Press gently.

BL. 23—These are on either side of the spine. They stimulate and regulate the Kidney Yin and yang, so important in Oriental medicine for keeping the menstrual cycle regular. Use finger pressure or moxibustion.

BL. 17—Is the main point used to disperse Stagnant Blood. Use finger pressure or moxibustion.

Female Infertility

Female infertility is defined as the inability to conceive after a year or more of regular sexual intercourse during the time of ovulation. It is also the inability to carry a pregnancy to full term. In Western medicine it is said to be caused by hormonal imbalance.

In women, obstruction of the fallopian tubes may prevent the eggs from reaching the womb. Or a woman may not be producing viable eggs. Or there may be physical defects in the womb. Often the problem is more a matter of anxiety, timing, and technique. Japanese books on the subject usually carry illustrations depicting positions during intercourse that most frequently lead to pregnancy.

Peter tells the story of a couple of old friends who tried unsuccessfully to conceive a child for five years. When they finally decided to give up and adopt a child, the pressure to conceive was alleviated, and the wife became pregnant within one year. Their story is not unfamiliar.

Oriental Medical Energetics

Oriental medicinal practitioners find several different patterns of imbalance in infertile women.

1) Kidney Yin, Kidney Yang, or Jing Deficiency

The Kidneys house the Jing, the reproductive energy necessary to give new life. In addition, in order for a woman to become pregnant, the Yin and yang of the Kidneys must be balanced. Out of balance, there is often Blood Deficiency, because the Kidneys cannot supply enough Jing to produce Marrow, which produces bone marrow, and bone marrow produces Blood.

Self-Help Strategies

—Tonify Kidneys.
—Supplement Regenerative Qi (Jing).

2) Insufficient Blood

Insufficient Blood in a woman results in symptoms such as irregular menstrual bleeding, light bleeding, dysmenorrhea, or amenorrhea. Accompanying signs might be excess urination, urinating at night, lower back pain, knee pain, cold feet, dizziness and fatigue, dry skin, sallow complexion, blurred vision, and dry, lifeless hair.

Self-Help Strategy

—Tone and increase the Blood.

3) Irregular menstrual cycles or amenorrhea prevents conception.

In *Endometriosis & Infertility and Traditional Chinese Medicine: a Laywoman's Guide*, Flaws writes, "The entire diagnosis and treatment of infertility in traditional Chinese medicine is the extension of the basic belief that 'When the father's semen and the mother's blood contact each other, they unite and congeal to become the fetus in the womb.'"[3]

The regulation of Blood as well as normal menstrual cycles are considered the keys to becoming pregnant in Oriental medicine. If you follow the basic principles of treatment listed below, you may take giant steps toward becoming able to conceive. Please use them in conjunction with professional care.

Self-Help Strategy

—Strengthen the Stomach/Spleen function.

4) Liver Qi Stagnation

The Liver is intimately involved in the menstrual process. Its job is to store Blood. If the amount of Blood in the Liver is ample, menstruation will be normal. If Blood is deficient, infertility and amenorrhea may result. Liver and Blood are mutually dependent upon each other. Abnormality in the Blood will affect the Liver.

But another important Liver function is that it promotes the free flow of Qi. It is the Liver's responsibility to move the Qi throughout the body smoothly and harmoniously. Stagnant Qi in the body is usually viewed as a Liver condition. Symptoms pointing toward Stagnant Liver Qi are dull, colicky pain or cramps in the lower abdomen, premenstrual breast distention, abdominal bloating, menstrual cramping, irritability, tightness in the chest, and headaches.

The Liver is the organ most affected by emotional upsets, according to Oriental medicine. In turn, many emotional problems can be traced to Liver imbalance. The Qi becomes sluggish or blocked when we are under stress or feeling or repressing a lot of anger and frustration.

Self-Help Strategies

—Activate the Qi and Blood by reducing stress and releasing pent-up anger and frustration.
—Tonify the Liver.

5) A Cold Uterus does not create a conducive environment for conception.

A cold uterus, or Cold Stagnation, is another energetic imbalance that affects conception. In Oriental medicine, life is warmth. Cold in the uterus restricts the development of life and the flow of Qi and Blood. This condition is related to a Deficiency of Yang energy in the Kidneys or an Excess of Cold in the uterus. The latter can be caused by ingesting quantities of iced drinks and frozen foods or by becoming chilled during menstruation. Take necessary precautions to keep warm inside and out.

The signs of a Cold uterus are extended but scant menstrual discharge mixed with dark clots, dark menstrual blood, and lower abdominal pain relieved by warmth are major symptoms. If there is Yang Deficiency there will be signs of Kidney dysfunction as described above, also.

Self-Help Strategies

—Preserve the warmth of the uterus by cutting out all iced and cold drinks and food.
—Move the Qi.

6) The accumulation of Damp prevents the natural movements of fluids in the abdomen.

Damp Accumulation is another common problem that affects Western women's fertility. Often, women with this problem are overweight. In Oriental medicine, excessive fat tissue is said to be caused by a dysfunction of the Spleen, which is unable to properly carry out its function of transporting and transforming food. Incompletely metabolized food condenses to become Damp and Phlegm, which then impede the healthy flow of Blood and Qi. The heavy dampness flows downward, taking the form of swollen feet and legs, leukorrhea, frequent urination, loose, inconsistent stools sometimes mixed with mucus, lower body obesity, delayed, scanty menses or sometimes cessation of periods.

Self-Help Strategies

—Tonify the Spleen.
—Remove Damp and Phlegm.
—Move the Blood and Qi.

Internal Applications

• Avoid or reduce Cool and Cold foods, iced beverages, and foods that create Damp (see Chapter 3).

• To warm and protect Kidneys and supplement Jing: pork kidneys are a traditional and powerful method of strengthening the Kidneys (see under Food Influences in Chapter 3 for more Kidney-tonifying foods. See also the recipes for properly cleaning and preparing fresh kidney meats under How to Prepare Organ Meats in the Appendix.)

• Azuki and kidney beans are important source foods for Kidney support. Eat them weekly. Drink Azuki Bean Broth three times a day, a few days a week (see recipe in the Appendix). See also the recipe for Pumpkin and Azuki Bean Stew.

• Include foods in the diet that help clear Damp and Phlegm (See Food Influences in Chapter 3).

• Prepare and drink Liver-Toning-and-Restoring Tea (see recipe in the Appendix).

External Applications

Acupressure for Stagnant Liver Qi
(See the BodyMap for the exact location of points and the meaning of abbreviations.)

> LIV. 3—Calms the Liver, promotes the flow of Liver Qi, eases pain inside and under the ribs, and calms the mind.
>
> L.I. 4—Can be combined with the above to promote circulation of Qi and Blood to ease pain.
>
> BL. 18—Promotes correct function of the Liver, eases pain in ribs and sides, and calms the mind.
>
> LIV. 14—Calms the Liver, moves obstructions, and eases pain in ribs and breasts.
>
> C.V. 17—Influential point for Qi. Aids in circulating Qi in general, pain and congestion in chest, breast pain, and distention.
>
> P.C. 6—Calms the Shen, the energy housed in the Heart, relieves depression and melancholia, and eases congested sensation in chest.
>
> SP. 6—Corrects menstruation, relieves menstrual pain, and harmonizes the Spleen, Liver, and Kidney channels.

• In cases of Blood Stagnation, acupressure to the entire sacral area is helpful. If this is due to Cold, or if there is Cold involvement, use moxa.

• Cycle-Regulating Wine

The color of safflower is a warm, beautiful red-yellow but not many women know what to do with this herb besides making tea with it. Try this cycle-regulating wine.

> 50 g dried safflower
>
> 1 liter 45° alcohol
>
> 100 g granulated sugar
>
> 100 g honey

Add ingredients together, let sit for one month, add 10 more grams of safflower, let sit 10 more days and filter into another bottle. Drink a *sake* cupful (20 ml) in the afternoon and/or evening after meals.

External Applications

• Yoga, tai'chi, and qigong: If you encounter a great deal of stress, have perfectionist tendencies, or lead a lifestyle that leaves no breathing room—and are not getting pregnant despite your best efforts—consider signing up for a classes in qigong, tai'chi, yoga, meditation, or stress management immediately. You may need to trim your schedule to do so. If that's a problem, perhaps it is time to reset priorities.

Endometriosis

Oriental Medical Energetics

There is no diagnosis "endometriosis" in Oriental medicine. It is understood to be an accumulation of Blood in the uterus and ovaries.

1) Stagnant Liver Qi

According to Oriental medicine, the Liver Qi is believed to be responsible for the smooth flow of Blood in the body. Smooth flow of Liver Qi is critical to alleviating this condition.

2) Qi Deficiency

Another cause of accumulated Blood in the ovaries and uterus is Qi that is so weak it is unable to "lead" the Blood, resulting in Blood Stagnation and endometriosis.

3) Depleted Qi with Weakened Liver Qi

The frequency of endometriosis seems to be related to modern women's busy, stressful lifestyles. High-pressure work situations and overwork deplete the body's store of Qi. Women's sense that they have to perform twice as well as men in the workplace to get anywhere also weakens Liver Qi.

Self-Help Strategies

—Relax.
—Make dietary changes to unblock Stagnant Liver Qi and tonify the Liver.
—Exercise to activate a sluggish metabolism.
—Regularize sleeping, eating, work, and rest habits.

Internal Applications

• Most importantly, avoid the regular or excessive intake of iced, chilled, and raw foods, drinks, fruits, and vegetables.
• Avoid excessive quantities of liquids, sugar, honey, molasses, maple syrup, and malt syrup, all of which cause Dampness and weaken the Spleen. They also weaken the body's capacity for creating Qi and Blood. The *Nei Jing*, a classic of Oriental medicine, says that that sweet flavor relaxes the Liver, and people with Liver Qi Congestion crave sugar. But when this craving is indulged, the difficulties are compounded.
• Nuts, oils, fats, chocolate, beef and pork, dairy products, eggs, citrus fruits, pineapple, apples and pears, salt, all hardened fats, fried foods, junk food, fast foods, coffee, and alcohol all exacerbate the problem.
• Caffeinated beverages—coffee, tea, and cola—and decaffeinated coffee are believed to be cooling to the body, and the negative effects of caffeine's volatile oils have been well documented in other publications. Women with a Liver Qi Stagnation problem, which is to say

anyone with menstruation difficulties, who is pregnant, or going through menopause, should try to cut down on caffeine.

• The basic Middle Burner warming diet of whole grains, legumes, small amounts of meat (particularly organ meats), fish and chicken, steamed and lightly cooked vegetables is indicated (see the Middle Burner warming suggestions under Food Influences in Chapter 3).

• Regularity is another element of life that many women have a hard time controlling. Its disappearance creeps up on us as easily as a few extra pounds and reintegrating regularity into our lives can be just as hard as taking those pounds off. Sensitive bodies do not function optimally without regular times for sleeping and eating. Of course women with babies and young children cannot help odd sleeping patterns. Try to do the best you can.

The rest of us can aim for regularity. Begin by writing out an ideal schedule, leaving room for time out in the day, that half hour of lost time in the morning before tea or your afternoon walk. Then put your schedule into practice. Allow yourself slips, but resolve to stay on track the next day.

If endometriosis is the problem, take a rest from sexual intercourse and strenuous exercise during your flow. Both can adversely affect the path of Qi and Blood. Sometimes it is suggested that women avoid sex during menstruation due to the belief that it reverses the flow of Qi and Blood from down and out to up and in, causing the formation of Stagnant Blood.

• Aerobic exercise is needed to clear up a sluggish metabolism, increase the production of Qi and Blood, and clear out stagnation and congestion. Begin with 20 minutes a day. This will greatly reduce the severity of symptoms related to Stagnant Qi and Blood.

• Relax. It is so important to the healthy functioning of the reproductive system. Many women's bodies register high levels of stress by locking up, blocking up, and filling up. Bodies like this deserve some consideration and a balancing break.

Leukorrhea

Oriental Medical Energetics

Oriental medicine categorizes two types of vaginal discharge. One is an inner Heat condition merged with Damp to produce the fluid. The other is a Cold Damp condition.

1) Damp Heat in the lower abdomen

A Damp Heat condition is signaled by a yellow discharge that is usually thick and sticky. It is sometimes accompanied by a stinging sensation, a strong odor, heavy period, and excessive bleeding.

Self-Help Strategies

—Clear Heat.
—Drain Damp.

2) Weak Spleen is not processing fluids correctly.

The Cold Damp condition, on the other hand, often results in the Spleen's inability to process fluids correctly, producing Dampness in the Spleen and Water Stagnation in the Stomach (conditions called Deficient Spleen Qi, Stagnant Blood, or an impaired Middle Burner). This, in turn, results in a clear or white odorless discharge; the menstrual blood tends to contain dark clots. Accompanying symptoms may include indigestion, weak appetite, fatigue or becoming easily tired, nausea, chronic diarrhea or watery stools, anorexia, headaches, fullness in the chest, watery skin eruptions, inflammation, trouble with the uterine lining, difficult pregnancy, liver problems, and hemorrhoids.

Self-Help Strategies

—Avoid foods that cool digestive Fire.
—Tonify the Spleen and Middle Burner.

Internal Applications

• In the first case, avoid foods that increase Heat and Fluid (see Chapter 3).
• Eat more foods that are cooling and assist Yin (see Chapter 3).
• Eat foods that assist Damp drainage (see under Food Influences in Chapter 3).
• In the second case, avoid Cool, Cold, and Damp foods (see Chapter 3).
• Eat warming foods that assist Yang (see Chapter 3).
• Foods that drain excess Damp are also recommended (see Chapter 3).

Yeast Infection, *Candida Albicans*, and Vaginitis

Vaginitis is defined as an increased volume of vaginal secretions of abnormal color or odor, accompanied by vulva and/or vaginal itching, burning or irritation, and sometimes burning urination. This is one of the most common reasons women visit a gynecologist. When there is painful urination present, a woman may think she has a urinary tract infection when the problem is, in Western terms, vaginitis. A urinary tract infection is painful inside while in this case urine passing over the inflamed labia causes the pain.

Oriental Medical Energetics

Damp in the lower abdomen

The discharges, unusual odor, and itching usually result from Stagnation in the Large and Small Intestine systems or Stomach/Spleen Disharmony leading to a Deficiency of Spleen Qi. Either case leads to an accumulation of Damp that moves down into the lower abdomen.

Acupuncture can successfully treat both conditions, aided by dietary therapy. Often people suffering from disharmony in the Spleen crave sweets; try extra hard to resist temptation while seeking treatment.

Self-Help Strategies

—Strengthen the Spleen Qi.
—Clear the Large and Small Intestines.
—Clear Damp.

Internal Applications

• Avoid Damp-producing foods (see Chapter 3), particularly peanuts and pineapple.
• Foods for Damp/Spleen complications: beet, black sesame, Chinese salted black soybeans, capers, dried ginger, Job's tears, turnips, mulberry, and pine nut.

• Whole grains, fresh, lightly steamed vegetables, some fruit, and legumes will help clear the Large and Small Intestines.

Fibroids and Cysts

Oriental Medical Energetics

1) Stagnant Qi and Blood

Fibroids and cysts are understood as symptoms of Stagnant Qi and Blood. This can be caused from Qi Congestion, leading to pain in the lower abdomen, dysmenorrhea, and infertility. Stress is the main cause of Qi congestion, involving the Liver and preventing the free flow of Qi. A prolonged stasis of Blood can give rise to masses or lumps—cysts and tumors in Western medical terms. Uterine fibroids, uterine hemorrhage with large clots, irregular, scanty, or suppressed menstruation, cervical dysplasia, or ovarian cysts and tumors develop when this Blood becomes congealed.

The patterns listed here are only some of the more common causes of cysts and fibroids. If you have this condition or suspect you might, see a practitioner immediately. Oriental medicine can be extremely helpful in finding a solution. (See also the section Dark Clots in Menstrual Blood, above.)

2) Excessive Cold

An Excess of Cold can also congeal Qi and Blood, causing it to stagnant in the uterus or pelvis. The cold may be from internal sources, such as ingesting quantities of cold drinks and salads, or may be due to a cold environment. Symptoms include cold, fixed pain in the lower abdomen relieved by warmth; dark, clotty menstrual blood, aversion to cold, late or absent menstrual period, lumps or masses, leukorrhea, lower back pain, soreness in the knees, tinnitus, frequent urination, and urinating at night.

3) Weak Kidney Yang

Weak Kidney Yang from congenital weakness, prolonged illness, extreme fatigue, sexual exhaustion, recreational drugs, or aging results in Cold in Spleen, Conception, Governor, and Penetrating Vessels (one of a group of eight energy channels beyond the meridians and organ networks covered in this book, the Penetrating Vessel—Chong Mai—is an energy channel that connects to the uterus and is very much involved in menstruation, fertility, and pregnancy).

Self-Help Strategies

—Reduce stress.
—Decongest Qi.
—Unblock Stagnant Blood.
—Warm the body. Strengthen the Spleen/Stomach function.
—Tonify Kidneys if Kidney imbalance signs are present.
—Exercise.
—See a practitioner.

• Women's Strengthening Brew
    150 g dang gui

50 g red dates
50 g lycium berries
50 g Chinese licorice
1 liter 45° alcohol
100 g honey
50 ml mirin

Add ingredients to $1^1/_2$ cups water in an earthenware pot or a Chinese herb cooker, and simmer to reduce water by one-third. Drink the warm, light-brown-colored preparation twice a day before or between meals to increase and revitalize Blood, regulate menstruation, support the function of the uterus, alleviate insomnia, anxiety, nervous energy, and light constipation, and supplement the body's warmth. Save the herbs and cook them again the next day.

Menopause

The Chinese call it the "third age" in a woman's life: what, exactly, is menopause? It can mean different things to different women (and men and families). For some women, it is a process that begins in midlife and is said to continue through their early 60s. For others, it is the symptoms: the night sweats and hot flashes, the mood swings and tearful afternoons that they go through as hormonal levels decrease.

Technically, menopause is a woman's last menstrual period. The ovaries gradually produce less estrogen, eventually dropping to such low levels that menstruation ceases altogether. About 80% of women experience menopausal symptoms, including irregular heavy bleeding, hot flashes, vaginal and urinary tract changes, psychological symptoms such as insomnia, irritability, anxiety, and depression. Dry eyes and visual disturbances, joint pain, and changes in libido may also occur. Osteoporosis is one of the most severe health problems that can occur after menopause.

Beyond menopause, there are other age-related changes that become more common in women after the menopause years. An increasing occurrence of breast, cervical, and uterine cancer, hypothyroidism, skin changes, and cardiovascular disease all seem to be somewhat related to the loss of hormonal support due to menopause.

A woman's change can proceed smoothly, but for those who feel stuck in mid-process, there are ways to treat yourself and find help to significantly alleviate difficult symptoms.

Internal Applications

• Avoid high-stress foods such as sugar, coffee, fat, and alcohol, which can exacerbate menopause symptoms.
• Cold, frozen drinks and raw food aggravate menopause symptoms.
• Although dairy foods are recommended as good sources of calcium, they create a condition of Damp in the body and promote the production of mucus; reduce or eliminate them from the diet. Better calcium-rich foods include asparagus, blackstrap molasses, broccoli, green leafy vegetables, oats, salmon, and tofu.
• Women who are pre-, during-, or post-menopausal, according to traditional Oriental medical theory, can often be helped by supporting or strengthening the Stomach/Spleen meridians and organ. When the Stomach and Spleen are healthy, the body has plenty of Qi,

regenerative energy (Jing), and Blood. This promotes the health of the Kidneys, the Heart, Liver, and Lungs.

• It is important to nourish the Kidneys, the House of Jing. Jing produces the matrix, Marrow, out of which the bones are formed. (see Chapter 3).

• Warming spices and seasonings in moderation can encourage the Stomach and Spleen: ginger, garlic, cardamom, nutmeg, and cinnamon.

• Why are cooked, warm foods better for a woman around the age of menopause? First, cooked foods are easier to digest, since they are in a sense predigested. If the Stomach breaks down food using less energy, it is able to absorb nutrients more efficiently. Raw foods require the Stomach to work harder. Light steaming or stir-frying is recommended; most of the nutrients remain intact while the Stomach function is aided. When the Stomach does its job efficiently, food moves on to the Spleen, in charge of the transformation and distribution of foods, which can then carry out its work smoothly as well. Cooked foods warm the body and prevent stagnation of energy. Eating the foods recommended here is good for the waistline, preventing an accumulation of stagnating Damp (read "fat") and promoting a trim, vital body.

• Eat foods rich in vitamin A; they can help protect against cervical and breast cancer. Supplements can be toxic over 20,000 I.U. a day. We believe it is safer and healthier to ingest foods containing vitamin A daily. Leafy greens—dandelion leaves, collard, and beet greens—can help protect against osteoporosis and excessive menstrual bleeding. Eat fruit sparingly, nuts and seeds in raw form (not roasted and salted), and purchase lean cuts of red meat from organically fed animals, trimming off all excess fat before cooking. Stay away from high-sodium cold cuts.

• Oils should be unsaturated: flax, sesame seed, corn, canola, safflower; or polyunsaturated: olive oil. Cold-pressed oils are purer and fresher. Wheat germ, soybean, and corn oils are excellent sources of vitamin E. Vitamin E has long been known to have important health benefits for the female reproductive tract. It has been shown to control hot flashes and heal the vagina and urinary tract, which can become dry and prone to infection after menopause.

• Menopausal women can benefit from Oriental medicine herbal treatment from a qualified practitioner. There are many herbal formulas to alleviate menopausal symptoms which, because they are prescribed for every woman individually, require a professional diagnosis to dispense.

• Adequate rest and an exercise program are also important. Exercise is vital to keeping bones strong and muscles firm. Light running and weight lifting are recommended, balanced with some strengthening and relaxing yoga or tai'chi. Peter adds that women can prepare for menopause best by exercising and taking care of their diets while still in the 20s and 30s. By taking care of ourselves now, we can make the symptoms and side effects that accompany the transition into menopause less apparent and uncomfortable.

Recipe[4]: Chicken Liver and Kohlrabi with Dates & Cinnamon

This dish is for toning and unblocking Stagnant Liver Qi. The chicken liver is Sweet and Warm, tonifies Qi and Blood, removes Blood Stagnation, expels Cold, sedates Yin, and is toning to the Liver and the Kidney.

Kohlrabi is Pungent, Sweet/Bitter, assists Yang, benefits Qi, tones Qi and Blood, dries Damp, and removes Stagnant Blood. Don't overeat it and do not eat if you have skin eruptions. Instead, use a more cooling leaf, like spinach.

(Serves 2)

> 10 Chinese red dates
> 10 g Chinese cinnamon

> 500 g liver
> salt & pepper
> 1 large red bell pepper
> $^1/_2$ bunch kohlrabi (or other green leafy vegetables)
> oil, and *sake* (or white wine), garlic, and ginger for frying

To prepare:

1. Wash and soak the dates.
2. Add dates and cinnamon to 2 c water and cook over low heat until the cinnamon softens. Add water as necessary until the consistency becomes fairly thick, as for sauce.
3. Slice the liver into $^1/_2$-inch-thick slices, and sprinkle with salt and pepper,
4. Slice red pepper into thin rings or lengthwise. Cut the stems from the kohlrabi and wash the leaves.
5. Fry the liver with a splash of *sake*, garlic, and ginger until cooked through.
6. Clean the pan, then quickly stir-fry the peppers and greens; add a small amount of water while cooking, and *sake*, garlic, and ginger to taste.
7. Cover the liver with the peppers and sauce; the greens can go to the side.

Recipe[4]: Lemon Sesame Eggplant with Shrimp

Eggplant builds and strengthens Blood, tones Qi, clears Heat, sedates Yang, removes Stagnant Blood, relieves pain, and heals swelling.

Shrimp is sweet and Yang, assists and tones Yang, tones Qi and Blood, benefits Qi, removes Blood Stagnation, expels Cold, and promotes lactation.

(Serves 4)

> 16 shrimp
> 2 tbsp. *sake*
> salt
> 1 tbsp. cornstarch
> 8 Japanese-style eggplants or two medium-sized American eggplants*

> 1 red or green bell pepper

> $^1/_2$ tsp. Sichuan peppercorns (sanshō)
> $1^1/_2$ tbsp. sesame oil
> juice of 1 freshly squeezed lemon
> 2 tbsp. soy sauce
> grated ginger

*If using American eggplants, cut, salt, and set aside for ten minutes, then rinse and use.

To prepare:

1. Clean, remove the shells and veins, and slice shrimp in half down the center length-wise. Marinate in *sake*, a dash of salt and 1 tbsp. cornstarch for 20 minutes. Then add to boiling water and cook until they change color. Drain and set aside.
2. Wash eggplants, remove the tops, cut in half lengthwise, then slice 3 or 4 times. Wash and dry pepper, remove the seeds, slice lengthwise.
3. Steam or stir-fry vegetables (women with Cold conditions and Blood Stagnation should be careful to eat eggplant well cooked but not overcooked, so the eggplant skins retain their color). Add peppers after the eggplants.
4. To make the sauce, crush or powder the peppercorns and add to a frying pan with 1$^1/_2$ tbsp. sesame seed oil, the juice of a whole lemon, and 2 tbsp. soy sauce. Cook over medium-low heat, being careful not to scorch the spices. Once they give off a fragrance, turn off the heat and add the grated ginger.
5. Place eggplant and peppers on round platter, add shrimp in the center, like an island, pour the sauce over and serve.

Recipe[4]: 8 Treasure Liver

Tones and activates Liver Qi and Qi in general.

(Serves 4)

3 g dang gui
3 g star anise
3 g dried orange peel
2 g Chinese licorice
3 g nutmeg
10 g Chinese cinnamon
3 g cloves

500 g chicken liver
1-inch piece ginger
2 cloves garlic
1 leek
2 cups herbal broth
4 tbsp. canola oil
1 tbsp. soy sauce
4 eggs
2 bunches yellow or green Chinese chives, or green garlic stems (if using garlic stems eliminate regular garlic from the recipe)
1 tbsp. *sake*
1 tbsp. mirin (if not using mirin, add 1 tsp. honey or a natural sweetener)
oil for wok
salt

To prepare:
1. Coat the liver well on both sides with salt and let sit covered overnight in the refrigerator. Rinse well before using. Cut into bite-sized portions. Slice the chives or garlic stems into inch-long pieces and set aside.
2. Place the first 7 spices in a handkerchief, tie the ends together, and add to 3 cups of water. Cook for 20 minutes.
3. Slice ginger and garlic, add to oil, and fry on medium-low heat for a minute. Then add soy sauce, leek, and liver. Cook over high heat for 1–2 minutes until thoroughly cooked. Add 2 cups herbal broth, along with the spice bag, and cook on medium heat. Add more water to the mixture as water evaporates.
4. When the water has fully evaporated, set the liver aside and wash the wok.
5. Add canola oil to wok, scramble eggs, set aside.
6. To cook the chives or garlic stems, add a little more oil, and a dash of salt. Add the greens, *sake*, and mirin, and stir-fry rapidly over high heat. While the greens are still softening but still quite bright in color, add liver and eggs. Continue to cook on high heat, stirring constantly for 1 minute. Serve immediately.

Endnotes

*1 Bob Flaws, *Endometriosis & Infertility and Traditional Chinese Medicine: a Laywoman's Guide*, Blue Poppy Press, Boulder, 1989; p. 60.
*2 Ibid, p.60.
*3 Ibid, p. 63.
*4 Note: Some of the recipes in this chapter include a few of the foods women have been advised to avoid. This section includes suggestions that should be used as guidelines but they are not hard-and-fast rules and should not be taken to excess. Cooling foods, for example, lend balance to the recipes where they appear. They can be eaten, but don't overdo it. Make sure to eat them warm and well cooked.

Hair

Nearly all practitioners agree: hair is a very clear barometer of general health. A measurement of essential trace elements and minerals, and the presence of excess toxic minerals, can be established through a process growing increasingly common in the West—hair analysis.

There are a number of common problems affecting the hair and scalp. Greasy hair is related to overactivity of the sebaceous glands. Dry, brittle hair occurs when these glands are underactive. Dandruff is the shedding of the skin of the scalp: dry, white flakes are produced when there is too little sebum, and yellowish, oily, sticky flakes are a result of too much sebum.

Oriental Medical Energetics

Disharmony in the Kidney, Lung, or Large Intestine

According to Oriental medicine practitioners, imbalance in one of the body's excretory systems—the Kidneys, Large Intestine, and the Lungs—is reflected in the condition of the hair on the head. Healthy Kidneys are essential to luxuriant, healthy hair. Thinning hair, except when due to hereditary baldness, may be related to Kidney problems. Too much sugar weakens the Kidneys and contributes to baldness.

The Lungs are associated with hair quality. Dry, brittle, lusterless hair may be a sign of Lung problems. But it may also be a sign of excessive cosmetic procedures applied to the hair. Bleaching, blow-drying, permanents, straightening, heated rollers, and curling irons are all irritants and can all cause dermatitis. Try to stay away from harsh shampoos and perfumed hair products. Environmentally and people-friendly hair-care products can be purchased at many health food stores. There is really no excuse for using harsh chemicals on hair anymore.

Self-Help Strategies

—Scalp and hair problems, like skin problems, can be effectively treated through dietary changes.

Internal Applications

• Avoid refined carbohydrates, dairy products, animal fats, and fried, greasy foods. These foods are notorious for clogging the digestive system. The skin and scalp are the body's secondary excretion outlets, so what the body cannot excrete through the digestive system will try to exit through the sebaceous glands.

Macrobiotic theory maintains that the intestines and the hair are connected, reflected in the structural similarity between the hair-like intestinal villi and the hair on the head. When the villi become coated with fats, the rate of absorption of saturated fats is reduced, resulting in release through the skin and scalp. Eating dinner immediately before bed exacerbates hair problems.

• For healthy hair, to restore graying hair to its regular color if caused by lack of nutrition or stress, and to retard hair loss, eat more cooked egg yolks, fresh fruits and vegetables, meat, poultry, soybeans and soybean products, whole grains, and yeast. These foods contain inositol and biotin, two vitamins necessary for healthy hair. They also help keep the digestion and elimination systems running smoothly.

• Sesame seeds, particularly black ones (commonly found in Oriental food shops), were recommended by the sages of old as a cure for baldness.

• For hair problems, stick to brown rice, eat quantities of hair-strengthening hijiki, kombu, nori, and black sesame, and chew your food well, advises Yuriko Tōjō, a well known macrobiotic and nutritionist in Japan.

• Scalp problems can be treated by ingesting unsaturated fatty acids contained in evening primrose or linseed oil. For brittle, dry hair, also try adding black currant oil or salmon oil to the diet. Follow dosages listed on the bottles.

• Daily intake of the herb ho shou wu (*Polygoni Multiflori Radix*) as a decoction (5 g to $1^{1}/_{2}$ c water) with lycium berries (5 g) and du zhong (3 g) or as a wine tonic made with the herb is said to restore hair to its natural color.

External Applications

• Remember that topical applications do not solve the problem but treat only the symptoms.

• Again, for balding and thinning hair, mix a warm decoction of ginger with sesame seed or camellia oil, cover the problem spots of the hair with the mixture, massage in well and wrap the head with a towel for a few minutes while the herbs stimulate and nourish the scalp. This can be shampooed out with a very gentle cleanser.

• For dandruff, rub aloe vera gel onto the scalp.

• Peter experienced the pleasant side effect of having his graying hair turn darker gradually after practicing his daily qigong and a set of Tibetan exercises called *The Five Rites* over a period of a few months. See Recommended Reading in the Appendix for more information.

Balding and Hair Loss

Hair loss can occur as the result of poor circulation, acute illness, surgery, radiation, skin disease, sudden weight loss, iron deficiency, diabetes, thyroid disease, drugs such as those used in chemotherapy, stress, poor diet, vitamin deficiency, and pregnancy. Peter has noticed that hair loss often occurs more frequently when the season changes. Male hair loss may be due to heredity, hormones, and aging. Most women lose some hair two or three months after childbirth due to hormonal changes during pregnancy that prevented hair loss.

Internal Applications
• Biotin, necessary for healthy cell growth and hair, is found naturally in cooked egg yolk, salt-water fish, meat, milk, poultry, soybeans, whole grains, and yeast. It is thought that biotin can deter hair loss in some men. Shampoos containing biotin are available at health food stores. It also promotes healthy sweat glands, nerve tissue, and bone marrow. A dry, scaly scalp or face in infants may indicate deficiency. Saccharin inhibits biotin absorption.
• Macrobiotics views hair loss as a symptom of an imbalance in the Liver organ and meridian. Naboru Muramoto, in *Healing Ourselves*, suggests avoiding alcohol, vinegar (other experts allow ume (plum) vinegar), chemicals, drugs, sugar, and large amounts of red meat, fried foods, and oil. Instead, eat more sea vegetables such as hijiki, wakame and kombu. Beans, particularly white broad beans, lima beans, and navy beans are good for Liver and contain less oil than other types of Liver-nourishing legumes, he adds.

External Applications
• It is also important to stimulate the scalp when you are losing hair. Lie down on a slant board for 15 minutes or learn to do a headstand properly in a yoga class and practice regularly to allow the blood to reach the scalp. (A headstand can be dangerous without adequate instruction.) Massage your scalp daily.
• Use commercial shampoos and conditioners with care. Allergic reactions to these products occur frequently. If you are not sure why you are losing hair, it might be a good idea to simply switch to a natural product purchased at your local natural foods store just in case.

Headaches

Headaches come in a number of varieties. Before reaching for your bottle of aspirin, try categorizing your headache to determine which type of self-help might be appropriate (and more healthful than a couple of aspirin) for you.

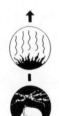

Oriental Medical Energetics

1) Liver Yang Rising

In Oriental medicine, a headache is often understood to be the result of Liver Yang (Fire) energy rising and becoming trapped in the head. The result is the pounding-head sensation typical of many headaches, along with a stiff neck and shoulders, possibly a red face or, more often, eyes. This type of headache is associated with anger.

Self-Help Strategies

—Cool the Fire.
—Take measures to reduce stress.
—See a practitioner for an expert diagnosis.

2) Blockage in the Stomach or Large Intestine systems

Different parts of the head are related to different organs and meridian systems in Oriental medicine. A headache in the forehead, sinus, and eye area indicates problems with the Stomach and Large Intestine channels, which run through these areas. The headache might be accompanied by chronic constipation and a blocked nose.

Self-Help Strategies

—Clear the Stomach and Large Intestine organ systems.
—Reduce stress levels where appropriate.

Internal Applications

• Avoid foods that clog or congest the Stomach/Spleen or the Lung/Large Intestine channels (see Chapter 3).

• Try not to overeat. This causes great stress to both the Stomach/Spleen systems and the Liver.

• Do try to incorporate more reasonably easy-to-digest whole foods that do not remain in the stomach or intestines for prolonged amounts of time.

• Also eat more foods with fiber and bulk that clear out the intestines.

External Applications

Acupressure for headaches

• For immediate relief, try applying acupressure by pressing and rubbing the following points with circular motions (see the BodyMap for exact location of points and meanings of abbreviations):

> Yin Tang/Indō—Rubbing the Third Eye, the point which lies right between the eyebrows, gives immediate headache relief.
> L.I. 4—Activates and disperses blocks of Qi in the entire body. It may be tender. Rub and press.
> ST. 36—Tonifies the whole body. Press and rub.
> T.H. 5—Clears Heat in head for red eyes, particularly recommended for migraine.

3) Blockage in the Gallbladder and/or Triple Heater meridian systems

Pain in the temple can be one-sided, as in the case of a migraine. This indicates trouble in the Gallbladder and Triple Heater channels. The Triple Heater has no corresponding visceral organ, yet it exists as a channel running into the temple area. It regulates the metabolism and the distribution of body fluids other than Blood.

Self-Help Strategies

—See a practitioner for acupuncture treatment, which can easily release a block in these channels.

—For immediate relief, try the following acupressure points:

• **Acupressure for a one-sided headache**
(See the BodyMap for the exact location of points and meanings of abbreviations.)

> L.I. 4—Activates Qi and Blood in entire body. Clears obstructions.
> Tai Yang—The temple depression. Press lightly with the thumbs and rotate.
> T.H. 5—Massage the point to clear Heat from the eyes and head; alleviates migraine headache.
> G.B. 43—A distal point, it is found by going down to the feet, to between the fourth and little toes; the point is between the two tendons where the toes begin to join. It may be quite tender; press and rub gently to relieve pain.

4) Tai Yang imbalance

Occipital pain, or pain at the base of the skull, is called a Tai Yang headache and could be the harbinger of a cold. This is a tested and true belief, as far as the authors are concerned. The headache is related to the Bladder and Small Intestine.

Self-Help Strategy

—Keep warm, drink warming drinks such as ginger tea, and go to bed.

External Applications
• Grate a daikon radish, wring out the juice, soak a clean cotton cloth in the juice, and hold it to the nostrils. This helps alleviate headache.

Acupressure for Tai Yang headache
(See the BodyMap for exact location of points and an explanation of abbreviations.)

BL. 10—Rub here for several minutes to relieve neck and shoulder pain and a Tai Yang headache.

BL. 60—Rub here to remove Qi blockages in the Bladder channel.

S.I. 3—The "Rear Ravine" of the Small Intestine channel can also be employed to alleviate headache.

The Heart and Circulation Problems

Heart disease is one of the most debated topics in Western medicine, as well it should be: it is still the single largest factor in premature death in the Western world. As the Japanese diet and lifestyle continue to incorporate increasingly more Western influences, the problem will likely become a major health issue sooner or later there, too.

The Heart in Oriental Medicine

The Heart is considered the ruler of the body in Oriental medical theory. It is the captain of the ship, aware of every movement, turn, response, and change in the body/mind. The Heart is represented by the element Fire. It is the body's center of wholeness. As the place where we exist in our most fully developed, integrated state, the Heart is the point from which we radiate the essence of who we are and who we are becoming.

The Heart is the seat of consciousness. The concept "Heart" is rendered with a character representing the heart *and* the mind in the Chinese language, signifying a lack of boundary between them. Mental activity as well as emotional experience are thought to take place in the Heart. The Heart holds awareness, the Shen, also described as the body's spiritual energy. The Heart organ and meridian channel affect consciousness and a person's responses to the world. Disturbed Shen results in unclear thinking, insomnia, a tendency to withdraw, mania, anxiety attacks, and a craving for drugs or alcohol. Prolonged emotional imbalance, conversely, can lead to a disharmony of Shen.

Disturbed Shen

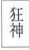

KUÁNG SHÉN
KI SHIN

The Heart controls circulation, blood vessels, and "body communication" in general. It manifests in the complexion. A person with a healthy glow about them has good circulation, while a pale, sallow, bluish complexion indicates a problem. Excess Heat in the body turns the complexion reddish.

The Heart also controls the tongue. Speech abnormalities are looked upon as Heart meridian system imbalance. A crack down the center of the tongue indicates congenital heart problems.

Oriental medicine can treat various disorders involving the Heart/heart. Following are a few typical patterns of Heart imbalances to give the reader an idea of the types of problems "Heart imbalance"—as the cause of illness in Oriental medicine—encompasses.

Hypoglycemia

Oriental Medical Energetics

Hypoglycemia is a relatively new term in the chronicles of Western allopathy but the syndrome has been a standard diagnosis in Oriental medicine for centuries. Low blood sugar, as we call it in the West, is understood as a deficiency in the Kidney or the Stomach/Spleen meridian systems, often involving a Liver Blood Deficiency as well.

1) Depleted digestive system

Worrying, improper diet, and overextension deplete the energies of the Spleen/Stomach functions of transformation and transportation of nutrients. Accompanying symptoms include abdominal pain, fatigue, nausea, and coldness in the limbs.

Self-Help Strategies

—Implement regular eating habits and nourish the Stomach/Spleen.
—Reduce worry and stress levels.
—Rest and try to work less.
—Smile more. Find ways to infuse life with humor and a sense of well-being.

2) Lack of Kidney Yang

Overwork or excessive sexual activity can deplete the Kidney Yang, resulting in a lack of energy, hair loss, loose teeth, a weak or chilled feeling at the waist, lower back pain, cold and aching knees, loose stool, frequent urination, and a diminished sex drive.

Self-Help Strategies

—Tone the Kidney Yang.
—Relax more, reduce stress levels.

3) Depletion of Liver Blood

Grinding the body down when it is already run-down results in serious depletion. Hemorrhage, chronic illness, worry, working while fatigued, and overusing the eyes depletes the stores of Blood in the Liver, resulting in blurred or failing vision, dry eyes, irritability, being easily startled, insomnia, pale lips and complexion, numbness in the limbs, light menstrual flow or amenorrhea and/or late menses, anemia, and hypotension.

Self-Help Strategies

—Tone and strengthen the Blood.
—Reduce worry, anxiety, and overwork.
—See a practitioner; moxibustion, acupuncture, and herbs are appropriate treatment.

Internal Applications

• Foods that aggravate the Spleen/Stomach should be drastically reduced or avoided altogether: alcohol, caffeinated beverages, cold and iced foods and drinks; greasy, oily, fatty foods.

• Also reduce foods that aggravate the Kidneys: same as above, plus chocolate and citrus.

• Avoid foods that aggravate the Liver: same as above, plus chemicals such as preservatives and food additives, over-the-counter drugs, and overeating.

• Begin to eat a warming diet that nourishes the Spleen and Stomach (see Food Influences in Chapter 3). And try the recipe for Anti-hypoglycemic Stew at the end of the chapter.

• Eat Blood-strengthening and -building foods (see Food Influences in Chapter 3).

• Eat Kidney Yang and Liver toners (see Chapter 3).

• To best treat the dizziness, weakness, sweating, and fainting that some people with this condition suffer from, reschedule meals to make several smaller ones throughout the day. This pattern of eating requires much less energy for digestion and keeps a constant supply of energy moving through the body from the food.

• Eat complex carbohydrates and soft-cooked grains. Whole-grain noodles and pastas are fine. These types of carbohydrates provide a much more dependable, sustained source of energy that won't result in sudden lows.

• Bancha tea with the meats of the umeboshi plum helps activate digestion and elimination.

• Try Saffron Wine, Essential Egg Oil, and the Four Things Vegetable Soup to build and tone the Blood and Qi (see the Appendix).

External Applications

• Ginger compresses on the lower abdomen and over the kidneys will warm and energize the body, stimulate the Kidney energy, and activate Qi.

• Take frequent ginger or daikon-radish-leaf hip baths.

• Light the body's "wick" by applying a ginger or salt-ring moxibustion treatment to the bellybutton. Moxa and acupressure are also good for SP. 6 and ST. 36. (See the BodyMap for location of points.)

• Try this self-massage technique to relieve excessive cravings for sweets:

—Sit comfortably.

—The left hand presses the point at the top of the inner side of the shoulder blade, 1 to 2 inches to the side of the spine. The point lies between the shoulder blade and the spine. This area may feel firm and resistant. The right hand presses the same point on the right side. Hold both, with pressure as hard as you can apply, for 3 minutes.

—Move the hands to the points at the top of the shoulder where the neck and shoulder meet. Press here on both sides for 3 minutes.

—Move the hands up the neck halfway so the fingers sit on the muscle next to the spine and press.

—Move the hands up to the base of the skull. Thumbs press the sensitive points 1 to 2 inches out from the spine.

Cardiovascular Disease

Hypertension

Hypertension has been called the "silent disorder" because the high pressure of blood pumping through the blood vessels has almost no symptoms. Silent, but deadly: it can eventually lead to a hardening of the arteries (arteriosclerosis or atherosclerosis) and heart attack. Early detection and proper treatment, however, can eliminate most of the risks.

High blood pressure is often called "essential hypertension," in Western medical terminology. According to Western medical models, a problem in the brain and the sympathetic nervous system causes the body to act as if it were reacting to an imaginary threat all the time. More blood is passed to the brain while peripheral arteries are constricted; the blood pressure remains elevated to levels that can damage the heart, kidneys, and other organs. Arteriosclerosis, atherosclerosis, cigarette smoking, stress, obesity, excessive dependence on stimulants, high sodium intake, and use of contraceptive pills can precede or trigger high blood pressure. Damage that appears first as palpitations and hypertension can develop into serious conditions such as angina if immediate steps are not taken to remedy it.

Atherosclerosis

Atherosclerosis is a degenerative disease of the arteries that is a stage of arteriosclerosis (a generic term for a number of blood vessel diseases characterized by thickening and loss of elasticity of the arterial walls). In the case of atherosclerosis, there is a build-up of fatty deposits along the vessel walls that have been weakened or damaged with lesions due to the high pressure. This results in the narrowing of the vessel passages and, ultimately, hardening and loss of elasticity. The causes are said to be unknown, although a mounting pile of evidence points to lifestyle and diet as prime contributing factors. As the condition progresses, insufficient blood flow can result in cell starvation, the formation of blood clots, and stroke or heart attack when a main pathway to the brain or heart is completely blocked.

Angina

Angina is a squeezing pain in the chest accompanied by a constant ache from the left shoulder down to the left hand. The pain is usually present with stress and high blood pressure caused by insufficient oxygen supply reaching the heart muscle, most often due to arteriosclerosis. Angina is a serious health condition that requires medical attention. An acupuncturist can help bring some balance back to the body, but please see a qualified practitioner.

Basic Guidelines

The bottom number of a blood pressure reading is called the diastolic pressure, and it is the measurement of the relaxed phase of the heart's pumping cycle. It is the more important number in determining health risks. If it is consistently above 100, try to get it down to around 80 or below by trying the following:

- Stop drinking coffee and all caffeinated drinks.
- Discontinue smoking.
- Try to stay within five pounds of your ideal weight.
- Decrease sodium (salt) and saturated fats intake.
- Increase potassium, calcium, and magnesium intakes. Calcium is found in large amounts in green leafy vegetables; magnesium is found in fish, meat, seafood, also blackstrap molasses, brewer's yeast, and brown rice. There are many other natural sources for these minerals.
- Begin a stress management program.
- Exercise regularly. A form of movement that combines stretching and strengthening with deep abdominal breathing and quiets the mind kills two birds with one stone. Yoga, qigong, tai'chi and other forms of martial arts fit the bill.

Oriental Medical Energetics

1) Heart and Kidney Disharmony combined with Heart Yin Deficiency

Imbalance created when a situation of long-term illness, excessive sexual activity, early childbirth or too many births, repeated miscarriages and/or abortions, or overwork or overstudy with insufficient rest drains the body fluids to create disharmony between Kidney (Water) and Heart (Fire). This combines with the Yin Deficiency of the Heart (caused by stress) to produce symptoms of insomnia, palpitations, dream-disturbed sleep, anxiety, and hypertension.

Self-Help Strategies

—Reduce work or study loads and sexual activity.
—Reduce stress.
—Nurture the Yin of the Kidney through diet.

2) Heat in Liver/Gallbladder

This imbalance is due to drinking excessive quantities of alcohol or coffee, eating excessive quantities of greasy, fried, fatty or rich foods, and/or smoking, activities that create too much Heat in the Liver/Gallbladder organs and channels. When imbalance in the Liver/Gallbladder is combined with excessive sexual intercourse or overwork, both of which tend to lead to deficiency in the Kidney organ and channel, the cooling energies of the Kidney Yin are depleted. The Kidneys become unable to keep Heat from the Liver in check. It rises to manifest as headache, dizziness, vertigo, redness in the face or eyes, blurred vision, irritation with outbursts of anger, insomnia, restlessness, constipation, in women menstrual difficulties, concentrated urine, nosebleeds, jaundice, a bitter taste in the mouth, hearing problems, poor memory, lumbago, and aching in the lower legs.

In addition, extreme amounts of stress could produce Excess Fire in the Heart, which combines with the Liver and/or the Kidney problems. Symptoms of this syndrome include the above-mentioned symptoms in addition to palpitations, dream-disturbed sleep, anxiety, and hypertension.

Self-Help Strategies

—Stop aggravating the Liver.

—Stop draining the Kidney, Liver, and Heart energy by working less, reducing stress, and abstaining temporarily from sex.

—See a practitioner. Acupuncture treatment is aimed at correcting these imbalances. In conjunction with herbal medicine it can be quite effective in controlling and in some instances clearing high blood pressure altogether. Changes in diet, moderate exercise, and practicing relaxation techniques are implicit in the treatment.

3) Depleted Heart Qi

This condition can arise out of prolonged emotional turmoil, mental irritation, or chronic illness. Arrhythmia, cardiac disease, and neurosis in Western terms, appearing with heart palpitations, a shortness of breath upon exertion, depression, vagueness, insomnia, and an irregular pulse, are symptoms of Heart Qi Deficiency.

Self-Help Strategies

—Relax; clear the mind.

—Treat any chronic illness.

4) Chronic illness, stress, hemorrhage, and prolonged Spleen Deficiency lead to anemia, neurosis, palpitations, etc.

Palpitations, dizziness, insomnia, having many dreams, a poor memory, anxiety attacks, irritability, a pale face and lips, and a weak pulse are commonly termed anemia, neurosis, or asthenia in Western medical terminology. These symptoms occur as a result of what Oriental practitioners call Heart Blood Deficiency.

Conventional allopathic doctors tend to treat heart disease with set diets and medicines, but the Oriental treatment is varied. Treatment will include dietary changes, acupuncture, and herbs, prescribed case by case.

Self-Help Strategies

—See a practitioner.

—Tone the Stomach/Spleen function.

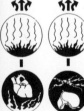
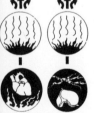

5) Flaring Liver Yang and Heart Fire

Here we see a new twist on Heart disorders with the involvement of the Liver Qi. Long-term stagnation of the Liver Qi due to excessive drinking of alcohol, smoking, eating quantities of greasy, deep-fried foods, chronic depression or extreme emotions, generates Liver Qi Fire. This manifests as a combination of some or all of the following symptoms: severe headache with dizziness, vertigo, menopause difficulties in women, redness in the face, red and painful eyes, tinnitus, irritability, a bitter taste in the mouth, vomiting sour or bitter fluids, insomnia, hypertension, constipation, nosebleeds, and coughing up blood in severe cases.

Self-Help Strategies

—See a practitioner.

—Cool the Fire.

—Dispel Liver Qi Stagnation, detoxify and tone the Liver Qi.

—Relax; alleviate stress.

4) Stroke occurs as a result of Liver Wind imbalance.

This is getting into some sophisticated Oriental diagnosis. (Review the concept of Wind in Chapter 2.) Wind moves around and affects symptoms that come and go. It is fast and changes quickly. Twitching is a good example of a Wind symptom. It is light and Yang and tends to affect the upper part of the body.

Wind can be generated if a vacuum in the Liver meridian is created when the Liver Yang rises and the Liver Yin is Deficient. Health depends on the presence of both Yin and Yang, but in this case, both have jumped ship.

The resulting imbalance is called Liver Fire Transforms to Wind. It can also rise and manifest as headaches, dizziness, and vertigo, a complete loss of balance, numbness and tremors in the limbs, involuntary twitching of the hands and feet, all of which can lead to a sudden loss of consciousness, stroke, coma, C.V.A. (cerebrovascular accident), and pseudo-C.V.A. Syndrome, with hemiplegia, facial paralysis, aphasia, or death as the final outcome.

Self-Help Strategy

—See a practitioner.

Internal Applications

• Avoid foods that Congest the Liver Qi: alcohol, caffeinated drinks, excessively spicy foods, heavy red meat, sugar and sweets, over-the-counter and prescription drugs, food additives and preservatives, and overeating.

• Avoid foods that are contraindicated for Heart imbalance (see Food Influences in Chapter 3).

• For Kidney involvement, also avoid citrus fruit and chocolate. Include more foods that tone the Kidney and Yin energy (see Chapter 3).

• Keep the diet limited to whole foods, fresh vegetables and fruits, legumes, whole grains, fish, and tofu. Eat Warming foods that strengthen the Stomach/Spleen function—orange and yellow vegetables, root vegetables, whole grains and cereals, legumes, and some chicken (see Chapter 3 and the section Adapting to Stress and Building the Immune System in Part II).

• Combine the above with some lighter foods that are clearing and dispersing: cucumbers, watercress, and alfalfa to cool the Liver Yang.

• The Doctrine of Signatures, or the theory of like-cures-like, indicates that eating heart organ meat nourishes the Blood and strengthens the Heart.

• For Liver disharmony, add foods that cool the Liver Yang and foods that relax the Liver. (See Chapter 3.)

• Porridge strengthens the digestive system; cooked with wheat berries (3 parts brown rice to 1 part wheat berries), it sedates and nourishes the Heart while calming the Shen. Celery rice porridge cools Heat and nourishes the Middle Burner and digestive function. Make the porridge with chrysanthemum infusion rather than stock or plain water. The chrysanthemum tea has cooling energy that will help extinguish the Heart Fire. (See the Appendix for instructions for preparing porridge.)

• Saffron, Sweet in flavor and Neutral in energy, promotes blood circulation and the digestive function, encourages sweating, has analgesic properties, and rejuvenates an exhausted condition. Add it to rice and simmered dishes.

• Oysters, in moderation, are believed to have a beneficial effect on the Heart. Sweet and Warm in flavor and energy, they help "extinguish" alcohol poisoning, contain an amino

acid that regulates blood pressure, and work to calm and soothe the Heart. They are indicated for high and low blood pressure and heart disease.

• Longan meats are indicated to soothe and calm the Heart. They can be purchased from a
Chinese grocer or pharmacist. Cook about 2 tbsp. of the dried meats in an earthenware pot
of water and eat the meats for breakfast with a little brown rice (which also has calming
effects). Drink the tea two or three times a day. Continue this for a week and watch for a significant change in peace-of-mind levels even before completing the course of treatment.

• A Japanese folk remedy for edema around the heart is to eat azuki beans with burdock
root. The azuki beans are indicated for removing excess fluid from the body, and the burdock is cooling and nourishes the Middle Burner. Put a pot of $^1/_2$ cup to 1 cup azuki beans
on the stove under low heat. The burdock is sliced, soaked for 10 minutes (discard the soaking water), then boiled with the azuki beans during the last 20 minutes of cooking. It is
done when the beans and burdock are cooked thoroughly (you will have to taste a little to
determine when they are soft). Add a little soy sauce to season, and eat a little with brown
rice twice a day.

• Tōchū tea, available at Japanese specialty stores (see Shopping in the Appendix,) is
believed to help lower blood pressure. In Chinese, this herb is called du zhong (*Eucommia
ulomoides*). It aids in the smooth flow of Blood, is considered tonic to the Kidney and Liver,
and is the subject of much research in China concerning its effects on the Heart. It can be
cooked as a standard decoction and drunk daily. It has a mild sedative effect in large doses,
but no symptoms of overdose have been recorded as far as we can discover.

• Chrysanthemum flower tea is said to have cooling properties and is often drunk in China
to help lower the blood pressure. It also prevents hardening of the arteries.

• The Japanese herb dokudami (*Houttuynia cordata*), a perennial of the family Sauru-
raceae, is constantly recommended in folk medicine in cases of heart trouble. Its use has
been documented for generations and appears in *The Detailed Guide to Family Health
Care*, better known as *The Red Book*, by Chikuda Tayoshi, which was the health manual for
Japanese families during the early Showa Period. Dokudami was drunk daily by people with
heart problems. It is believed to flush toxins out of the body, aid the stomach and digestive
tract, improve skin problems, and preserve health. It can be found as an ingredient in
health teas imported from Japan and sold at Japanese food stores in the States (see Appendix). Strong tea made with the leaves is recommended for heart trouble: 30 g dokudami
leaves to 1 $^1/_2$ cups water, simmered until the water is reduced by a third. Drink 3 warm cups
a day.

• Go for greens, particularly if your diet has been rich in animal proteins until now. Juice
green leafy vegetables and drink a cupful everyday. Or lightly steam dandelion, kale, mustard green, Swiss chard, spinach, and bok choy regularly and eat with a liver-cleansing
dressing of lemon juice, olive oil, and cayenne pepper.

• Fish oils contain EPA and DHA fatty acids. These are involved in the formation of
prostaglandins, which are known to inhibit the development of blood clots, to lower the
blood viscosity and help the blood flow more smoothly, and to reduce blood fat levels. The
best types of fish to eat are the red meat fish—sardines, salmon, and mackerel. EPA breaks
down during cooking; sashimi (raw) is the best way to eat these fish. Be careful to eat only
the freshest fish, and avoid sashimi on Sundays—the fishermen's day off.

• Vinegared Rice and Soybeans

The vinegar is believed to counteract toxic amines that constrict blood vessels in the intestinal tract, while the oxidation of soybeans is said to promote the breakdown of fats that clog the arteries.

$^1/_2$ c dried soybeans
white or rice vinegar

Soak the beans, drain, rinse with cold water, and cook well. When thoroughly cooked, keep in a wide-mouth jar and cover with vinegar. Eat a little daily. This also helps clean out the colon.

• Kombu and Shiitake Mushroom Drink

Kombu has long been recognized as a preventative for hardening of the arteries. It is contraindicated for those with thyroid trouble and digestive problems.

50 ml water from soaking dried shiitake mushrooms
100 ml water
3 pieces of "silver" kombu (coated with white powder)

Mix ingredients and let sit overnight. Use them in a simmered dish (remove the kombu before eating), or strain the following day and drink the liquid. Heat well before serving.

• Onion Peel Broth

Onions are well known in the Far East for their laxative properties. Often added to miso soup, they also help prevent a rise in blood pressure by clearing the intestines and alleviating constipation.

Peels of 2–4 white onions
1–2 liters water (depending on amount of peels)

Add the peels to water and bring to a boil. Turn off the heat and infuse for 10 minutes. This can be used as a base for simmered dishes, stews, miso soup, and rice porridge. The active ingredient in onions also helps strengthen capillary walls.

• Pickled shallots have long been considered an angina preventative folk remedy. This recipe comes from China: soak shallots in a diluted vinegar solution overnight and eat within the following day or two to prevent heart trouble.

• Pine nuts were used as a cure for hardening of the arteries. Add 100 g to a 750 ml of *sake* or 45° clear alcohol and let sit until the alcohol begins to evaporate, becoming very sticky. Drink 20 ml a day after meals.

External Applications

• To improve circulation, take frequent foot baths with ginger water or apply ginger compresses to the soles and tops of the feet, with a hot-water bottle placed on top to keep the compresses warm.

• Follow this with a foot massage, paying particular attention to the arches of both feet, which are related to the Heart and Kidney. Then massage the fingers, especially the middle (related to circulation) and ring fingers (autonomic nervous system). Also turn the ankle to the left and right with one hand while bending and flexing the toes with the other.

• Begin to practice some form of meditation or slow, meditative movement, such as slow-moving qigong or yoga, that incorporates deep-breathing and the body/mind unifying principle. These are excellent tools to facilitate the recovery of the stressed-out, over-achieving, Type A personality who suffers most from heart disease.
• Moxibustion for the Heart was traditionally applied to the
—big toe, 4 mm below the bottom of the nail, on the joint
—middle of the arch of the foot.
Burn 3 balls of moxa on each point every day.

Acupressure for the Heart
(See the BodyMap for exact location of points and the meanings of abbreviations.)

> ST. 36—Tonifies the whole body and regulates the heartbeat and rhythm of the heart.
> SP. 6—Stimulates circulation, eases the throat, supports the following HT. 7 point and relieves insomnia.
> HT. 7—Regulates the Heart and calms the Shen.

Recipe: Anti-hypoglycemic Stew

That's what we call it in Tokyo. Make this weekly for chronic low blood sugar and low energy.

> 1 c azuki beans
> 2 2-inch pieces of kombu
> $1/2$ onion
> 1–2 garlic cloves
> 1-inch piece ginger
> 6–8 Japanese peppercorns (sanshō), lightly crushed (optional)
> 2 tsp. canola oil
> 1 whole winter squash: Hokkaido pumpkin, buttercup, butternut squash, or large turnip, peeled and chopped into bite-sized pieces
> 3–4 c water, or vegetable or chicken stock
> 1 tsp. lycium berries (optional)
> 3 dried Chinese red dates (optional)
> $1/4$ c walnuts, chopped (optional)
> 1 tbsp. honey (optional)
> 1–2 tbsp. soy sauce or 1 tbsp. miso paste with 1 tbsp. soy sauce
> 2 tsp. canola oil
> slivered scallions
> 1 tbsp. sesame seeds or black sesame seeds

To prepare:
> 1. Precook the beans with the kombu with a liter of extra water, and add more as the water evaporates. When the beans are soft, drain, reserving the liquid in a pitcher. Drink once or twice a day for several days.
> 2. Chop the onion, crush garlic, slice ginger, crush the peppercorns, and add to a stewing pot with 2 tsp. canola oil. Sauté until the onion is soft.

3. Add kabocha, squash, or turnip, enough stock to cover completely, the berries, dates, chopped walnuts, and/or honey if you desire (pumpkin and buttercup squash are naturally sweet, however, so keep a light touch), and cook on simmer.
4. Add 2 tbsp. soy sauce, or 1 tbsp. soy sauce and 1 tbsp. miso paste, and mix well.
5. Add the beans when the squash or turnip are soft.
6. Top with slivered scallions and sesame seeds and eat with brown rice.

Recipe: Glorious Green Oysters

Oysters and mushrooms have a calming effect on the mind; spinach is cooling, the onion stimulates Blood circulation, and pine nuts tone Qi and Blood, remove Stagnant Blood, and expel Cold and Wind.

(Serves 4)

$^1/_2$ kilo oysters
$^1/_2$ onion
10 shiitake mushrooms
1 bunch spinach
1–2 tsp. olive oil
2 cloves garlic, crushed
$^1/_4$ c pine nuts
saffron
white wine

To prepare:

1. Wash the oysters in salt water, drain and set aside.
2. Dice the onion, slice mushrooms. Wash spinach well and spin- dry, cut into 2-inch sections.
3. Coat the pan with olive oil, add the crushed garlic and the onion, and sauté on low heat until onion is transparent.
4. Crush the pine nuts slightly and add to onions. Cook for a minute.
5. Add oysters, mushrooms, saffron, and wine. Cover, to steam-cook the oysters.
6. When the oysters are nearly done, add the spinach and lightly steam.
7. Serve with long-grain brown rice.

Recipe: Heart O-hitashi

O-hitashi is a side dish commonly found on traditional Japanese tables. This one is for the easily irritated who also have nasal inflammation, dry or chapped lips, dry mouth, redness in the face, athlete's foot, a tendency toward infection, high blood pressure, peritonitis, and inflammation in the stomach.

(Serves 4)

$^1/_2$ cup napa cabbage
$^1/_4$ lb chrysanthemum greens
$^1/_4$ lb dark leafy greens (except mustard greens)
$^1/_4$ lb spinach

4-inch slice daikon radish, grated
tomatoes (optional)
cucumber (optional)
bonito flakes (optional)

Dressing

2 tbsp. soy sauce
juice from 1 lemon
1 tbsp. light miso
1 tsp. sesame oil

To prepare:

1. Wash and spin-dry the leaves, cut in 2-inch sections, and steam.
2. When the greens are cooked but still retain their fresh color, remove from heat, and rinse with cold running water until cool.
3. Pick them up with your hands and wring out the excess water, forming the greens into a ball. Or wrap them in a bamboo sushi roller to remove water and mold into a cylinder.
4. If you rolled the greens, place on an oblong dish and cut into 1-inch sections, like a sushi roll. This step is optional.
5. Grate daikon very finely, squeeze out the excess water, and add a dollop over the greens, along with diced tomatoes and cucumbers if you like, just before serving.
6. Mix dressing ingredients together and add to the greens. Sprinkle the bonito flakes on top, if desired.

Hemorrhoids

Oriental practitioners treat hemorrhoids as they do any condition: according to the accompanying symptoms and collective signs of disharmony.

Oriental Medical Energetics

1) Stagnation in the Intestines

A person who tends to be overweight and who eats quantities of rich, spicy, or greasy foods, overconsumes alcohol, and lacks ample dietary fiber in the form of fresh vegetables and whole grains may create Heat and Damp Stagnation in the Large and Small Intestines. Obstructed or Congested Qi manifests as generalized discomfort, fullness, pressure in head, hands, chest, limbs, and abdomen, belching and flatulence, constipation, wheezing, difficulty swallowing, and a fullness under the ribs. Hemorrhoids usually manifest as ulcerations and sores in the inner walls of the anus. In this case the practitioner would prescribe herbs to disperse Qi and ease elimination.

Self-Help Strategies

—Move and tone the Qi.
—Reduce Heat and Damp.

2) Accumulation of Heat and Depleted Moisture

This is a more severe Heat scenario. Symptoms pointing to the acute Accumulation of Heat include fever, heat associated with infection, inflammation, pain with a sensation of heat or burning, sores or infections with green or yellow pus, yellow or green discharges from anus, and extreme thirst with cravings for cold liquid. In this case the practitioner would prescribe herbs to purge Heat.

There may also be signs of Depleted Moisture—dry, parched mouth, skin, and throat, a dry stool, scant urine, and unstable blood sugar. Due to the lack of moisture, the patient strains during bowel movements and stresses the anal wall.

Self-Help Strategies

—Dispel Heat.
—Restore Moisture.

3) Depleted Qi resulting in organ prolapse

While patients with Excessive Heat conditions may tend to be active, tense, warm, and gregarious, practitioners at times see hemorrhoid patients whose Qi is Deficient; they are physically weak and tend to worry. They are under stress or depressed. This could be for any number of reasons: overwork, recent childbirth, or insufficient diet. Symptoms may also include a general sensation of coldness in the body, cold hands and feet, shortness of breath, lassitude, sallow complexion, dizziness, lack of appetite, prolapse of organs or rectum, and hemorrhoids extending from the anus. In this case, the central Qi is weakened and cannot hold the organs and muscles in place. They sink, creating pressure at the anus, which results in stagnation in the area.

Self-Help Strategies

—See a practitioner to strengthen the Stomach/Spleen Qi.
—Eat a nourishing diet of easy-to-digest foods—rice porridge and well-cooked grains, chicken and vegetable broths.
—Relax more and try to express your emotions.

Internal Applications

• Avoid refined sugar, caffeine, alcohol, and tobacco.
• Foods that increase Heat—black pepper, cayenne pepper, heavy red meat (especially lamb), fatty foods, dairy products, excessively spicy foods, and hot and warming spices—should be drastically reduced.
• Heat-types should include foods that cool the body and dispel Heat (see Chapter 3). This is not for Cold or Deficient types.
• Foods that support the Middle Burner and the Stomach/Spleen function should be eaten regularly by Deficient types (see Chapter 3).
• Take in more foods that get Qi and Blood moving (see Chapter 3).
• Foods that lubricate and add moisture can help smoothen the feces and facilitate peristalsis and evacuation: taro, yamaimo, konnyaku, and nattō.
• Calming foods help reduce stress—try longan, mushroom, oyster, rice, rosemary, wheat, and wheat germ.
• The regular ingestion of porridge made with 1 c brown rice, $^1/_4$ c chestnut flour, 2 tbsp. pine nuts, and $^1/_4$ c each of chopped daikon radish and celery added during the last half-hour of cooking, can help tone and clear the intestines, clear Heat, and stimulate the Qi. Chestnut (ground) is useful in the treatment of anal hemorrhage. It tonifies Kidneys and strengthens the lower back and knees. Daikon radish is a digestive and cools Hot problems of the digestive organs. Celery is cooling and helps lower the Fire in the early stages of Liver Yang Rising. Pine nut moistens the Heart and Lungs, harmonizes the Large Intestine, and is helpful for constipation. Top with cooling grated spinach if you like.(See the Appendix for instructions for making porridge.)
• Take 10 to 15 grams of dried lotus root (if using fresh, use the area around the joint. If

using dried lotus root, don't worry about using the joint). Boil in 2 cups of water until reduced by half, and drink three times a day. This remedy helps stop the bleeding of the rectal area. It is also good for the bleeding from a stomach ulcer, blood in the urine, and aids the cessation of other forms of internal bleeding. Lotus root has constrictive properties that cause its hemostatic effect. Start the lotus root remedy as soon as you begin to have a problem with constipation that causes bleeding.

External Applications

• A lotus root plaster is indicated to stop bleeding due to hemorrhoids: Cut very thin slices of room-temperature lotus root, enough to cover the affected areas, and wrap in gauze that has been dipped in a lotus root infusion (see under Internal Applications, above) so the juice permeates the fabric and reaches the skin. Apply to the outer anal area. This should effectively stop the bleeding.

• When you have hemorrhoids, frequent and proper cleansing of the area is important. Anal washes and baths are particularly effective ways to treat hemorrhoids because they warm the area, providing physical comfort and an increase in circulation. It is helpful to use a low stool in the bath, the depth of your tub permitting, and let your rear end hang off to keep direct pressure away from the sensitive areas.

• In cases of anal prolapse (when the muscles collapse and the colon/rectal area feels like it has fallen in), apply absorbent cotton dipped in a light sea-salt solution to the anus and hold in place while you bathe.

• Make a salve using oils of comfrey, plantain, calendula, and goldenseal by soaking 4 oz of the fresh or 2 oz of dried herbs in bottles of 1 c olive, sesame, or almond oil for 2 weeks. Keep the oil is a dark spot and shake every day. Strain the herbs, reserving the oil, and add 1 tsp. vitamin E oil to it. Then melt beeswax (in a pot especially for this purpose, because it won't be usable for anything else afterward), add to the oil, and mix well. You will have to experiment with the proportions to make a consistency that is soft and spreadable, yet not runny. Pour into a storage container (glass or tin) and cover. Makes about 4 oz of salve. To use, rub directly onto skin.(See the Appendix for F.D.A. information on comfrey.)

• For hemorrhoidal pain, apply moxa to the tailbone (GV. 1). (See Chapter 4 for instructions on using moxibustion.)

• A daikon radish leaf bath is a folk remedy from Niigata, the north country of Japan. Use dried leaves. Boil down in an infusion for 5 minutes and add to the bath. Soak until your body is quite warmed through. Once you are out, cut a small portion of leaves, wrap in a layer of gauze, and apply directly to the affected area. The bath is also believed to improve the quality of the skin.

• Frequent bowel evacuations help this condition. You don't want feces sitting in the colon for too long, or bacteria to further infect the hemorrhoids.

• Lack of tone in the rectal muscles can result in rectal prolapse and chronic constipation. If hemorrhoids and constipation are chronic, the Kegel exercises can help retrain the function of the muscles of elimination.

To do the exercises, first you must locate the PC muscle (pubococcygeus), which is the muscle that tightens when you voluntarily stop urinating. It also tightens the anus. To strengthen the PC muscle, tighten it and release, first slowly, then quickly. Build up to 200 contractions a day. The exercises can be done anytime and anywhere: while walking, sitting at your desk, and so forth.

Acupressure for hemorrhoids

(See the BodyMap for location of points and the meaning of abbreviations.)

BL. 30—The "hemorrhoid point" in Oriental medicine. It is located right on the tailbone. Use moxa or acupressure here.

LU. 6—The Large Intestine is often treated through its Yin partner, the Lung. This point on the arm is used for acute conditions and Blood-related conditions, such as when blood is found in the sputum.

GV. 1—Pressing and rubbing the tip of the tailbone is also effective for stimulating the Qi in the lower body.

GV. 20—This point at the tip of the head is a well-known point for hemorrhoidal relief.

SP. 6—Regulates the flow of Qi in the entire body.

Acupressure to build Spleen Qi

ST. 36—Increases digestive function.

SP. 6—Aids in the breakdown and transport of nutrients; strengthens the Spleen Qi.

GV. 20—The tip of the crown of the head is usually needled (pulls the Yang energy to crown). This is the main point for prolapse, and moxa can be used on it at home.

Insomnia

Thirty percent of the American population complains of being affected by insomnia at least once a year; an estimated 50% of those occurrences are related to stress or psychological factors. But in Peter's experience, insomnia is also one of the first symptoms to disappear with acupuncture treatment.

Oriental Medical Energetics

1) Weak Kidneys cannot control Heart Fire.

This type of insomnia is accompanied by lower back pain, afternoon fever, and Heat in the palms, soles, or center of the chest, restlessness, and night sweats. Very likely the Kidney Water is unable to control the Fire aspect of the Heart, resulting in restlessness and sleeplessness. (The Kidney Water controls the Heart Fire in the Control Cycle of the Five Elements.)

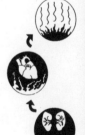

Self-Help Strategies

—Tone and strengthen the Kidney Yin.
—Calm the Shen.

2) Liver imbalance keeps the body awake from 11 p.m. to 3 a.m.

A stiff neck and shoulders, irritability and bursts of anger, an inability to make decisions, headache, and inability to sleep between 11 p.m. and 3 a.m., the times when the Liver and Gallbladder energy is at its strongest and the Liver renews itself, point to an imbalance in the Liver meridian.

Self-Help Strategies

—Calm the Liver.
—Calm the Shen.
—Relax.

3) Imbalance in the Spleen

If insomnia is accompanied by obsession or excessive contemplation of a problem, there may be an imbalance of Spleen (Earth) energy. If there is insomnia with gastric problems, the problem is probably overeating before bed.

Self-Help Strategies

—Tone the Stomach/Spleen.
—Relax and take steps to reduce anxiety and stress.
—Leave time between eating and bed.

4) Yang cannot enter Yin.

Irregular sleeping patterns might include difficulty getting to sleep and lack of sleep, insufficient length and amount of sleep, interrupted sleep, restless sleep, and waking too early. The diagnosis is easy to understand. Think of the day as a continuum between Yin and Yang, Yin being the most sedate and yang being the most active. At the end of the day one is unable to stop and unwind, the Yang continues to be fired up, not approaching the lower end of the continuum. Waking up too early and interrupted sleep are variations of the pattern.

Self-Help Strategies

—Take measures to wind down at night before bed.
—Quit working earlier.
—Avoid strenuous exercise before bed and overexercise.
—Avoid thrilling television shows and the evening news right before bedtime.

Internal Applications

• Avoid eating large meals before bed. This puts an enormous strain on the digestive system: the Stomach/Spleen is forced to break down and transport foods and thus takes away energy that ought to be with the Liver in the hours between 11 p.m. and 3 A.M.

• Eliminate stimulants such as tea and coffee completely if insomnia is a chronic problem. Many people are unable to drink caffeinated drinks after 4 p.m.

• Eat foods that calm the Heart as part of your regular diet (see Chapter 3).

• Foods that support the Stomach/Spleen will help reduce the worry and obsessive thinking that characterize some forms of insomnia (see Chapter 3).

• When the nervous system is disturbed, the body could be lacking in vitamin B. Foods rich in vitamin B are whole grains, beef and chicken liver, desiccated liver tablets, and brewer's yeast.

• There are several types of commercially prepared herbal formulas that help balance disorders manifesting as insomnia—inability to get to sleep, waking up in the middle of the night, inability to fall into a deep sleep. Ask your practitioner about them; they are nonaddictive.

• Try ingesting the following foods every day to regulate the autonomic nervous system and calm the nerves: dandelion tea, a small amount of onion (cooked), pumpkin seeds toasted with black sesame seeds, and/or a cup of miso soup with toasted brown-rice mochi.

• A Chinese herbal infusion to treat sleeplessness related to stress, hysteria, and nerves is made of equal parts of Chinese licorice, dried Chinese red dates, and wheat berries. Combine to make a total weight of 2 ounces, boil with 3 cups of water, then turn down the heat and simmer until the water is reduced to one cup. Drink a cupful in the morning and evening.

• Red Date Wine

Red dates are a traditional tonic nutrient and guiding herb. Energetically Sweet and Neutral, they are said to "clear the Nine Openings" of the body, and improve circulation; they are slightly sedative and relax the smooth muscles.

1 cup red dates, pitted or unpitted
750 ml 45° clear alcohol
$\frac{1}{2}$ cup honey

Add the ingredients to a wide-mouth jar and store for one month in a cool, dry place. Shake regularly. Drink 20 ml, or a *sake* cupful, once a day in the afternoon after a meal for insomnia, headache, anxiety, neurosis, restlessness, depression, and general nervousness. Contraindicated if headache is accompanied by constipation. Do not drink if you have any problem with gallstones.

External Applications

• The establishment of new bedtime habits is crucial to teaching your body to sleep regularly. Habits that relax the mind and muscles—leisurely walks, warm baths, foot baths that move blood from the head down to the feet to promote relaxation and sleep, massages, soft music (rather than *Terminator II* before bed), quiet meditation, deep breathing, and a glass of warm milk—facilitate a smoother transition to sleep.

• Massage can be extremely helpful when the insomnia is a direct result of musculoskeletal pain or physical tension. Have the entire back massaged with repetitive, soothing strokes.

• Here's an old one for insomnia. In Japan, sleeping on a pillow filled with azuki beans is actually a very old traditional remedy for sleeplessness. Simply fill a small pillow with beans instead of down or foam. Azuki are quite expensive in Japan, so this is considered a luxury, but even during times of famine people went hungry rather than lose sleep—they left the beans in their pillows instead of eating them.

Kidney Disorders and the Urinary Tract

Includes: frequent urination, excessive nocturnal urination, urinary blockage, concentrated urine, nephritis, kidney stones, bladder stones, sensitive bladder, edema.

In the West we usually associate the kidneys with kidney stones, nephritis, urinary problems, and retention. These are all acute, serious medical emergencies. Seek immediate help for them all.

Oriental Medical Energetics

In Oriental medicine, imbalances involving the Kidneys are not limited to symptoms revolving around the kidney organ. The Kidneys, when understood in terms of their function in the body, are seen as having a much wider sphere of influence than their Western medical-concept counterpart.

The Kidney organ and its network govern reproduction, sexual maturation, fertility, and regeneration through the energy of the Jing that is housed there. The Jing begets the structural elements of the body and regulates physical and mental growth. The Kidney balances fluids in the body and plays a vital role in the healthy functioning of the joints, particularly in the lumbar region and the knees. Hair on the head, the ears and hearing, and the correct functioning of the brain are regulated by the Kidney.

The Gate of Life

MÌNG MÉN
MEI MON

The Kidneys are considered to represent the Water essence (Yin) of the body, but they also store the spark of life in the body, the *Ming Men*. The Ming Men is defined as activated Kidney essence (Yang) that energizes the entire body and holds the organism's hereditary blueprint. The Ming Men is not an actual organ in the Western sense, but is a combination of substance and energy (form and function = essence) said to be produced out of the dynamic interaction between the right and left Kidneys. Traditionally, the right Kidney was believed to hold the essential Fire of the body, while the left was said to contain the essential Water. Their interaction is usually illustrated as a pot of water (Kidney Water, or Yin) over a fire (Kidney Fire, or Yang), which produces steam (essence). Incidentally, the Chinese ideogram for steam contains the character Qi, which means energy.

Once this energy is produced, it is carried by the Triple Heater to the body's three main energy centers, the Upper, Middle, and Lower Burners, and distributed throughout the system. It warms the entire body and supplies the organs and their systems with vital energy.

One more function of the Ming Men is to release the activated Kidney energy, or vital energy, to the genitals when the body is sexually stimulated.

Other organs are directly affected by the Kidney's energy. The Spleen depends on the Kidney Yang energy to warm it. The Liver depends on the Kidneys to keep it moist. The Kidneys extend to the spinal column, the brain, the sexual organs, and the bones.

Problems involving the Kidney meridian may include a lack of proper physical development or mental retardation in children, and improper or slow sexual maturation during puberty. Infertility, impotence, poor memory, lack of concentration, and the emotion of fear may be problems in adults. Urinary excess or retention, pain in the lower back and knee joints, loss of hair (not related to hereditary baldness), tinnitus (ringing in the ears), other hearing problems, and failing vision may all be related to Kidney imbalance.

Kidney conditions are usually imbalances of Deficiency, generally caused by overworked organs further worn down by prolonged illness, stress, a diet consisting of too much greasy or oily food, excessive consumption of cold beverages, coffee and caffeinated drinks, and alcohol, and a high intake of drugs. The kidney organs are kept busy filtering these out of the system.

1) Depleted Yang energy

When the Kidneys are Deficient in warm, Yang energy, the body feels coldness in the waist, lower body, or sometimes the entire body. Frequent urination, excessive nocturnal urination, or urinary blockage may be accompanied by all or some of the following symptoms: lower back pain, cold and aching knees, a lack of energy in general, withdrawal, dizziness, tinnitus, pallor, loose teeth, hair loss, anorexia, amenorrhea, infertility, diminished libido, edema, enuresis, a lack of concentration, poor memory, and hypothyroidism. Possible causes include long-term illness, congenital weakness, excessive sexual activity, and eating excessive amounts of cold foods and drinks.

Self-Help Strategies

—See a practitioner for herbal and moxibustion treatment. Acupuncture can be used as an adjunct therapy.
—Tone the Kidney Yang.

2) Deficient Kidney Yin

Deficient Yin or cool energy in the Kidney results in a rise of body temperature in the late afternoon accompanied by a flushed face, night sweats, dark and concentrated urine, constipation, a restless or irritable mood, insomnia, ringing in the ears, lower back pain, and pain in the heels. Chronic nephritis, diabetes mellitus, or chronic ear and hearing disabilities could also develop. Possible causes include long-term illness, excessive sexual activity, overwork or overstudy, and an improper diet.

Notice that the same conditions that cause a Deficiency of Kidney Yang in some people can cause a Deficiency of Kidney Yin in others. The form a deficiency will take depends on the tendencies of the individual. Be aware that a polarity exists between the two manifestations that can sometimes result in the condition changing into its opposite. Peter has treated people who exhibited Deficient Yin symptoms, which progressed so far that they suddenly switched into Deficient Yang symptoms, and vice versa.

Self-Help Strategies

—The symptoms can be effectively treated with acupuncture and herbs.
—Tone the Kidney Yin.

3) Lack of Jing

The regenerative energy of the body is stored in the Kidneys. When it is lacking, the Yin will be affected, Blood generation inhibited, and the Yang drained. Symptoms may include signs of both Yin and Yang deficiency, premature aging, gray hair, poor memory, loss of teeth, senility, weakening of the bones, and impotence without the Heat signs (concentrated urine, afternoon fever, constipation), lower back pain, Blood-related problems, and presenile dementia. In children, a lack of Jing is manifested as mental or physical retardation, slow or incomplete closure of the fontanel, bed-wetting, poor bone development, and retarded sexual development. Possible causes include chronic illness, excessive sexual activity, and a lack of Jing from weak parents.

Self-Help Strategies

—Relax, work and study less.
—Abstain from sex until fully recovered.
—See a practitioner to tone the Kidneys and discuss ways you can augment treatment.
—Adopt the general tonifying diet recommended in Chapter 3.

Internal Applications

• Avoid foods that irritate the Kidneys (see Chapter 3).
• Include foods in the diet that tone the Kidney Yin or Yang, depending on your symptoms (see Chapter 3).
• Free-range chicken meat, organs, and eggs are warming and tonifying.
• Mussels have warm energy and are considered an effective Yang tonic. These shellfish are believed to be especially good for lumbago and for raising the temperature in the genitals. Oysters have warm energy, but clams are cooling and tone the Yin.
• Animal kidneys are highly recommended Yang tonics and are said to aid in weight loss. According to the principle of the Doctrine of Signatures, weak Kidneys are nourished by dietary kidney supplements—beef, pork, chicken, or lamb kidneys. Make sure to eat animal protein from animals that have been organically fed and free-range grown. (For cooking instructions, see the section on Preparation of Organ Meats in the Appendix.)
• Lycium berries, also called wolfberries, are small, red, slightly sweet berries that can be added to soups and stews as a general Kidney tonic. Or decoct 1 to 2 tbsp. in 2 cups of water, reduce by a third, and drink half a cup 2 to 3 times a day.
• Try a healthful drink of water from cooked azuki beans to strengthen the Kidneys (see Recipe in the Appendix).
• The sticky white root called nagaimo or yamaimo is also beneficial.(This is *not* taro, or albi.) Purchase it from larger international grocery stores or Oriental markets, or buy it in its dried form (called dioscorea, from Oriental medicine pharmacies) and add to soups and stews. To use the raw potato, peel and grate to a soupy consistency and pour on top of soba

noodles. Or slice into julienne strips and eat as a salad, covered with radish sprouts and a lemon and sesame-oil vinaigrette.

• Yin Deficient types can try a decoction made with 5 to 10 g watermelon seeds to a cup and a half of water. Simmer and reduce by a third. Drink warm 3 times a day.

• Yang Deficient types can try dried daikon-radish slices, sold at Japanese specialty shops, for water retention. Soak to reconstitute and eat with a small amount of ume (plum) vinegar. Sprinkle black sesame seeds, carrot shavings, or a touch of chopped watercress on top. Eat miso soup with cooked daikon to increase water elimination. Or grate daikon and cook with water and 5% soy sauce to promote sweating or to expel liquid from the bowels.

Kidney Stones

Internal Applications
• If you have ever had kidney stones, drink plenty of liquid and prevent fluid loss by avoiding profuse sweating. Regulate the bowel function by adopting a whole foods diet, and avoid purgatives.

• Steer clear of anything containing oxalic acid, such as spinach, beet root, rhubarb, chocolate, vitamin D-enriched foods, dairy products, alkaline mineral water, and fluoridated water.

• To prevent and diminish the pain of gallstones and stones in the urinary tract, Yuriko Tōjō recommends drinking dokudami tea (20 g fresh or dried in 1 liter of water, reduce by one-third) for its diuretic properties. It also clears the blood of excess amino acids due to overeating red meat.

• Peach Wine

Peach wine is a traditional recipe for Kidney inflammation, mucus emissions with the urine, and fatigue; it supplements vitality and strength.

$^3/_4$ kilo fresh peaches
100 g rock sugar
1.8 liters 45° clear alcohol

Place ingredients in a wide-mouth jar and let mature for three months to a year. Drink 20 ml after dinner.

External Applications
• Hot ginger compresses applied to the abdomen and lower back warm and stimulate the Deficient Kidneys and the Liver.

• Hot mustard foot baths will encourage sweating for cases of Yang Deficiency. After the foot bath, wipe the body down with ginger compresses. This treatment increases circulation and improves the metabolism.

• Dried daikon-leaf hip baths stimulate the metabolism.

• Exercise: anything to move the inner organs helps the Deficient Kidneys. Yang Deficient types in particular can use a good sweat to rid the body of water toxins. Yin Deficient types should concentrate on building the Yin reserves before they begin exercising. Try yoga or qigong.

• Moxibustion for night urination can be applied to the top of the big toe between the nail and the joint. Use a moxa stick or 5 small grain-sized balls of moxa, wipe the area with Tiger Balm, and light with an incense stick. Repeat this treatment daily for a week.

Acupressure for Kidney-related problems
(See BodyMap for location of points and the meaning of the abbreviations.)

•**Chronically full or sensitive bladder**

Urinating too frequently can lead to a sensitive bladder that becomes incapable of holding anything. There is also a feeling of having to urinate all the time. To relieve an oversensitive bladder and frequent urination:

> C.V. 3—Reflex point for the Bladder. Press lightly 5 to 10 times or use ginger moxa on this point.
> BL. 23—Regulates the Kidneys, regulates Kidney Qi, relieves lumbar pain.
> Entire sacral area—Use acupressure and a moxa stick to warm and stimulate the entire area.

• **To strengthen the urinary function**

> C.V. 3—The reflex point for the bladder. Press here with medium-to-light pressure.
> BL. 23—Stimulates the Kidney, the Bladder's Yin partner.

• **Edema and tired legs**

This combination of points relieves pain and numbness, improves blood circulation, lightens the sensation in the feet, and improves swelling in the ankles. Press and rub the following points:

> SP. 6—Balances the Kidney and Liver energies, tones the lower Yin channels, and invigorates the circulation of Qi and Blood. Press with medium-hard pressure five to six times.
> C.V. 9—Clears fluids, promotes urination. Light pressure or moxibustion are fine.
> BL. 23—Regulates the Kidney and body fluids.
> KI. 3—For edema, afternoon fever, and night sweats. Press with fairly heavy pressure for a minute. Relax and repeat.

Edema

Edema is also called "water cyst" in Oriental medicine; in other words, it is thought of as a build-up of toxic water, reflecting imbalance in the body. If you press the swollen area and the shape immediately goes back, follow the remedies here; the condition should improve soon. If the skin stays depressed, the condition is quite Deficient and is much harder to bring back to balance. See a practitioner.

Internal Applications

• Edema can be helped by cornsilk (*Zea mays*) tea, which encourages urination; drink this instead of tea and coffee.

• For edema and Damp Heat in the Lower Burner with painful urinary function, drink dokudami tea, which is an Acrid, Cool herb. It is contraindicated for patterns of Cold Deficiency.

• Celery and watermelon juice is believed to improve Kidney function. Juice a 20 cm section of fresh celery with a quarter of a small watermelon, seeds removed. The juice is said to help flush toxins, promote urination, and increase vitality.

• When you want to urinate but cannot, eat a small piece of brown rice mochi—without soy sauce or any seasonings—before you go to bed. If you wake up in the middle of the night and feel a need to urinate, force yourself to stay in bed. Do not urinate until you wake up in the morning. Eat more of the mochi during the day. Repeat until the urinary tract is conditioned to urinate upon waking in the morning.

Recipe: Kidney Yin Deficiency Rice Porridge

The pork kidneys tone and supplement the Kidney, the cornsilk promotes urination, and walnuts have a tonifying effect on the Kidneys, as do lycium berries. (See How to Prepare Organ Meats in Appendix.)

200 g pork kidneys
1 cup brown rice
20 g cornsilk
20 g lycium berries
$^1/_4$ c walnuts
10–12 ginkgo nuts
7–8 cups water
sliced ginger and scallions

To prepare:
1. Prepare the kidney meat by slicing in half, removing the white cartilaginous middle, and steaming for 30–40 minutes.
2. Wash rice and add all ingredients, except for kidneys, to the porridge pot. Cook on lowest heat possible.
3. Slice the kidneys when cool enough to do so and add to the porridge. Cook until creamy, and top with sliced ginger and scallions. Do not add salt.

Recipe: Kidney Tonifying Porridge

Particularly recommended for edema.

1 c brown rice
$^1/_4$ c chopped almonds
7–8 c water
$^1/_2$ c azuki beans
$^3/_4$ c green string beans
scallions
1-inch piece ginger

To prepare:
1. Wash the rice and add to the porridge pot along with almonds and water. Cook on low heat.
2. Cook azuki beans separately until almost soft, remove from heat, drain.
3. Wash, trim, and cut string beans into 1-inch pieces.
4. Half an hour before the porridge is done (it should begin to be turning creamy), add the azuki beans.

5. Add the string beans 15 minutes before serving.
6. Serve topped with slivered scallions and slivered ginger.

Liver Problems

Includes: hepatitis, sluggish liver (cholestasis), alcohol-induced fatty infiltration of the liver, cirrhosis, and gallstones (cholecystitis).

In Western terms, the liver serves four basic functions: to detoxify the body, to metabolize foods so they can be used by the body, to store nutrients, and to manufacture bile, heparin (to prevent blood clotting), and the proteins found in blood plasma. Protecting the liver from overexposure to toxins and taking measures to strengthen the organ increases the body's metabolism and its overall vitality.

Western medicine identifies a number of hepatic conditions, such as hepatitis, which is caused by viral infection; a fatty liver and cirrhosis are clearly related to excessive consumption of alcohol; the formation of gallstones is related to a diet high in cholesterol in combination with other factors such as other diseases that are present, sex, race, obesity, and drugs. Oriental medicine does not contain any of the diagnoses listed above, nor does it identify specific pathogens or causes that lead to the formation and development of a single pathology. Rather, an Oriental medicine practitioner would examine the patient and make a diagnosis based on the individual's unique pattern of symptoms, the pulse, the tongue, color of the eyes, and other relevant information. An Oriental practitioner is also aware of the interconnection of the organs and pathways of the body, and knows that when there is Liver imbalance, other organs and symptoms will most likely be involved.

Oriental Medical Energetics

Remember that the Liver in Chinese medical theory is the "Wood organ" (see Chapter 2). Blood flows through the Liver, where it is detoxified. The Liver also stores the Blood while the body is at rest and releases it when the body resumes movement. The Liver system also includes the peripheral nervous system and plays a large role in controlling neuromuscular activity. It is in charge of the smooth flow of Qi energy in the body. In order for the body to fully relax the Liver must be balanced and Qi in its meridians flowing freely and smoothly.

Creativity, the sexual urge, and the will to grow are influenced by the Liver. The libido is governed by the Liver, and having sex can temporarily relieve the build-up of anger associated with Liver imbalance. Be careful with this mechanism; in the long-run excessive sexual activity could damage the Kidney Regenerative energy, resulting in premature aging, memory loss, fatigue, aches and weakness in the knees, and urinary irregularity. It bodes better for one's longevity to learn to cope with the stress and emotion in other ways and preserve the Regenerative Jing.

Stress and emotional upsets can throw this sensitive organ off balance. Since this is the organ responsible for the smooth flow of Qi, the entire body is immediately affected by Liver imbalance. Many liver diseases are greatly affected by and sometimes even caused by stress and other extreme emotions experienced for prolonged periods.

Hepatitis

Allopathic medicine diagnoses two main types of hepatitis caused by viral infections: hepatitis A and serum hepatitis B. Both are considered highly contagious. Hepatitis A is spread through personal contact and through polluted or contaminated food and water. Travelers are particularly vulnerable to the virus; travel-weary and budget-minded, one might be tempted to eat food or drink water from questionable sources, but extra caution is advised. Hepatitis B is spread through the blood, therefore through blood transfusions, contaminated syringes and needles, bloodsucking insects, and sexual contact. Symptoms include fever, weakness, nausea and vomiting, fatigue, drowsiness, headache, abdominal pain, and jaundice.

The virus is very contagious from two to three weeks before and one week after the appearance of jaundice. The virus is active in the feces; isolated treatment and careful attention to hygiene is recommended.

Oriental Medical Energetics

There is no diagnosis called "hepatitis" in Oriental medicine. A weakened Liver manifests patterns of imbalance that could anticipate and lead to the development of jaundice and the set of symptoms that typify hepatitis.

1) Blocked Liver Qi

Repressed anger, frustration, and stress are said to be the main causes of this condition. Symptoms include pain and distention in the sides and below the ribs, a congested feeling in the chest, a tendency to sigh, depression, mental anxiety, irritability, and sudden outbursts of anger. In women, there is irregular menstruation and distention in the breasts. This condition precedes or could make one more vulnerable to developing the hepatitis virus.

2) Stagnant Liver Qi invades the Spleen/Gallbladder.

Blocked or stagnant Qi in the Liver rises and invades the Spleen and Stomach; if the Spleen is weak, this could disrupt the digestive system. Symptoms include pain in the epigastrium, burping with acid reflux, nausea and vomiting, anorexia, gastric-duodenal ulcer, diarrhea, and the symptoms listed in 1) above. Qi Stagnation in the Liver/Gallbladder could interfere with the flow of bile, to produce a bitter taste in the mouth, constipation due to the lack of bile in the intestines, gallstones, and pain in the lower back and sides. Hepatitis could fall under this pattern of imbalance.

3) Damp Heat in the Liver

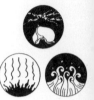

Jaundice, in Oriental medicine, is seen as a manifestation of imbalance in the Spleen. In this case, Damp Heat in the Spleen, usually understood to be the result of a pathogen that has entered the body through the digestive system, affects the Liver first. Damp Heat accumulates, inhibits the flow of bile from the Liver, affecting the Gallbladder and Spleen, and causes the yellow tinge of the skin.

Accompanying symptoms may include a bright yellow face and eyes, a bitter taste in the mouth, fever or alternating fever and chills (indicates struggle between the Protective Qi and an invading pathogen), thirst, cloudy urine, digestive difficulties (especially a lack of appetite), nausea, vomiting sour fluid, fullness and distention in the area under the ribs, a tendency toward anorexia, abdominal distention, dark and concentrated urine, diarrhea with mucus in the stool, and a bright orange-colored stool. In women, there may be a thick, yellow, strong-smelling discharge. In men there may be pain, swelling, and a burning sensation in the testicles.

Damp Heat may be due to a prolonged consumption of alcohol, greasy or deep-fried foods, and excessive consumption of sugar. It could also arise from being in a damp or tropical environment—such as that of tropical countries. In Western terms it is diagnosed as acute hepatitis, acute pancreatitis, cirrhosis of the liver, or cholecystitis.

Self-Help Strategies

—Unblock the Liver Qi.
—Harmonize and strengthen the Gallbladder and Spleen.
—Clear Damp and Heat.
—See a practitioner.

Internal Applications

• Avoid foods that aggravate the Liver: alcohol, coffee and other caffeinated beverages, excessively spicy foods, heavy red meat, fats, deep-fried food, sugar and sweets, refined flour, chemicals and over-the-counter drugs.

• Avoid taking antibiotics for a prolonged period; this creates more stagnation in the Liver.

• Do not overeat. It puts unnecessary stress on the Liver.

• Include foods to relax, clear, and tone the Liver (see Chapter 3).

• Also include some foods in your diet that clear Damp and Heat (see Chapter 3).

• Brown rice porridge with barley and azuki bean strengthens the digestive system and helps drain Excess Damp. Adding lycium berries, a little pork, beef, or chicken liver from a free-range animal can tone the Liver (see the Appendix for instructions for preparing porridge and organ meat).

• Light vegetable soups, such as chicken broth with carrot and leeks to disperse Liver Qi Stagnation, balanced with cooked daikon radish and garlic to drain Damp, are recommended.

• Try a Blood-cleansing dressing of olive oil, the juice of half a lemon, and a dash of cayenne pepper to activate the Liver Qi.

• Dandelion, dokudami, gentian, mugwort, and Foetid Cassia seed (*habu-cha*) teas are recommended to cleanse the Liver.

• Sour foods are astringent and drying. In moderation they can be eaten to help dry mucus, stimulate the digestion, aid in the breakdown of fats by stimulating bile, and aid in fat absorption. Lemons, dried orange peel (purchase at Chinese food shops), vinegar, raspberries, blackberries are recommended.

External Applications

• Of all the organs, the Liver is the most dependent on the strict maintenance of balance: emotional, dietary, and work/study related. Treatment for any Liver condition in Oriental medical terms begins with relaxation.

• Bed rest and sufficient sleep are necessary to the treatment of an imbalance as serious as Damp Heat in the Liver/Spleen.

Sluggish Liver, Fatty Liver, and Cirrhosis of the Liver

Cholestasis, also referred to as a sluggish liver, refers to a condition of diminished bile flow. The causes of blocked bile ducts include gallstones, alcohol consumption, toxins, pregnancy, hereditary disorders, steroidal hormones, various chemicals and drugs, viral hepatitis, and hyperthyroidism. Symptoms may include fatigue, lassitude, digestive disorders, allergies and chemical sensitivities, constipation, and premenstrual syndrome in women.

Fatty liver is a build-up of fatty deposits in the liver organ. In some individuals, the ingestion of only 25 g of alcohol can lead to the development of fat deposits in the liver. This results in impaired liver function and an increased risk of further liver damage.

Cirrhosis is described in allopathic terms as a degenerative, inflammatory disease characterized by a scarring and hardening of the liver tissue, which can prevent the flow of blood through the organ. Early symptoms include constipation, diarrhea, fever, nausea, and jaundice. Later stages may include anemia, bruising, and edema. Excessive intake of alcohol is the main cause of cirrhosis; viral hepatitis can also cause the disease.

Oriental Medical Energetics

1) Stagnation of Qi

When the Liver Qi stagnates, it may invade the Stomach/Spleen and disrupt digestion and elimination processes. Symptoms may include pain in the epigastrium, belching with acid reflux, nausea and vomiting, anorexia, pain and distention in the abdomen, sides, and under the ribs, borborygmus, diarrhea, anorexia, depression, anxiety, irritability, outbursts of anger, and in women irregular menstrual cycles and dysmenorrhea.

2) Damp Heat in the Liver (see under Hepatitis, above).

Self-Help Strategies

—Eliminate alcohol.

—Clear stagnation to ease the pain and promote the free flow of Liver Qi.

—Reduce stress.

Gallstones (Cholecystitis)

Gallstones are stones that form when a normally soluble component of bile (often cholesterol) cannot be dissolved due to bile super-saturation within the gallbladder, caused by an increase in cholesterol or a decrease in bile salts. This initiates the formation of the stone, which may then increase in size. The stones may exist without causing symptoms, or they may cause excruciating, stabbing abdominal and back pain at irregular intervals, as well as abdominal bloating, gas, and nausea and discomfort after rich, fat-laden meals. The intake of fats can trigger an attack of gallstones; for some individuals, just the smell of fats alone can make them nauseous. The presence of gallstones must be verified by an ultrasound test.

Oriental medicine treatment, including acupuncture—to reduce pain, increase the flow of Qi, and augment the flow of bile in the Liver/Gallbladder—herbal therapy, and diet modification, can often be very effective in moving the stones. Very large stones or large quantities of stones may require surgical removal, however. Even if stones have been surgically removed, acupuncture treatment is recommended to help the patient turn around the root condition that caused their formation in the first place.

Oriental Medical Energetics

The Oriental medical diagnosis of gallstones falls under **Stagnant Liver Qi invades the Spleen/Gallbladder** of Hepatitis (see above). There are many herbs specific for this condition. See a practitioner for a proper diagnosis and individualized treatment.

Self-Help Strategies

—Reduce or eliminate intake of fats in the diet.
—Reduce or eliminate refined, simple sugar.
—Eat less animal protein, while increasing intake of fish and whole grains.
—Follow other recommendations under Hepatitis (see above).

Liver Imbalance in Oriental Medical Terms

Rather than identifying illness as the progression of a specific pathogen in the body as allopathic medicine does, Oriental medicine recognizes imbalances that are made up of sets of symptoms. Each organ and meridian channel is susceptible to a number of typical imbalances, which make up the problems that affect each organ (and interrelated organ systems as well). When we speak of Liver problems in an Oriental sense, we speak of something very different from the specific illnesses that are recognized as liver disease in the West. Besides the imbalances listed above, common Liver imbalances according to Oriental medicine include the following:

1) Throat obstruction caused by Spleen Deficiency and Congealing Liver Qi

A weak Spleen, disturbed by the overconsumption of cold and raw food, and chilled or iced food and drink, is unable to break down and carry away food and fluid. The fluid accumulates to become a thick, sticky Phlegm. The Stagnant Qi and Phlegm combine and rise, creating a feeling of having something stuck in the throat. This is called a "plum seed obstruction" in Oriental medicine. In Western medical texts this is considered a figment of the neurotic mind, called *"Globus hystericus."* (See Lump in the Throat in the Colds section on page 156.) The condition usually worsens with increased emotional upset or intense stress.

2) Stagnant Liver Qi causes Blood Stagnation.

While a layperson might think of stagnant blood as the blood that remains as a bruise after injury, an Oriental medicine practitioner refers to Stagnant Blood also in an energetic sense. This Blood congests the lower abdomen, causing menstrual irregularities such as amenorrhea and dysmenorrhea, cold feet, "liver spots" on the face, and dry skin. A worsening of the condition can result in a congealing of Stagnant Blood to form tangible masses, such as ovarian cysts, uterine fibroids, and cervical and breast cancer. (For a more extensive explanation, see *Endometriosis, Infertility and Traditional Chinese Medicine* by Bob Flaws or *The Breast Connection* by Honora Wolfe, listed in the Recommended Reading section in the Appendix.)

3) Liver Yang Rising

Hypertension and migraine headaches can appear in cases of long-term Liver Qi Stagnation. In this pattern, the Stagnant Liver Qi transforms to a very hot condition, Fire, from the prolonged overconsumption of alcohol, tobacco, or of fatty or deep-fried foods, and from emotional influences such as frustration, chronic depression and extreme emotions. Migraine headaches and hypertension may be accompanied by anger, red or painful eyes, tinnitus, irritability, menopause symptoms and complications, thirst, a dry bitter mouth with a bitter taste, vomiting sour or bitter fluid, insomnia, restlessness, constipation, nosebleeds, coughing of blood, or vertigo.

4) Liver Yin Deficiency

Neurosis, hypertension, menopause complications, menstrual disorders, Ménière's syndrome, and eye disease can result from a lack of Liver Yin. This lack of Liver Yin can arise out of a lack of Kidney Yin or deficient Jing. The lack of either is caused by stress, overwork with inadequate rest, excessive sexual activity, too many childbirths, repeated miscarriages or abortions, ingesting quantities of difficult-to-filter foods, and long-term illness that depletes Yin fluids. The Liver Yang may then rise up and cause a throbbing headache, dizziness, blurred vision, tinnitus, dry throat and mouth, (possibly with a bitter taste), insomnia, irritability, and palpitations—all signs of Heat in the upper body.

5) Cold Stagnation of Liver Qi

Hernia, intestinal spasms, male genital disorders, and prostatitis may result from Cold Stagnation of Liver Qi. This condition is caused by an invasion of Cold, which contracts the Liver channel, resulting in blocked Liver Qi and Blood that congest the lower abdomen and genitals.

Internal Applications

• Aloe vera is an important Liver tonic and helps reproductive difficulties. It cools Fire, which is appropriate for a Flaring Liver Fire condition. Take 2 tsp. of the gel in warm water 2 to 3 times a day.

• Wonderfully delicious coffee-like dandelion coffee is available from natural foods stores in

Japan (see Shopping in the Appendix). Grind it in a coffee grinder and use 1 tbsp. to 2 cups of water, bring to a boil, and let simmer for 5 minutes. Strain, pour into a thermos, and take it to work with you.

• See Chapter 3 for foods that have specific actions on the Liver organ and channel.

External Applications

• See a practitioner if you have symptoms for any of the imbalances above. Even a few trips to the acupuncturist for treatment will include a discussion of a diet appropriate for your condition and other self-help measures that can significantly alter the state of your health.

• Consider a Liver imbalance an invitation to change your life in pleasant ways. It is the excuse you have been waiting for to give yourself a break, work less, cut back on perfectionist tendencies, laugh, play, dance, and indulge much, much more. Consider a class in yoga or meditation not as work, but as time to create a space for yourself that the rest of the world cannot invade. Competition, ambition, family demands, and being the best do not enter these doors once you begin.

Male Health Difficulties

In the self-care field, an ever-growing wealth of information on women's health issues is available, but very little information for men has reached the public. Our emphasis in this section is on the prevention of imbalances affecting men.

Male Impotence

Many men experience impotence for at least a short period in their lives. "Most people I see have impotence in combination with an overall lack of vitality associated with lifestyle," comments Peter. These men do not realize that not eating well, not getting enough sleep, overworking, having sexual intercourse too often, drinking alcohol, and smoking contribute to impotence. "Cigarettes are the worst because they cut the supply of blood and oxygen to the penis," comments Peter.

Oriental Medical Energetics

1) Kidney Yang Deficiency or Jing Deficiency

"Overindulgence in alcohol causes the energy to rise to the head. If intercourse is attempted, the energy will not be in the right place and the Kidney Qi will be drained, causing damage and degeneration of the lower back," said the ancient physician, Qi Bo, to the Yellow Emperor.[1] According to the Chinese medical model, male impotence reflects a dysfunction of the Kidney organ and meridian system. The Kidneys store Jing—generative energy—and Yang (Fire) essence, a Deficiency of which is caused by the lifestyle habits mentioned above. Accompanying symptoms may include chronic nephritis, hypothyroidism, chronic lumbago, and urinary dysfunction. A Deficiency of both Yang and/or Jing will certainly cause underperformance in the sexual function. Pushed to extremes, this condition could literally burn a man out.

Self-Help Strategies

—Warm and tone the Kidney Yang.
—Strengthen the Jing.
—See a practitioner.
—Abstain from sexual emissions until recovered.

2) Kidney Yang Deficiency with Liver imbalance

The Kidney Yang Deficiency often appears with a Liver component. The Liver meridian encircles the genitals, manages the Blood, and metabolizes testosterone, an androgen produced in the testes that can be used in the body only after it has been metabolized in the Liver. Thus, as Peter points out, "An impaired Liver may equal an impaired libido." Symptoms of Liver imbalance may include anxiety, a congested feeling in the chest, depression, distention and pain in the sides and ribs, headache, irritability, red eyes, and sore neck and shoulders.

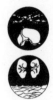

Self-Help Strategy

—See a practitioner for an expert diagnosis of the nature of the imbalance.

3) Emotional factors

Impotence can have an emotional aspect, as well. A deteriorating relationship can be one factor in a man's lack of arousal, and treatment for an impotence problem includes addressing relationship difficulties. The Taoists believed that "the brain is the most important sexual organ." To them, a loving partnership of mutual caring and regard played a vital role in healthy sexual functioning.

Self-Help Strategy

—Consider counseling if emotional factors are beyond your control.

4) Adult onset of diabetes

The adult onset of diabetes, which inhibits circulation, is another major cause of impotence. Doctors speculate that as many as 70% of diabetic men are impotent.

Self-Help Strategy

—See a practitioner; acupuncture treatment could help increase circulation.

5) Use of drugs blocks the parasympathetic nervous system.

Some prescription drugs for high blood pressure block the parasympathetic nervous system, which can affect erection. Impotence is in some cases a side effect of Tagamet, a drug treatment for ulcers.

Some antihistamines and decongestants have blood-constricting effects that inhibit erection. Ask your doctor to prescribe another drug: there are some without those side effects. Chinese herbs can also be used effectively to treat allergies, high blood pressure, and ulcers, conditions for which medications with impotence-causing effects are prescribed.

Internal Applications

• Avoid tobacco.
• Also try to stay away from foods that aggravate the Kidneys and Liver, and avoid overeating in general (see under Food Influences in Chapter 3).

• Eat warming foods to tone Kidney Yang (see under Food Influences in Chapter 3).

• Also eat more foods that cleanse, tone, and relax the Liver (see under Food Influences in Chapter 3.)

• A diet that is toning to the Middle Burner is recommended. The Middle Burner, an energy center in the thorax, is the source of all postnatal Qi (see Chapter 3 and the section Adapting to Stress and Building the Immune System).

• Have Four Things Vegetable Soup (see the Appendix).

• Try adding these strengthening herbs to your diet: Siberian ginseng, Korean ginseng (to increase the body's natural steroids), sarsaparilla root, and dioscorea. Mix in 2 to 3 g Chinese licorice with 3 to 5 g of any of the herbs just listed and decoct. Drink once a day.

External Applications

• To begin treatment, it is recommended that men abstain from sexual activity for at least 100 days in order to cultivate reserves of newly accumulating sexual energy.

• Adequate exercise encourages the development of strength and stamina that can extend from the track, field, court, or dojo to the bedroom. Another positive effect of stretching and unifying exercises (those that incorporate deep breathing) is that they also improve sexual performance.

Prostatitis

The prostate gland is a walnut-sized organ surrounding the urethra at the neck of the bladder in men. Its secretions are one component of semen. Prostatitis, or inflammation of the gland, is a common ailment of men who are prone to urinary tract infections. This condition easily becomes chronic and is difficult to treat.

Symptoms of prostatitis include pain in the perineum area, pain when sitting, difficulty in urination and ejaculation, a feeling of never being able to empty the bladder, dribbling urine and occasionally blood, and lower back pain. This condition is difficult to treat because the gland has a poor blood supply, making it hard for the immune system to defend it against infection. Conventional allopathic medicine can do little for the condition beyond treating it with antibiotics—a dubious course of action because the antibiotics have trouble reaching the site, again due to poor blood supply.

Oriental Medical Energetics

Stagnation of Cold in the Liver

Cold Stagnation in the Liver channel causes the contraction of the channel, with the Stagnation of Qi and Blood in the lower abdomen and genitals. Pain in the perineum area, distention and a cold sensation in the lower abdomen, swelling or contraction and pain in the scrotum, cold limbs and a general dislike of cold accompany urination difficulties; hernia and intestinal spasm are other symptoms that could accompany prostatitis.

Self-Help Strategies

—See a practitioner. Cold needs to be dispelled from the Liver channel and lower trunk area.

—Eliminate all prostatic irritants.

—Reduce stress and stop overworking.

—Try to exercise in adequate amounts.

Internal Applications

• Coffee, decaffeinated coffee, all sources of caffeine, alcohol, tobacco, red pepper, and excessively spicy food irritate this condition.

• A diet of fresh, organic fruits and vegetables (lightly steamed), sea vegetables such as kombu, hijiki, and nori; nuts, seeds, and whole grains. In particular, bee pollen, yellow and orange vegetables such as Hokkaido pumpkin, winter squashes, and turnips; sunflower seeds, and walnuts (grind the nuts and use as a powder) are said to benefit the prostate gland.

• Include more foods that tone the Kidney/Bladder (see Chapter 3).

• Cornsilk (*Zea mays*, diuretic and tones the Kidneys), dandelion leaf (slightly diuretic, cleanses and tones the Liver), parsley, and raspberry leaf (a urogenital tonic) teas are full of minerals and have diuretic properties. They are nonaddictive.

• Dehydration puts tremendous stress on the prostate; drink ample quantities of fluid—hot tea and room-temperature water—every day. Sip continuously.

• Add a little safflower or wheat germ oil (they are polyunsaturated), to your daily diet. Evening primrose or borage oils are also recommended.

External Applications

• Try hot and cold packs over the perineum in the following order: begin with a hot pack for 4 to 8 minutes. Follow with a cold pack for 1 minute. Repeat this process 2 to 3 times.

• The Kegel exercises, which were developed for pregnant women who lose control of urination, can benefit men with prostatitis. To do them, first locate the pubococcygeal muscle that runs from the pubic bone to the coccyx. This muscle stops the flow of urine. To exercise it, try clenching it as if trying to stop the flow of urine. Now release. Clench again for a count of 3, relax for 3. Repeat this 10 times. Then push out as if trying to urinate, 10 times. Repeat the whole sequence 2 or 3 times.

• A daily massage to the perineum area helps to prevent prostatitis. A monthly self-exam is also recommended.

Prostate Enlargement

Enlargement of the prostate gland is a complaint of 50 to 60% of males over 40 years old in the United States.[2] The prostate grows larger, surrounding and compressing the urethra and subsequently the bladder itself. Early symptoms include a thin urine stream, an increased urge to urinate, inability of the sphincter muscle to relax, and difficulty starting and stopping the flow of urine. Most people remain at this stage. If the condition progresses, however, complications such as cystitis, uremia, and kidney infection arise because the bladder does not empty completely.

Internal Applications

• Regulate the diet according to the recommendations listed under Impotence, above.

- Men in the first stage of prostate enlargement can benefit greatly from herbal treatment. A visit to a qualified acupuncturist who also practices herbalism is highly recommended.
- Take cornsilk, dandelion leaf, parsley, and raspberry leaf teas to ease inflammation and reduce the frequency of and discomfort when passing urine.
- In addition, men with prostate enlargement should try eating "super foods:" Korean ginseng, Siberian ginseng, and bee pollen. Sea vegetables such as kombu, hijiki, and nori are "super" in that they contain all the necessary trace elements.
- Increasing your intake of vitamin A and beta-carotene will increase sperm count: eat yellow vegetables such as kabocha pumpkin, butternut squash, and carrot, apricot, leafy green vegetables (especially dandelion greens), sweet potato, red pepper, and broccoli.
- Spirulina, a blue-green algae, is one of nature's original whole foods. It is a complete protein, contains the entire B-complex, and is rich in beta-carotene and minerals including calcium, iron, phosphorus, zinc, potassium, magnesium, and selenium. It is also an immediate source of energy.

Endnotes

[*1] *The Yellow Emperor's Classic of Internal Medicine*, Chapter 3, trans, Moashing Ni (Boston: Shambhala Publications, 1995), p. 11.
[*2] Michael Murray and Joseph Pizzorno, *Encyclopedia of Natural Medicine* (Rocklin, Ca.: Prima Publishing, 1991), p. 480.

Memory and Brain Function

Until now Western science has accepted the degeneration of brain function as normal in its elderly population, but research on aging has produced substantial evidence that the aging process itself is not responsible for many of the disorders we associate with it. Memory loss and Alzheimer's disease are among the most feared symptoms of old age.

Oriental Medical Energetics

Memory, according to Oriental medicine, is related to the body's vital, regenerative essence, Jing. Jing is responsible for correct growth and development, proper sexual maturation, reproduction, a healthy pregnancy, normal aging processes, bone and hair development, and the formation of the brain. Out of the Jing also arises the Marrow, which, again, is that insubstantial substance out of which the spinal cord, bone marrow, and Blood are created. Jing resides in the Kidney. Abundant supplies of Jing are believed to foster a long, healthy, full life, while a lack of Jing results in physical or mental retardation in children, premature aging, fatigue, and sexual dysfunction.

1) Depleted Jing

Loss of memory occurs as we get older and deplete the Kidney Jing regenerative energy. Symptoms of aging, such as hair loss, graying hair, wrinkles, loss of teeth, weakening of bones, a gradual worsening of hearing and sight, impotence, lack of vaginal secretion, lack of interest in sex, poor memory, inability to think clearly, and poor concentration are due to a loss of Jing. We deplete this vital essence by overworking, overstudying, excessive sexual activity, eating a poor diet full of chemicals and preservatives, excessive spices, and caffeine, and by drinking alcohol.

A weakness of Kidney Jing may also occur if the parents are aged and not in good health when children are conceived, as we see in the case of children born with congenital defects. Childbirth can deplete a woman's supply of Jing, but not always; everyone knows radiantly healthy mothers of large broods. It simply depends on one's physical constitution and lifestyle, and on how one replenishes one's supply of Jing.

Self-Help Strategies

—Maintain a Jing-nurturing diet.

—Take Kidney-tonifing herbs and foods.

—Practice meditative techniques that build the energy of the *hara* (the hypogastric plexus, a ball of nerves located about two inches below the navel).

Internal Applications

• Refined sugar negatively affects the brain; avoid simple sugars—white, refined sugar, brown sugar, and corn syrup—in favor of complex carbohydrates. Try malt as a natural sweetener, and reach for fruit rather than sugary foods when you have a relentless sugar craving.

• Allergies to dairy and wheat products could cause or contribute to memory loss. Nutritionists suggest cutting them out for a month and then, if no memory improvement occurs, slowly putting them back into the diet.

• The B vitamins—particularly choline and B_6—and amino acids play an important role in maintaining or increasing memory power. A lack of these nutrients or the overconsumption of processed, refined, fried, and junk foods are bound to affect the concentration and memory. All food contains small amounts of vitamin B_6; those with the highest amounts are brewer's yeast, carrots, chicken, fish, meat, peas, spinach, sunflower seeds, walnuts, and wheat germ. Significant amounts of choline are contained in egg yolks, legumes, meat, milk, and whole grain cereal.

• Include foods that tone the Kidney Yang and Jing (see Chapter 3).

• Superfoods such as ginseng, bee pollen, lecithin, and ginkgo nuts (*Ginkgo biloba*) are highly recommended for memory improvement. (See the section Adapting to Stress and Building the Immune System and the Glossary.)

• The ginkgo tree is native to Japan; its power of resistance is legendary there. It was the first plant to blossom in Hiroshima the spring after the atom bomb was dropped. The leaves have attracted much attention for their ability to increase blood flow to the brain. The extract and capsules can be purchased in most health food stores. For memory enhancement, try taking two capsules twice a day for a two-month trial period. It is nontoxic.

External Applications

Keeping the mind active and participating in the world are two very important ways of keeping the mind functioning longer. Practice remembering games, such as repeating words of a language studied in one's youth, to help keep the memory aspect of the mind supple.

When you have to memorize information that you will have to pull out very soon, such as for an exam, studying in the morning is better than in the evening, say students of memory. If you are studying for something you will need weeks or months later, study during the afternoon when your long-term powers are at their peak.

The real secret to good memory, moreover, may be lodged in how much attention one pays to what one wants to remember. If you do not think remembering a certain piece of information is important, low motivation will certainly hinder your memorization of it. Also, developing concentration through meditation practice fosters the power of attention and is probably the best memory enhancer of the lot.

2) Heart imbalance disturbs the Shen.

Traditionally in Oriental medicine there is little discussion of the brain organ itself. Rather, we talk about the mind or Shen (Heart or spirit energy), which resides in the Heart. The Shen is "the organizing force of the self, reflected in the mental, emotional, and expressive life of an individual," writes Ted Kaptchuck in *The Web That Has No Weaver*.[1] Strong Shen in a person is identifiable through clear eyes, vital energy, emotional and physical balance, clarity of expression, and the existence of concerns beyond the personal.

The connection between the brain and the Heart functions is intimate, according to Oriental medicine. The Heart function closely resembles that of the cerebral cortex, the part of the brain that gives rise to thought, perception, sensation, speech, communication, and memory. The sharpness of the brain's functioning very much depends on the condition of the Heart and the Shen it houses.

Healthy spirit (Shen) depends on an abundance of Qi and Jing. Together, these three energies make up the Three Treasures, the three vital energies of the body without which we would not be living, thinking creatures. The Three Treasures exist in dynamic relation; a lack of any one of them will affect the others. A lack of Qi and Jing may result in unhealthy or disturbed Shen, which manifests as muddled thinking, poor memory, confused speech as a result of unclear thoughts, and restless, jumpy eyes that are unable to focus on one object.

Overwork, long-term emotional upset, and exceedingly high stress levels or other forms of mental irritation can throw the Heart organ and channel off balance, affecting the Shen or even evicting it from the Heart.

A person can have plenty of Qi and Jing, however, and still have disturbed Shen. In the cases above, the depleted Shen is manifested as palpitations, shortness of breath upon exertion, fatigue, lethargy, depression, a dull spirit, and vagueness. The quick, clear functioning of the brain will be reduced as well.

Self-Help Strategy

—Cultivate the Shen through meditation, stress reduction, and working or studying less.

Internal Applications

• Alcohol, cigarettes, drugs, excessive sexual activity and other compulsive behaviors should be avoided.
• See the Internal Applications for depleted Jing, above.

External Applications

• Qigong, tai'chi, zazen, Taoist Shen meditation, yoga, prayer, and conscious cultivation of compassion refine the Shen. Practicing these techniques dramatically improves the power of concentration. Increased mental strength, clarity, willpower, and perception improve the function of the brain. A realization of your connection to the world around you, a feeling of oneness of body and mind, connection with other people and concern for others' well-being, calmness and joy, among other things, can result from the consistent cultivation of these practices.
• Exercise helps the body get rid of excess stress, and it increases the body's intake of Air Qi, or oxygen, which increases vitality, energy levels, and brain function.

• Talking to trusted friends, a teacher, or a therapist can help by releasing stress, excessive and confusing emotion, and fostering a sense of calm and relief.

• Challenge the brain with stimulation: read, do crossword puzzles, play memory games or chess, study a new language.

Endnote

*1   Ted Kaptchuk, *The Web That Has No Weaver* (New York: Congdon & Weed, 1983), p. 45.

Motion Sickness

No matter how much one loves to travel, a serious bout of motion sickness can definitely spoil the ride. In motion—or travel—sickness, nausea and vomiting are induced by traveling in a car, boat, or plane. It affects adults and children alike, although children are more susceptible.

There are two causes of motion sickness. Physically, weak muscular activity in the stomach slows down or prevents digestion—a situation that could be caused by stomach acids that are not strong enough to digest foods—and then the motion triggers nausea or regurgitation (most frequent in children or elderly people), along with constipation, anxiety, and "nerves."

Functionally, one's sense of balance may not be working properly, as happens when the balance organs inside the ears and the balance mechanism of the eyes send different messages to the brain. For example, if the inner ear senses the rocking of the boat but the eyes are looking at the inside of the boat, which appears to be level, the brain becomes confused. This affects the nervous system and may cause vomiting.

Internal Applications

• Over-the-counter drugs for motion sickness are best avoided. Use the ginger remedy instead. Peter recommends that this universal remedy for motion sickness be taken *before* traveling. Grate about a square-inch chunk of ginger into a cup, pour boiling water over it, and steep for 10 to 15 minutes. Drink while still warm. Put the remainder in a thermos, and during the trip, drink a little whenever you feel queasy. Add a little crushed cardamom and fennel for more of a digestive-system boost—they address symptoms of nausea, stomach cramps, dyspepsia, and flatulence.

• Long-distance travelers may prefer dried ginger capsules. The dosage is two #00-sized capsules at intervals when needed. Do not swallow the ginger without the capsule coating, which protects the esophagus. Chewing fennel and cardamom seeds can help control feelings of nausea during travel.

External Applications

• Good posture is essential to countering motion sickness. Curling up on the car seat or slumping down into it prevent energy from reaching the stomach. Avoid reading or playing games that involve looking down. It is far more helpful to keep the eyes looking out the window. If traveling in a car, keep the windows open at least a crack at all times. If you are at sea and can take walks out on deck, do so frequently.

• Try the Nei Guan (P.C. 6) wrist massage, which has been used for thousands of years in China to treat nausea. The point lies between the two tendons about 2 inches up the inner arm from the wrist crease. Massage here for a couple of minutes or apply pressure with a fingernail or the blunt end of a toothpick.

Respiratory Problems

Includes: asthma, bronchitis, bronchial problems related to pneumonia.

Western medical doctors diagnose asthma as an episodic constriction of the bronchial tubes resulting in wheezing and a difficulty in exhaling. Childhood asthma occurs in allergy sufferers. It may also be accompanied by eczema and hay fever. Late-onset asthma is thought to be less a response to the environment than one set off by something within the body.

Asthma can be triggered by external stimuli such as dust, pollution, pollen, feces of the house dust mite, foods containing sulfites and other additives, the behavior of another person, exercise, a sudden change in breathing pattern (breathing heavily or laughing), or respiratory infection. Sometimes it has no obvious cause. It can come and go without warning.

Severe cases can be fatal. The strong drugs that doctors prescribe to treat it are often addictive, very toxic, and ineffective. In most cases they are aimed at treating the symptoms and not the underlying cause. They tend to perpetuate asthma and reduce the chance that it will disappear on its own. Many inhalers contain steroids.

One note on terminology: Phlegm has been capitalized in the text to mean an condition of congealed mucus that creates a chronic, deeply rooted energy block in the body. This condition is different from mucus, which has not congealed or not yet created a deep-rooted, difficult-to-disperse energetic block in the system.

Oriental Medical Energetics

There is no diagnosis "asthma" in Oriental medicine. It is understood to be a symptom of an energetic imbalance or a combination of imbalances in the body. Bronchial problems and pneumonia are understood as part of the same syndrome.

1) Wind invasion

Bronchial asthma and chronic and acute bronchitis result from a Wind attack. Wind, as you remember (see Chapter 2), is associated with sudden change. Wind can be literal, as

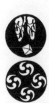

with the weather, or it can occur on a physiological or emotional level in the body. Wind attacking the Lungs results in an itching throat, nasal congestion, sneezing, headache, body aches, and a dysfunction of the dispersing and descending functions of the body, which means that the Lungs are unable to send the accumulation of mucus and fluid that is building down to the Kidneys, where fluids are further processed. (For a description of how the Lung acts on the Kidney, see the Five Elements Theory, Chapter 2.)

One is most susceptible to External Wind invasion during the change of seasons, says Peter, when the weather is capricious and erratic. Other factors that could anticipate an attack of Wind are sweating after working or partaking in recreational activities outdoors. Wind enters the body through the pores, which open when the body sweats. As the body cools, the pores contract, trapping the Wind inside. External Wind attacks frequently occur when the immune system is weak and the Protective Qi cannot provide a barrier to defend it.

The energetic manifestation of change (Wind) combines with Heat or Cold. Chills, a watery nasal discharge, white sputum, and a lack of sweat indicate a Cold Wind attack.

A fever, sore, dry throat, and thick yellow nasal discharge indicate an attack of Heat and Wind.

Self-Help Strategies

—Clear Wind and Heat or Cold through a combination of acupressure, herbs, moxibustion, and ginger baths.
—Balance and strengthen the whole body.
—Avoid drafts when the body is wet.

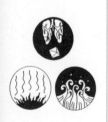

2) Qi is blocked by fluid in the Lungs that turns to Phlegm. The body fluids are exhausted by Heat.

Asthma, bronchitis, pneumonia, and pulmonary abscess result when Qi is blocked by fluids stuck in the Lungs that turn to Phlegm, and body fluids are exhausted by Heat. The above condition of Wind/Heat or Wind/Cold has progressed to create a chronic condition of Heat in the Lungs. The Lungs, meanwhile, have lost their ability to rid themselves of mucus, and the mucus-like fluid builds up and congeals—much in the way mulch and rotten food in a compost pile will combust if left to lie long enough—to become a hard, thick Phlegm (a physical condition and an energetic principle). The Phlegm blocks the passage of Qi as Heat exhausts the body fluids.

Self-Help Strategies

—See a practitioner. This is a serious condition. The practitioner will work to clear the Heat and eliminate Phlegm, correct the Lung function, clear toxins, and soothe asthma.

3) Kidney Deficiency leads to fluid accumulation in the Lungs.

Mucus and coughing occur when fluids accumulate in the Lungs because the Kidney, which is supposed to receive fluids and Qi from the Lung, is Deficient. The point here is that the root of the illness is the Kidney rather than the Lung. The practitioner will work to balance the Kidneys as well as to clear the mucus.

Self-Help Strategies

—Reduce overwork and excessive studying.

—Tone the Kidney.

4) Stagnant Liver Qi lies at the root of fluid in the Lungs.

This is a complicated situation. Mucus and phlegm build up in the Lungs because the Liver Qi Stagnates, moves up into the subcostal region, makes movement in the diaphragm difficult, then invades the Spleen and hampers its ability to transform foods and fluids. These accumulate and become Dampness that rises to create sticky mucus in the Lungs. See the adjacent diagram for a clearer picture of the relationships among the organs.

Self-Help Strategies

—Tone the Spleen.
—Clear Stagnant Liver Qi.

Internal Applications

• Avoid alcohol; coffee and caffeinated beverages; cold, iced, and raw foods; drugs, chemicals, food additives and preservatives; excessively spicy foods; heavy red meats; overeating and excessive intake of fluids.

• Refrain from eating foods that produce Phlegm (see Chapter 3).

• Eat more warming foods that nurture the Spleen and aid its function of transporting fluids (see Chapter 3).

• Include foods that tone the Kidney and aid elimination of excess fluids (see Chapter 3).

• Ingest foods that clear Phlegm (see Chapter 3).

• Job's tears, soaked until soft and then cooked by itself or with brown rice, is an excellent Lung-toning agent. Alternately brew roasted hatomugi to make a tea for the same purpose.

• A decoction of black beans is said to help eliminate mucus. Add 2 tbsp. black beans to 600 ml of water, cover, soak for eight hours or overnight, and boil in a heat-resistant earthenware pot until the water is completely black. Add a small amount of barley malt to sweeten, if necessary, and drink the liquid twice a day. Eat the beans.

• Eat several baked garlic cloves a day to help eliminate the cough and mucus. Folk remedy users also recommend squeezing the stems and leaves of fresh garlic plants and taking 20 drops of the essence to break down phlegm. If the garlic odor is too strong, try Kyolic garlic capsules, which are odorless.

• Ginkgo nuts are said to be good for coughs and breathing difficulties. Traditionally they were used in treatments for tuberculosis. Eat 5 to 10 ginkgo nuts a day, cooked in simmered dishes or stir-fries, or roasted.

• To alleviate bronchial coughs, grate lotus root and ginger and place in a pot with 5 to 6 times the amount of water as vegetable; add a dash of salt and bring to a slow boil. Turn down the heat and cook for 15 to 20 minutes. Drink 2 or 3 times daily between meals.

• **Ginkgo Nut Anti-Asthma Oil**
    100 g shelled and skinned ginkgo nuts
    rapeseed or canola oil

Place the nuts in a glass bottle or earthenware container, then fill to the top with the oil. Wait 100 days before using. Use like ordinary cooking oil, whenever you feel an attack of asthma coming, following an asthma attack, or during bouts of bronchitis.

• Daikon Radish and Lotus Root Energy Cooler
   For yellow mucus coughs such as in acute bronchitis.
   $^1/_4$ c grated daikon radish
   $^1/_4$ c grated lotus root
   1 tsp. grated ginger
   dash of tamari or naturally fermented soy sauce

Mix the ingredients and simmer in $^3/_4$ cup water. Reduce liquid to $^1/_2$ cup and drink quite warm. Children can have this beverage with a little honey instead of the ginger.

External Applications

• A traditional folk remedy to alleviate asthma is the hot red pepper plaster, a mixture of flour, water, and pepper that is spread and wrapped up in a light cotton fabric to protect the skin, and placed on the chest. When the wheezing and coughing start, add flour to ground red pepper in a proportion of 10 parts flour to 1 part pepper. Add water, knead, and spread onto half of a piece of fabric that is two times bigger than the entire chest area. After spreading, fold the clean side over the gluey spread and apply to the chest area. Occasionally lift the plaster to see if the skin has turned red, and once it has, remove the plaster and wash the area with tepid water.

• A tofu plaster over the respiratory organs can help draw out the internal Heat of acute bronchitis. Wrap a standard-sized block of tofu in a towel and squeeze out the liquid. Then place the tofu in a mixing bowl, add 1 to 2 tbsp. flour, and mash with a fork using a light cotton cloth; follow the rest of the directions for a grated red pepper plaster, above.

• A pickled plum (umeboshi) plaster is recommended for a bad cough. Mix 5 parts umeboshi meats with 1 part flour and 1 part water, spread on a thin cotton fabric, fold over, and apply to the sternum and lungs. See also the section on Colds, Coughs, and Sore Throats for more cough remedies.

• Friction applied twice a day to the throat, shoulders, chest, upper and lower back with a dry towel is said to reduce the severity of asthma attacks.

Acupressure for bronchial asthma, acute bronchitis, and other forms of Wind attack
(See BodyMap for exact location of points and the meanings of the abbreviations.)

   L.I. 4—Activates Qi in the entire body, dispels Wind/Heat and Wind/Cold, and warms the Lungs.
   LU. 7—Activates the dispersion function of the Lungs, combines with L.I. 4 to clear Wind/Cold, and promotes sweating.

Sexuality

Without the basic harmony of Yin and Yang, neither medicines refined from the five minerals, nor the most potent aphrodisiacs, will be of any use.[1]

Classic of the Plain Girl

In Oriental medicine, an aphrodisiac is defined as a practice or potion that increases sexual potency in males (we include females). Three legendary women were instrumental in teaching the Yellow Emperor how to increase his longevity through proper sexual practice: Su Nu, the Plain Girl, Hsuan Nu, the Mysterious Girl, and Tsai Nu, the Rainbow Girl. Records of their dialogues with the Yellow Emperor and Peng Tze, a Taoist adept who is said to have lived for 800 years, date from the third-fourth century B.C.

Traditionally, the Chinese viewed sexual relations between men and women as the primary earthly manifestation of the universal principles of Yin and Yang, or polar energies of light and dark, hot and cold, dry and damp, summer and winter. As such, sex was believed to be necessary to human health and longevity.

The Complete Classic of Su Nū

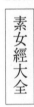

SŪ NŪ JĪNG DÀ GUÁN
SO JŌ KEI TAIZEN

Oriental Medicial Energetics

1) Lack of Jing

The trick was to partake in healthy sexual relations without spending too much sexual, regenerative energy—Jing—which in Western terms amounts to the biochemical nature of the body, including the endocrine system. It is this generative energy that determines basic growth patterns and body constitution, and the ease with which one develops and ages. The body's supply of this energy can be depleted through overwork, illness, nervousness, lack of sleep, poor nutrition, drugs, liquor, and "improper thinking." Premature aging and sexual difficulties are two problems that result from an imbalance involving Jing.

There is a Taoist theory that women have an endless supply of sexual energy because they do not release their sexual juices and essence during sexual climax. That is why ancient Chinese aphrodisiacs and sexual rejuvenators were basically for men. The authors have found, however, that women who have menstrual disorders, who tire easily, feel a general coldness in their bodies, and have low self-esteem hardly possess the healthy sexual appetites that our Taoist forefathers and some contemporary Taoist male peers assume they have. Therefore in this section, we will also discuss ways to increase female sexual energy.

There is no quick fix for impotence, lack of sexual desire, or other sexual dysfunctions, says Peter. Although Oriental medicine is famous for its aphrodisiacs and sexual enhancers, they should be used with discretion, he warns. One's purpose for taking them must be clear.

If a person wants to have sexual intercourse with many partners and to increase sexual performance, taking aphrodisiacs will help in the short run by stimulating the energy of the Liver meridian, which Oriental medicine says is necessary to vital sexual performance. But doing this for an extended period results in depleted Kidneys and Jing, which can lead to premature aging, impotence, and other serious health problems.

Self-Help Strategies

—Relax, reduce stress; calm the mind.
—Tone the Kidney Yang and Jing.
—Increase general vitality.
—Abstain from sex until fully recovered.

2) Other lifestyle factors

A weakened sex drive, says Peter, is often indicative of problems in other areas of one's life, such as strained marriage relations or a dissatisfactory relationship, a lack of physical exercise, inadequate nutrition, overwork, stress, or a combination of any of the above. Simply reaching for the turtle's blood tonic, or going to see a practitioner for herbal and acupuncture treatment, will not take care of the problem.

Self-Help Strategy

—Take an honest inventory to discover whether any of the above-mentioned factors apply to you. Take measures to resolve the situations where applicable.

3) Imbalance in the Pericardium meridian system

The Pericardium meridian does not have a corresponding organ in Western medicine. Nevertheless it plays a major role in the dynamics of healthy sexual appetite and function.

Correlated to the heart's protective sack, the pericardium, this meridian is in charge of protecting the Heart from emotions generated by other organs. (In Oriental medicine, each organ is said to release specific emotions, such as anger originating from the Liver and fear from the Kidneys.)

The sex role of the Pericardium channel is related to the powerful, hot, Yang energy of the Kidney organ and meridian, which provides a great deal of vital, sexual energy to the body and mind. Oriental medicine says that the feeling of love expressed through sexuality comes from the Pericardium meridian, which unites physical desire with emotional love from the Heart. A balanced Pericardium meridian contributes to equilibrium between sexual desire and emotional love.

Self-Help Strategies

—Restore balance to the Pericardium and the Kidneys by reducing stress, working less, and resolving personal and relationship difficulties.

—Reduce foods and beverages that strain the Kidneys (see Chapter 3).

External Application

• A pressure point on the Pericardium meridian helps balance this energy channel. Pericardium 6 is located on the inner arm, three fingerwidths up the arm from the wrist crease between the two thick tendons. Pressing in here for several minutes on each arm helps to calm the mind and opens a restricted chest, releases the diaphragm, calms the Stomach, and relieves nausea. It will relieve the feeling of neediness that may arise when one's emotional needs are not being met and that may lead to using sex as a means to fulfillment.

Chinese Aphrodisiacs

The most potent Chinese aphrodisiacs are derived from medicinal plants and certain animal parts. Sexually tonifying herbs include Chinese lycium berries, ginseng, dang gui, Chinese cinnamon, *Cornus officinalis*, and Chinese licorice. Aphrodisiac ingredients from animals read like a Shakespearean curse: deer horn or antler, red spotted lizard, and the dried genitalia of certain animals, for example. Parts from these and other animals were and are still being used due to the phallic shape they share, or because they are believed to contain some "essence" of that animal's virility. Many of these animals are on the Endangered Species List and are being hunted to extinction for their aphrodisiac properties. We do not condone the use of animal parts as medicine or as aphrodisiacs. The body can be nurtured to a state of optimal sexual arousal and function through a combination of diet, botanicals, and exercise.

In Oriental Medicine, the theory of "like cures like" is based on the Chinese cosmological view of the world. Humans are considered to be a microcosm of the universe, which works according to the principles of growth, change, and development. All things are manifested according to these principles, and things that look similar or share similar structures embody similar energies, the Chinese reasoned. In the West during the medieval era, this idea was called the Doctrine of Signatures. According to the doctrine, a root that looks like a man will be tonic for the whole person. Ginseng is exactly that.

Internal Applications

• Oysters, which may look like testes to some people, are said to tonify Yang energy and sexual energy. Oysters, beef and sheep testes, and turkey are all used in Oriental medicine as sexual strengtheners. Women eat them as well for a surge of strength and vitality especially after giving birth.

• To tone the Kidneys, eat pork kidneys; (see the section on Preparing Organ Meats in the Appendix). Kidney meat porridge, with a sprinkling of Chinese cinnamon, cooked rehmannia (di huang), lycium berries, chestnuts, walnuts, red dates, dang gui, and poria, is prescribed for Deficiency symptoms such as impotence, a lack of sexual interest, spermatorrhea, lumbago, and premature ejaculation. (See Chapter 4 for directions on making porridge. Add the herbs to the rice from the beginning of cooking and put them in a cheesecloth or tea filter bag so they can be easily removed after cooking.)

• Chinese Cinnamon is a strong Yang tonic, especially for Kidney Yang energy. It is famous in China as a strengthener and sexual tonic. In general, the thicker the cinnamon bark, the better. It has a full-bodied rich taste, much fuller than Western culinary cinnamon. Do not take cinnamon unless you have a Cold constitution, polyuria, frequent night urination, impotence, aching knees, and lumbago. It is contraindicated for Hot types.

• Bee pollen, ginger, ginseng, pumpkin seed (for men), dang gui (for women), sesame seeds, and Siberian ginseng are all recommended to increase general vitality and sexual energy. For specific formulas, we refer the reader to Ron Teegarten's book, *Chinese Tonic Herbs*. (See Recommended Reading in the back of the book.)

• Ginseng decoction is recommended for enhancing sexual vitality, but add other herbs to the decoction to make it a more balanced and effective tonic. Recent studies have shown that Chinese licorice combined with ginseng is a specific pituitary tonic improving overall hormonal functioning. Chinese licorice and Chinese dried red dates are "guiding" herbs, which take the herb where it is most effective in the body. Add a little of both when you make ginseng.

• **Ginseng Toner**
> 5 g ginseng
> 2–3 g Chinese cinnamon
> 2–3 Chinese red dates
> 2–3 g Chinese licorice

Add herbs to 1½ cups of water and decoct in an earthenware pot or traditional Chinese herbal cooker. Drink a few times a week or more if the constitution is weak.

• **Female Toner**
> 3–4 slices dang gui
> 2 red dates
> 2–3 g lycium berries
> 2–3 slices dried Chinese licorice
> 10–20 g chicken meat (the meat from a drumstick or wing), or a chicken's egg (in shell)

Decoct in 1½ cup of water in an herbal cooker until reduced by one-third. Drink daily for up to one month (eat the meat or the egg) after childbirth, for anemia, or for a general feeling of cold in the body until the body is strengthened and warmed. The decoction also increases libido. Healthy women can drink it once a week, but should leave out the licorice periodically. Stop drinking the toner while menstruating—dang gui increases the flow of menstrual blood. The dates and berries can be eaten, as can the dang gui, but most people find dang gui's distinctive taste unpleasant. The herbs can be recooked once, then thrown away. Start from scratch the next time.

• Codonopsis can be substituted for ginseng in any formula, when ginseng has too strong or aggressive an effect on the system. Codonopsis has Neutral energy, a Sweet taste, and it tones the Yin in cases of Yin Deficiency. It has vigor-restoring properties similar to ginseng's but does not make one jittery or hot, side effects of taking ginseng. It is also tonic to the Middle Burner (the Lung and Spleen energy), and thus strengthens the whole system. It balances False Fire symptoms such as stiff neck and shoulders, headaches, and high blood pressure, and it can be taken every day. (Leave out the licorice occasionally.) Use it as the

Chinese do—add one or two 2-inch roots to soups and stews in winter, along with 1–3 g each of lycium berries, dioscorea, Chinese red dates, and astragalus (if you have some).

External Applications

Solitary walks, deep abdominal breathing, meditation, or a meditative and physical practice such as qigong or yoga will all help calm the mind. To increase vitality a regular, well-balanced diet, sufficient sleep, and regular exercise are essential. See Chapter 6, Pain and Vitality, in Part I of the book.

The reader may hesitate at sexual abstinence, the third Self-help Strategy. But if and when you abstain, do so completely. The Taoists believe that sexual energy resides in the area called the Gate of Life, along the spine around the adrenal glands and kidneys. Sexual stimulation of any kind, including reading erotic books or magazines or watching videos, will cause energy to descend to the genitals, and upon sufficient sexual stimulation, the energy will stay there and be discharged whether one has intercourse or not. This is the energy you want to conserve, for a while at any rate.

Once you start to regain the sexual vitality you were lacking, it is extremely wasteful and nonsensical to dissipate it before making a full recovery. Waiting will not only help to correct the dysfunction and strengthen the whole body and sexual vitality but will also allow the mind and the consciousness to see the role that sexuality can play in one's life and general well-being.

A Ginseng Aside

Ginseng, or *Panax ginseng*, the "King of Herbs" in Oriental medicine, is perhaps, of the Chinese herbs, the best known to Westerners. It is the most effective sexual tonic in the Chinese pharmacopeia. "Ginseng" means "sacred person" root and it is estimated to have been known in China for 5,000 years. The Chinese say it replaces Qi energy to meridians and organs. Both men and women can use it with beneficial tonic and energy-enhancing effects.

Western and Eastern scientists have researched ginseng extensively. The root is a proven stimulant, affecting mental and physical activity. It strengthens and protects the body under strain, improves the function of brain cells, stimulates the function of the endocrine system, and protects the organism from radioactive elements. It contains steroids similar to the human sex hormones testosterone and estrogen. Ginseng's active ingredients also regulate the endocrine system, mildly increase metabolic activity, and stimulate the circulation and digestion.

There are several species of ginseng (genus *Panax*; family *Araliaceae*), four of them indigenous to China—Wild Manchurian Tung Pei (white), Yi Sun (also white), Shiu Chu (red), and Kirin (golden yellow). Tung Pei ginseng is the best and extremely expensive. It is very rare and and almost never used. It is fat, white, and some roots are up to 200 years old. Yi Sun ginseng, which looks much like Tung Pei, is also wild. Chinese Taoist master Share K. Lew, a 77-year-old herbalist, qigong and tui na massage teacher, and priest from Canton, China, who now lives in the United States, cautions that wild ginseng could cause an adverse reaction if taken for tonic purposes and should be used only as a medicine, prescribed by a practitioner.

Ginseng

RÉN SHEN
NIN JIN

Red Ginseng

HÓNG SHĒN
KŌ JIN

Kirin Ginseng

KI RIN
NIN JIN

Red ginseng nurtures Yin energy and sedates False Fire symptoms—anger, high blood pressure, tension headaches, and excessive sexual desire. Kirin ginseng has a slightly mellowing effect and can be taken by Yang types who find Korean ginseng too strong and heating.

Korean ginseng (also *Panax ginseng*) is indigenous to Korea. It is considered more Yang than the Kirin; Tierra attributes this to the Koreans' practice of steaming the roots to preserve them from insects. The steaming turns them red and adds warmth, thereby producing a better sexual tonic. On the other hand, people with high blood pressure, or other heart or liver problems, should stay away from it. The active ingredients in American ginseng (*Panax quinquefolium*; Araliaceae) are similar to Chinese ginseng, as are its uses, although its effects are said to be milder. It also increases body fluids. People who find Chinese ginseng too strong may prefer American ginseng's more subtle effects.

Siberian ginseng (*Eleutherococcus senticosus; Araliaceae*) is an herb with properties similar to Panax ginseng. The bark of this root is used to treat lack of vitality and low endurance. It is given to athletes to improve performance, is antirheumatic, reduces swelling and edema, and aids poor circulation and general coldness in the body. (See the section Adapting to Stress and Building the Immune System.)

Avoid instant ginseng products, such as ginseng tea. These products contain too little ginseng to be of any significant use to the body, and the quality of ginseng in them is usually poor.

Cook ginseng in an enamel, glass, or earthenware pot. Before cooking a root, Chinese herbalists often cut the top off. Master Lew says this is because the top negates the effect of the rest of the herb. Cooking and ingesting the "head" acts as an antidote, canceling out any adverse reaction to the ginseng. To cook, bring an ounce of herb to boil in $1^1/_2$ to 2 cups of water, turn down the heat, and continue cooking until the water is reduced by one-third to one-half. Drink warm, before meals. The root may be recooked and drunk again.

Western Barbarian
Ginseng

XĪ YÁNG SHĒN
SEI YŌ SAN

Endnote

*1   Daniel Reid, *The Tao of Health, Sex, & Longevity* (New York: Fireside, 1989), p.263.

Skin Disorders

Includes: acne, boils, eczema, rash, rough skin due to exposure to detergents, warts; miscellaneous tips for clear, smooth skin.

The mutual correspondence among one's complexion, the movement in one's vessels, and the condition of one's skin... is comparable to the mutual correspondences among the beating of a drum and the sound produced, and also to that of an object and its shadow, or a sound and its echo. They cannot be separated from each other![1]

The Yellow Emperor's Classic of Medicine

Chronic problems with the skin are among the most difficult to treat, regardless of the therapy employed, but Oriental medicine can significantly improve chronic skin problems such as acne or eczema. Treatment consists of adjusting the balance of the entire body, not simply focusing on attacking and ridding the system of visible symptoms. Eradicating the symptom without treating the underlying imbalance will force that imbalance to manifest itself in another, often more serious, way.

Oriental medicine usually treats skin problems with herbs and dietary changes. Shingles, or herpes zoster, can be cured with acupuncture alone. The Japanese have a long tradition of treating skin diseases with moxibustion.

Why is Oriental medicine often effective in treating skin problems where other treatments fail? The primary adjustment of the balance of energy and the regulation of the Blood are probably the most important reasons. Skin eruptions due to stress also benefit greatly from the calm that acupuncture induces. Acupuncture, herbal medicine, and moxibustion strengthen the immune system, increase white blood cell count, strengthen the body's anti-inflammatory function, and stimulate the release of antihistamines naturally if that is what the body requires. Oriental medicine treatment will also accelerate the repair of damaged tissue and improve blood circulation, promoting a faster replacement of skin cells and tissue healing.

Oriental Medical Energetics

Skin disease is understood in the West to be the result of an allergic reaction, a fungal, bacterial, or viral infection, or a problem with the nervous system. The Eastern view, on the other hand, sees skin problems as an attack by Wind and Heat blocking the channels, which in turn affects the Blood and pushes Damp lodged in the body out the pores, creating a rash or other eruptions.

Acne

An outbreak of pimples is not confined to our teen years. Acne occurs when changing levels of sex hormones (androgens) stimulate the increased activity of the sebaceous (oil) glands, which then produce more oil than necessary and block the pores. Blocked pores appear as blackheads and whiteheads. If the pimples become infected by bacteria, acne can turn into fiery red pustules.

1) Excessive Heat Imbalance

In Oriental medicine, a case of acne is diagnosed as a Heat Excessive condition resulting from improper diet, stress, and the body's inability to eliminate excess Heat from the system.

Holistic healers uniformly agree that diet is related to the outbreak of acne. Says Peter, "A doctor had one of my patients on antibiotics for years for his chronic acne, while another doctor told him his pimples were the result of excessive sweat produced during athletic training. No one asked him about his diet, which consisted of a high proportion of alcohol and sweets, and a very low proportion of grains and vegetables." The patient's treatment consisted of a combination of acupuncture, herbal medicine, and topical applications of aloe vera. This course of treatment was accompanied by dietary changes. He was asked to cut out all Heat-producing foods—red meat, fried foods, sweets, and alcohol—which he did. He then went on a diet incorporating steamed vegetables, fish, white chicken, whole grains, some fruit, herbal teas, and water. His skin cleared up within six months and has stayed clear, though he has relapses of acne whenever he drinks alcohol.

The school of macrobiotics holds that the location of the outbreak of pimples on the face indicates where mucus deposits and fatty acids are occurring in the body. Acne on the cheeks indicates problems with the Lung and upper respiratory tract. Acne between the eyebrows indicates Liver and Gallbladder trouble, while a pimple above the upper lip and on the chin points to the prostate gland or sexual organs; and acne on the forehead suggests intestinal problems.

Self-Help Strategies

—Clear Heat.
—Cleanse the body's elimination channels.

Internal Applications

• Avoid alcohol, coffee, tea and cola, cold foods and beverages, chocolate, oily deep-fried foods, red meat, and oily fish such as tuna, yellowtail, and shellfish. (The last is controversial. Many Oriental-style therapists suggest avoiding it, while many Western-style nutritional therapists say to include it. Try your own controlled experiments with shellfish.) Also avoid saturated fats, ice cream, refined white sugar, honey, maple syrup, white flour, sweet rice, and mochi made from polished sweet rice.

• Eat more cooling, clearing, fiber-rich foods (see Chapter 3).

• Include foods full of fiber, including most vegetables and whole grains, and sticky or gelatinous foods that encourage elimination, such as taro potato, yamaimo potato, kanten (agar), nattō, and konnyaku (yam cake).

• An allergy to dairy products can trigger skin outbreaks. Consider testing for an allergic reaction to dairy products by going off all dairy products for one month. After a month, gradually add one item at a time to determine whether you are allergic. A food allergy can manifest immediately or can have a delayed adverse effect. Sometimes chronic symptoms for which no explanation can be found are the result of a food allergy. Acne, dark circles and puffiness under the eyes, chronic diarrhea, malabsorption, chronic infections and chronic inflammation are common signs and symptoms. For more information on food allergies, see Recommended Reading in the Appendix.

• Strengthen the Kidneys, the organ primarily involved in the body's elimination of wastes. Tired or overworked Kidneys can lead to acne. (See the section on Kidney Tonics in Chapter 3.)

• When cooking azuki beans add about 1 liter extra water while cooking, cook the beans until soft, and reserve this water. Let cool slightly before drinking. The liquid can be refrigerated and warmed before ingesting, three times a day, to strengthen the Kidneys.

• Lycium berries are indicated to tone the Liver and the Kidneys, two filtering organs of the body. These small, oblong berries can be purchased in dried form and added to soups and stews. You can reconstitute them in hot water, *sake*, or wine and add them to salad dressings or sauces. They have a sweet, pleasant taste and add wonderful color to tofu or greens.

• Roasted Job's tear (hatomugi) tea and dokudami tea cool and cleanse the Blood and clear out toxins exiting from the skin.

• Fish liver oils have been found to aid skin in its tumultuous teen years. Take 2,500 I.U. of vitamin A in the form of fish liver oil to reduce sebum production and the thickening of skin around the oil follicles.

Fish and fish livers with high vitamin A content include angler fish (20,000 I.U. per 100 g), dried yatsume eel (25,000 I.U.), eel liver (15,000 I.U.), cod (6,300 I.U.), squid (5,000 I.U.), grilled eel meat (4,700 I.U.), tuna (954 I.U.), and bonito (832 I.U.).

External Applications

• Regular applications of aloe vera gel or vitamin E oil can help reduce scarring. Apply directly onto the skin morning and evening.

• Rice bran can be applied over red, fiery acne to help take the redness out and relieve inflammation. Place about 1/4 cup onto a handkerchief, then tie the ends to make a small pack. Add to a quart of water and boil until the water takes on a warm beige color. Let the water cool slightly. Use the liquid as a facial wash, and daub the rice bran pack onto acne patches. Repeat daily until the red clears.

• Fresh or dried dokudami leaves that have been heated in a skillet the same way as fresh saxifrage, above, can be applied to the skin. The treatment should begin to take effect in two or three days. Or make a rinse with infusion of dokudami tea (10 g dried leaves to 1 liter water, bring to a boil, turn down heat and simmer 5 minutes. Cool until safe to use. This will keep in the refrigerator for several weeks; warm gently before using.). Daub onto skin during a bath or after a shower when the pores are open, leave on for a few minutes, and rinse off with warm water.

Boils and Other Skin Eruptions

A boil is the painful inflamed swelling of a hair follicle and the skin around and underneath it that becomes infected to form a red, raised nodule. As the condition progresses it spreads, becoming localized pus pockets with white centers. It is sometimes accompanied by a mild fever. Boils are most often seen on hairy parts of the body that are frequently exposed to friction, pressure, or moisture. Several of these in one location join together to form a carbuncle.

Oriental Medical Energetics

Oriental medicine views boils as a build-up of Toxic Heat and Damp in the body that in treatment is most often cleared with herbal medicine.

Self-Help Strategy

—Clear the Heat and Damp.

Internal Applications

• Avoid sugar and simple carbohydrates that tax an already depressed immune system.

• Reduce foods that increase Damp in the body (see Chapter 3).

• Allergies, usually to food, play a role in the formation of boils. See a nutritionist to discuss the possibility of trying a rotation or elimination diet to determine which foods, if any, are allergens to your system. For a brief introduction to food allergies, we refer the reader to Murray and Pizzorno's *Encyclopedia of Natural Medicine* (see the Bibliography).

• Try to incorporate foods into the diet to clear Damp (see Food Influences in Chapter 3). Shrimp is on the list, but stay clear of it in this case.

• Also eat more foods to clear Heat (see Food Influences in Chapter 3).

• Blood-cleansing foods aid the efficiency of the circulation system. Try to make a serious effort to eat more chlorophyll-rich and other blood-cleansing foods (see Chapter 3).

• Di huang (rehmannia) decoction is indicated for cleansing and supplementing Blood. See a practitioner for a proper diagnosis and prescription.

• Burdock root is recommended for cooling and cleaning impurities from the Blood. You can add burdock root to simmered dishes; soak it for 10 minutes in cold water before cooking. Or make a tea: cut it up or grate it, add $1^1/_2$ liters of water, and boil down until fairly dark. Drink several times a day.

• Take goldenseal (15 to 20 drops in a cup of warm water) to fight infection. Or try comfrey, fresh is best but the powder or tincture is fine (250 to 500 mg daily or follow the dosage listed on the bottle) once a day for up to (but no more than) 10 days. The American Food and Drug Administration has issued a warning on comfrey. See the Appendix for more information.

External Applications

• Burdock root (*Arctium lappa*, *A. majus*) grows wild in many parts of the world, from Asia to Europe and North America, and its seeds and roots have been used in Chinese medicine for hundreds of years. The wild roots can be used for medicinal purposes (although they are said to be difficult to dig up) but are not recommended for eating. The burdock root has antibacterial and antiseptic properties. Make a poultice for the skin by grating a piece of root—the amount depends on how large and how many boils you have—together with the leaves if you can get them, straining the liquid, and dipping a piece of cloth in the solution. Wrap this around the affected area, cover the cloth with gauze, and tape on to hold in place overnight.

• Burdock root and Chinese licorice make an effective rinse for boils. Add 3 g Chinese licorice to freshly grated, finely chopped, or dried burdock root, in a cup of hot water. Let the water cool to lukewarm (about 15 minutes), soak a small piece of clean cotton fabric in the infusion and apply directly over the affected area.

• Kuzu, available at Oriental and natural food stores, is sometimes misidentified as arrowroot starch. The two are separate entities. Mix kuzu root powder with some warm water and apply directly over boils and blisters. This helps drain accumulated fluid.

• Diluted ginseng extract painted over boils is said to help drain them without breaking the skin.

Eczema

Eczema is the most common form of chronic skin disease, making up nearly 40% of the skin complaints that Peter treats. Typically, eczema appears as small, itchy skin lesions that give off a yellowish fluid. The itching is so bad that gloves are often placed on babies' hands to prevent them from scratching. After a while the skin begins to turn thick and brown. In acute stages, the skin becomes swollen, itchy, crusty, and cracked. New tissue that grows from affected areas is thick and dark. Often the skin is overgrown with *Staphylococcus aureus*.

Eczema is seen a lot in Japan. It usually appears on the face, neck, upper trunk, wrists and hands, the folds of the knees and elbows, and the groin. It is commonly found in people with a personal or family history of allergies and asthma.

Oriental Medical Energetics

The eczema/Lung connection is logical in Oriental medicine terms when we consider that the Lungs are said to control the skin. An imbalance in the Lung organ or meridian could affect the skin's condition. Internally, in addition to a Lung imbalance, Kidney inflammation, gastrointestinal difficulties, or gynecological problems could be related to the appearance of eczema. All of these can be caused or exacerbated by stress and emotional tension. External causes may include soap, cosmetics, shampoo, or synthetic clothing. There is no single known cause of eczema.

Acupuncture treatment aims to clear Wind, Damp, and Heat, or toxins lodged in the organ channels. These influences affect the Blood. Nearly all the patients Peter has treated for eczema have had either a Lung complication, signifying trouble taking things in, or a

Large Intestine problem, which means trouble putting things out. Eczema responds fairly well to acupuncture treatment, although it is generally slow to clear. It is important to be patient and not give up after a couple of weeks or even months of regular treatment. There is no instant cure.

Self-Help Strategies

—Use natural skin-care and health products.
—See a practitioner.

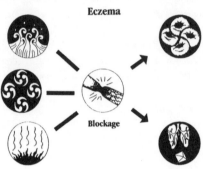

Eczema

Blockage

Internal Applications

• Avoid foods that produce Damp and increase Heat (see Chapter 3).

• Determine and eliminate food allergens. If you suspect that you have food allergies, consult a qualified practitioner to help you work out an elimination or rotation diet to discover and control them.

• Eat foods rich in vitamin A (see Adapting to Stress and Building the Immune System in Part II).

• Incorporate into your diet foods that have a cooling effect on the body (see Chapter 3).

• Foods rich in zinc, including brewer's yeast, egg yolks, fish, legumes (particularly lima and soybeans), mushrooms, poultry, seafood (especially oysters and sardines), soy lecithin, pumpkin and sunflower seeds, pecans, and whole grains are also indicated. Take zinc supplements with caution. Daily dosages of more than 100 mg can depress the immune system. Less than that can improve its function. The proper zinc/copper balance must be maintained, which is why we suggest increasing your zinc intake through food rather than by taking supplements.

• Eat foods that clear up Phlegm in the Lungs when eczema is accompanied by an asthmatic condition: daikon radish, garlic, fresh ginger, kohlrabi, marjoram, mustard greens (see Food Influences in Chapter 3).

• Fresh burdock root can be chopped and boiled to make a tea, or mix burdock root powder 4:1 with warm water and drink. Inulin is the primary active ingredient in burdock root. It helps correct the underlying defects of the immune system that are commonly found in people with eczema. It also fights staph infection.

External Applications

• Grate burdock root and strain so that much of the liquid is removed. Spread the pulp onto a piece of clean cotton fabric to make a plaster and place directly onto affected areas. Leave on for several hours. Do this once a day. If no positive results appear within a week, discontinue the treatment.

• Herbal formulas containing Chinese licorice or German chamomile may be effective topical applications for temporary relief of itching.

• Steep 2 tbsp. of cooling chrysanthemum-flower tea and strain. Add a touch of naturally fermented vinegar to the infusion and apply to rash. This is also useful for rashes that appear on babies' heads. Naturally fermented vinegar contains no artificial ingredients that might trigger an allergic reaction. It can be found in your local natural foods store.

• Be careful with cosmetics. Chemicals and toxins in your cosmetics could aggravate the condition. Natural shampoos, make-up, and hair sprays (nonaerosol type) can all be found at health food stores. Baking soda makes a good shampoo for sensitive scalps.

Acupressure for eczema
(See BodyMap for exact location of points and the meanings of abbreviations.)

—To help control the itching and allergic reaction, rub and massage below the 7th cervical vertebra—the large protruding bone at the base of the neck—and points to either side of it. Press fairly hard so that you feel a ringing sensation under the skin.

GV. 20—Helps control allergic reaction, clears Wind and Heat in the head.

Rash

Rashes are commonly seen along the pathways of a meridian or nerve, usually signifying Heat or Damp lodged in that channel or along the nerve. But how can you decipher which it is? To start with, check an acupuncture chart to see if the rash follows along the lines of a particular meridian. See a practitioner for chronic rashes.

1) Heat lodged in the channels
Heat problems may be accompanied by a fever, redness and swelling, heat and itching in the affected area, thirst, and perhaps constipation, depending on whether the heat is blocking only certain meridians or the whole body.

2) Damp lodged in the channels
Dampness is recognizable by a lack of appetite, nausea, and perhaps abdominal bloating and indigestion, if it is affecting the entire body. When the condition is compounded by Wind, the rash will spread, or disappear, only to reappear in another area. You might have the sensation that something is trapped under the surface of the skin. Rashes are difficult to treat by oneself. Seek professional help for chronic rash.

Most of the patients Peter has treated for rash have had Lung, intestinal, or Liver problems in addition to the rash. The skin is called the "second Lung" in Oriental medicine, referring to its function of taking things in and out. Trouble in the intestines suggests difficulty in elimination. The Liver is one of the primary filters of toxins from the system.

Self-Help Strategies

—Clear Heat/Damp.
—Cool the Blood.

—Control itching.

—Follow up with treatment to clear the Liver, Intestines, and Lung.

Internal Applications

• Foods that create Damp interfere with digestive and eliminative processes. Dairy products are prime examples. They also aggravate a mucus condition in the Lungs. Greasy, oily, deep-fried foods and junk food are big trouble, as is ice cream. Avoid them.

• Spicy foods affect and sometimes damage the Lungs. The Heat can exacerbate itching. These, too, are best avoided.

• Cut down on Hot and Warm foods such as lamb, dairy products, black pepper, red pepper (see Chapter 3).

• Incorporate foods that drain Damp (see Chapter 3).

• Roasted Job's tears (hatomugi) tea helps clear the Lungs and is a cooling agent for the rest of the body.

• Chrysanthemum and Chinese green teas are cooling teas.

External Applications

• Aloe vera is one of the best topical applications for skin problems. First check to see whether you have a reaction to it—dab a little on a test patch of skin before smearing it over the rash area. It cools the skin and promotes tissue repair, and encourages the growth of healthy new skin cells.

• Use a rice bran poultice rather than soap to wash. Or place rice bran in a small fabric bag or on cheesecloth or a handkerchief, the ends fastened with a twist tie, and add to the bath. You can add an infusion of loquat leaves to the rice bran bath for relief of rash, scabies, and other skin diseases.

• Use moxa on the point Uranaitei for rash.

Skin Irritation from Exposure to Detergents

Tap water containing high amounts of chemicals is so bad in some cities that fashion models routinely wash their skin in bottled distilled water rather than risk destroying their complexions. That, along with the use of harsh and environmentally unfriendly detergents, has contributed to what the Japanese call "housewife rash," or red splotches and eruptions on the skin due to overexposure to water and detergents. The fingers and backs of the hands become dry and itchy; if the condition is left untreated, the inside of the hand will become chapped and cracked.

The following suggestions are effective in eliminating dry skin, which is understood to be a problem with the circulation in general.

Internal Applications

• Avoid cooling foods—raw fruits and vegetables, iced or chilled drinks, melons and nightshade fruits and vegetables (tomatoes, eggplants), millet, sugar, and sweets.

• Eat Blood tonifying foods (see Food Influences in Chapter 3).

• The herbs mugwort and dang gui tone the Blood. Mugwort can be drunk as a tea, dang

gui as a decoction and added to soups, stews, and broths.
• If the condition includes lower back pain and dark circles under the eyes, add Kidney-nourishing foods and di huang (see Chapter 3).

External Applications
• Wear rubber gloves every time you put your hands under water.
• Aloe vera is probably the best topical application, followed by vitamin E oil. Just prick a capsule open and squeeze out as much oil as you need. Do this two or three times a day until the dryness clears up.
• Sesame seed oil is also high in vitamin E. You can rub this onto the skin directly from the bottle.
• Eggplant tips were traditionally used in Japan to help smoothen and soften the skin.

Common Warts

Warts are rough, irregular, flat, or raised skin growths caused by a virus. They tend to appear when the immune system is weakened. They can be found on the hands and feet, forearms and face, or anywhere on skin that is exposed to continual friction or rubbing. In general, warts do not cause pain or itching. Since they are highly contagious, it is best to leave them alone unless they begin to cause problems.

Self-Help Strategies

—Strengthen the immune system.
—Try to avoid constant friction to the same areas on skin.

Internal Applications
• Avoid foods that are difficult to digest, iced drinks, and cold foods that weaken digestive functioning, which in turn weaken the immune system. Deep-fried, greasy-oily foods, red meat, and dairy products also fall into this group.
• Eat easy-to-digest foods that strengthen the digestive function: green leafy vegetables, root vegetables, squashes, whole grains, and legumes are recommended.
• Eat to strengthen the immune system. (See the section Adapting to Stress and Building the Immune System in Part II.)
• Foods that detoxify Blood and improve circulation are also indicated (see Chapter 3).
• Brown rice porridge made with Job's tears (1:4) and sesame seeds can be eaten once a week as a general Blood tonic.
• Job's tears is also indicated in cases of flat or common wart. Boil 40 g in $1^1/_2$ c water and drink the decoction twice a day, or cook 60 g with 200 g rice and eat daily. Add some sliced dried shiitake while cooking, for flavor and an immune system boost. The root of the wart may become red and more inflamed, but then it dries up and disappears.

External Applications
• Crushed fresh mugwort leaves (*Folium Artemisiae*) placed over warts and changed several times a day will encourage them to drop off in anywhere from 3 to 10 days.
• A traditional Oriental remedy for warts is to place a ball of moxa (dried mugwort leaves)

the same size as the wart directly over the wart, light it, and burn it down. Use 5 to 7 balls and do this for two or three days. It should kill the root of the wart, which will turn black, dry up, and drop off within a few days.

• Also try burning moxa on L.I. 4 (see the BodyMap) to help remove the toxic build-up in the body. This treatment does not hurt. (See the section on moxa in Chapter 4, for instructions on its use.)

• A castor oil compress can be applied to warts. The oil not only heals warts, it stimulates the body's circulatory system and detoxifies the body in general. To make a castor oil compress, soak cheesecloth in the oil, then heat the cloth in the oven. Place over the affected area, wrap in gauze or plastic wrap, and fasten with medical tape. Keep on for several hours or overnight.

Clear, Supple Skin

Although aging skin is a natural phenomenon, martial artists and yogis, for example, are famous for smooth, glistening, vibrant skin that accompanies them well into old age. While there may be little we who are not martial arts masters or yogis can do to reverse the aging process of our skin, we can slow it down considerably.

Part of the secret is to improve the metabolism. When your body processes foods and eliminates toxins briskly and effectively, your skin reflects that condition by remaining supple and smooth. Again, a healthy metabolism results from a balanced diet, regular exercising, proper rest, and the efficient elimination of wastes.

Internal Applications

• Smoking cigarettes is especially detrimental to skin quality.

• Lightly steamed fresh vegetables, whole grains, legumes, a regular intake of Job's tears, roasted Job's tears tea (hatomugi-cha), soybeans and soybean products will improve the tone and quality of the skin. See the basic dietary guidelines in Chapter 3.

• Soybeans are beauty beans, say the Japanese. The legendary smooth skin of Oriental women is often attributed to their high intake of soybeans and soybean products such as tofu, miso, nattō, soymilk, and fermented black soybeans. In ancient Japan, "smelling of rice bran miso" was a common description of court women whose kitchens were full of aged miso used to make pickles. The women who actually plunged their hands into the paste were known for their young-looking hands.

Soybeans are high in malt, which slows down the formation of melanin in the skin. They are also rich in lecithin, and are known as "edible make-up" in Japan for their ability to break down unusable fats. They increase the body's metabolic rate and enhance its efficiency in excreting toxins while helping it maintain a balanced fluid level.

• Walnuts, according to ancient Chinese medical records, "keep a person healthy, the skin young-looking, and the hair black." Walnuts warm the Lungs and tone the Kidneys, Qi, and Blood. They have been considered important beauty supplements in China for centuries. Some Chinese practitoners say they are more effective if ground to a powder first and then ingested.

• Sitz baths are indicated to clear toxins from the Liver and the Kidneys. The baths strengthen the function of both organs and their channels, promoting the detoxifying function of both. See Chapter 4 for directions.

External Applications
• Loquat leaf, fresh soybeans and roasted Job's tears infusions (hatomugi-cha) make good facial rinses. Often in herbal medicine, what is good for the inside is also effective applied externally. Cucumbers, for example, when applied topically, will cool itchy, hot skin. They also work to cool internally.

Freckles and Liver Spots

Dark spots on the skin are usually attributed to Stagnant Blood as a result of Stagnant Liver Qi. When this manifests without forming a lump or mass, symptoms such as dysmenorrhea, amenorrhea, chronic vaginitis, emotional imbalance, dry skin, chapped lips, dark spots on the skin, yellowish complexion, thirst, a tendency to have cold hands and feet, constipation, and chilblains result. If several of these symptoms occur in addition to spots on the skin, please see a practitioner.

Self-Help Strategy

—Activate the Liver Qi and clear Blood.

Internal Applications
• Reduce—or better—eliminate foods that irritate the Liver: alcohol, coffee, sugar, and excessive sour foods such as sauerkraut and pickles.
• Avoid foods that depress the Stomach/Spleen functions: greasy, oily, deep-fried foods, dairy products, iced foods and drinks, fruit juices. Stay away from quantities of sweets, especially if you crave them. They cause Stagnation in the Stomach/Spleen, weakening an already weakened Earth element function, which weakens the body as a whole.
• Rice porridge with ginger, Chinese red dates, fennel seed, long green onion (leek), or azuki beans help clear Stagnant Blood. (Contraindicated for those with polyuria and nocturia.)
• Dokudami tea, habucha tea, and senna tea can all replace regular tea or coffee. Dandelion tea and coffee are also good for tonifying the Liver.

External Application
• A sitz bath is recommended to promote the clearing of toxins from the Liver and Kidneys. Strengthening the functioning of both these organs does wonders for the skin.

Endnote
*1 Paul Unschuld, ed., *Introductory Readings in Classical Chinese Literature* (Netherlands: Kluwer Academic Publishers, 1988).

Stiff Neck and Shoulders

The causes of chronic stiff neck and shoulders, a condition that starts as pain and swelling and develops into numbness and a gradual loss of movement in the arm, are myriad. Initially the pain can be due to negligent postural habits, such as sitting for too many hours in front of a computer or a television set, but even shivering with cold can start it. Muscle strain can occur with the sudden lifting of heavy objects. Athletic training can also cause soreness and stiffness if one overworks muscles one has not used in a while.

Oriental Medical Energetics

Internally, the pain could be rooted in imbalances in the circulatory system, the Liver organ network, or the Stomach/Spleen system. It could be a nerve problem, or it could be related to a problem with the throat and ears or with the teeth, or even, in women, to gynecological imbalance.

1) Imbalance in the Liver

One common scenario of neck and shoulder pain occurs when there is imbalance in the Liver meridian. Overwork, to begin with, strains the Liver, which is in charge of the body's "sinews," the tendons and muscles. Stress, large quantities of coffee and alcohol, and overeating contribute to the formation of a Heat condition in the Liver that rises and eventually manifests itself as a stiff neck and shoulders accompanied by red eyes, irritability, headaches, redness in the face, and perhaps hypertension. The situation has now become chronic and a challenge to rebalance. Simple massage might prove an effective palliative but would do nothing to prevent the pain from coming back; acupressure can be administered effectively to help treat the root of the imbalance.

Self-Help Strategies

—Eliminate the Heat.
—Clear Stagnation from the Liver.
—Reduce work and stress.
—See a practitioner of acupressure *and* acupuncture.

2) **The location suggests implication of the Lung meridian.**

Pain in the shoulder area in general indicates a relation to the Lung organ and meridian system. If sometimes one experiences pain in the shoulders, sometimes in the lower back, sometimes down the backs of the legs, the traveling pain is known as Wind. A dull pain on a cloudy or rainy day suggests a problem with Damp.

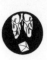

Self-Help Strategies

—Clear the Lung and its complementary Yang organ, the Large Intestine.
—Protect the body from cold and damp weather.
—See a practitioner to clear Damp.

3) **In women, Blood and Qi Stagnation in the Liver causes Heat to rise during menstruation.**

Shoulder pain due to menstruation is common. Oriental medicine diagnostics attributes this to Qi and Blood Stagnation of the Liver.

Self-Help Strategies

—Relax the Liver.
—Avoid overwork, stress, and anger.
—See a practitioner to clear Stagnation.

4) **Heart Blood Stagnation**

Pain shooting from the left breast to the shoulder and upper back and down the left arm to the little finger, accompanied by palpitations, tightness in the chest, fatigue, Cold extremities, and blue or pale complexion, lips, or nails may be due to Heart Blood Stagnation. This condition is known as myocardial infarction or angina pectoris in allopathic medicine.

No Self-Help

This condition is extremely serious—consult your doctor and a practitioner; complementary treatment may yield positive results.
Any pain, tightness in the chest with accompanying pain, or tingling in the arm should be checked by a doctor.

General Guidelines

Self-Help Strategies

—In nearly all cases of internally rooted stiff neck and shoulder pain, the most effective way to get rid of the pain is to eliminate fluid toxins and stagnation from the body.
—Improve eating habits, eliminate or reduce Hot foods.
—Reduce work and stress.
—Exercise consistently.

Internal Applications

• Foods that stress the Liver and overeating should be avoided (see chapter 3).
• Blood-cleansing and -toning foods are recommended (see Chapter 3).
• Qi-activating foods will aid Stagnant Qi and Blood conditions (see Chapter 3).

External Applications

• Hot baths followed by massages using Tiger Balm or camphor-containing creams can immeasurably alleviate back and shoulder pain. Take a hot bath nightly after half an hour of abdominal deep breathing and light exercise to increase circulation and aid the removal of lactic acid. A massage whenever possible is recommended.

• Ginger or daikon radish compresses can stimulate circulation in the painful area. To make, grate about $1/4$ cup of ginger root or daikon radish root, add to $1^1/_2$ cups water and cook over medium heat for 10 to 15 minutes. Strain the solution, return the liquid to the pot, and when just cool enough to handle, soak cotton towels in it. Wring well and place over the affected areas. (This is lovely if someone does it for you.) Cover with a dry towel or a sheet of plastic and a heating pad. The trick is to keep the compress warm for a while. If the heat treatment feels good, follow it up with some stick moxa. Gentle massage along inflamed areas will feel heavenly. Avoid a deep, intense massage: not all the toxins need to be pushed out at once.

Acupressure for neck and shoulder pain

(See BodyMap for the exact location of points and the meanings of the point abbreviations.)

S.I. 3—Press and rub for several minutes.

BL. 10—Press and rub to relieve neck and shoulder pain.

BL. 60—Press to relieve blockages in entire Bladder system, which stretches up into the head.

L.I. 4—Activates Qi and Blood in entire body.

Varicose Veins

Oriental Medical Energetics

Varicose veins are discolored, twisted, and dilated veins in the legs resulting from Blood Stagnation. The condition is seen in four times as many women as men, and up to 50% of adults in the West are affected by them. Imbalance in the Liver and Spleen meridians leading to Blood Stagnation is the primary cause of this condition. These two meridian systems run around the insides of the legs around the veins. The Heart channel, in charge of Blood circulation, may also be involved.

The condition can sometimes be accompanied by fatigue, dull ache, pain, discomfort, and a feeling of heaviness.

1) Sudden weight gain and lack of exercise

Sudden weight gain, pregnancy, and too little exercise increase blood volume in the body and weaken the walls of the veins in the legs. The veins collapse against gravity. Once the veins collapse, the valves that push and pump blood up from the legs to the heart are unable to function and the blood stagnates. Obesity and lack of muscle tone puts people at higher risk of developing varicose veins.

Women with varicose veins often have a history of menstrual problems, headache, stiff neck and shoulders, and pain in the lower abdomen, pointing to Liver Qi and Blood Stagnation. These symptoms commonly appear with varicose veins and are related. Breathing difficulties and varicose veins are also often seen together, which may have something to do with the fact that the Lung Qi helps the Heart to move the Blood.

Self-Help Strategies

—Avoid sudden weight gain.
—Implement an exercise routine.
—Move the Qi.
—Tone the Liver and the Spleen.

2) Constipation

Interestingly, varicose veins are rarely seen in cultures in which high-fiber, unrefined diets are eaten. We rarely see the problem in Japan and China, for example. People who eat few unrefined foods tend to strain more at the toilet, a suggested cause of varicose veins. The straining increases pressure in the abdomen, which obstructs the flow of blood up the leg. The increased pressure may, over a long period of time, weaken the vein walls in the lower legs. The straining could also weaken the wall of the large intestine and produce diverticula in the large intestine, leading, eventually, to hemorrhoids. Dietary measures can help control the formation and spread of varicose veins.

Self-Help Strategies

—Disperse the blocked food.
—See Constipation in the Digestive Problems section of Part II.

Internal Applications

• Foods that aggravate the Liver and overeating should be avoided. Alcohol, caffeinated drinks, dairy products, heavy red meat, refined sugar, tobacco, food additives and preservatives, and over-the-counter drugs are the worst offenders.
• Try to reduce your intake of foods that injure the Stomach/Spleen: iced drinks, cold or chilled food, caffeinated beverages, refined sugar, and heavy red meat.
• Include more foods to move Liver Qi Stagnation and tone Qi (see Chapter 3).
• A high-fiber diet is most important. Load up on whole grains, vegetables that are lightly steamed rather than raw, fruits, and legumes. The vegetables, fruits, and legumes add liquid to the digestive tract and promote peristalsis, while the high-fiber foods attract water to the tract, keeping the feces soft, gelatinous, and smooth. Smooth feces indicate an absence of straining.
• Eat plenty of garlic, onions, chives, and long green onion (leeks). All members of the allium family, they help maintain elasticity of the veins and capillaries.
• Eggplant tones Qi and Blood, removes Stagnant Blood, and heals swelling; it is commonly used to treat anal hemorrhage, carbuncle, skin ulcer, and breast inflammation.
• Other foods that remove Blood Stagnation are marjoram, mustard greens, onion (and many others listed in Chapter 3).
• Most people could benefit by increasing their intake of lecithin and vitamin E. Lecithin keeps the walls of cell membranes flexible. Vitamin E is active in cell repair and improves circulation. Adequate supplies of these nutrients are necessary in the prevention and repair of varicose veins. Whole grains, dark green leafy vegetables, nuts and seeds, and cold-pressed oils are rich suppliers of vitamin E. Soybeans are an excellent source of lecithin.

External Applications

• Movement, to increase circulation and maintain muscle tone, is extremely important. Both cardiovascular exercise—running, bike-riding, swimming, and hiking—and "soft" exercise—tai'chi, yoga, and walking—are fine. Pregnant women who want to be gentle on their bodies and are experiencing varicose vein problems may want to consider practicing these softer movements. Those with a history of thrombophlebitis would probably benefit from softer forms of movement, as well. The motion will produce a contraction in the leg muscle that pushes the pooled, stagnating blood back into circulation.

• Deep breathing also helps increase blood circulation and promotes a return of blood to the heart. Anyone with a heart problem could benefit from deep breathing exercises for at least 30 minutes a day. Consult with your physician before beginning any sports regimen. The half-hour of exercise can be separated into 15 minutes in the morning and 15 minutes in the evening if that is more do-able.

Weight Fluctuation and Weight Problems

Sudden shifts of weight upward and downward can be alarming, particularly when the cause is not understood and the problem feels out of control. Weight issues are complicated matters in terms of their relation to psychological factors. Once conventional allopathic medicine has ruled out any serious or life-threatening condition, Oriental medicine may be able to locate a solution. Rather than attempting to analyze the specific psychological make-up of a patient, the practitioner of Oriental medicine deals with the issue on a holistic level, considering energetic, physiological, and psychological factors part of the complete picture of disharmony.

Peter notes that many overweight people do not necessarily eat large quantities of food. Recent tests indicate that overweight is due more to the way foods are processed in the body (addressed by Oriental medicine Spleen therapy) or to the ingestion of certain combinations of foods.

Oriental Medical Energetics

Oriental medicine views unexplainable weight fluctuations as an imbalance affecting the digestive function, primarily the Stomach/Spleen system. The Stomach is said to receive the food and break it down, and the Spleen then receives the broken-down food, transforming it into a nutritive substance that combines with Air (oxygen) taken in from the Lungs, to produce Blood and Qi. This nutritive substance is then distributed to the rest of the body. An imbalance in the Stomach/Spleen function can result in both weight gain and weight loss.

1) Sudden weight gain or loss is due to a Deficient Spleen.

Weight loss or gain—combined with a gastric or duodenal ulcer, gastric neurosis, chronic gastritis, chronic enteritis, chronic dysentery or chronic hepatitis, a sallow complexion, anorexia, fullness and distention in the abdomen and epigastrium, abdominal pain relieved by pressure, tiredness in the limbs, nausea, loose stool, and a pale, flabby tongue with teeth marks—may be due to irregular eating habits, excessive worry, mental strain, or long-term illness.

At times, no matter how much one eats, if one can eat at all, no weight gain is possible despite a serious effort to gain. The body is not able to convert the food to energy and transport it to the tissues.

2) No matter how much you eat, you are still hungry due to Heat in the Stomach.

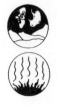

The previous condition can combine with Heat in the Stomach, which feels like no matter how much one eats, one is never satisfied. This symptom could be accompanied by bad breath, dry mouth, stomach pain until meals, and constipation or a stool on the dry side.

Some years ago, a friend who was in training for the competition of the Australian karate team came to Peter for help. He was training very hard, and reported that even though he was eating large quantities of steak, eggs, milk, and other dense, full foods, he was unable to gain weight. In fact, he was losing it. (He was tall, on the slim side, but had a large bone structure and wide shoulders.) Western doctors could find nothing seriously wrong with the man.

Upon further questioning, it was found that he was anxious about his karate training and university studies, and felt generally restless. Physically, he had a pain beneath the ribs in the solar plexus area, which could be temporarily relieved by eating. Shortly after meals he suffered from heartburn and was again soon hungry. He also had bad breath, frequent mouth ulcers, a sour taste in his mouth in the morning, a strong thirst for cold drinks, a dry stool, his muscles felt tight, and he complained that his flexibility was worsening.

Emotional anxiety and Heat-producing foods (heavy red meats, dairy products) can lead to extreme Stomach Heat manifesting as some or all of the symptoms listed above. Acupuncture, appropriate herbs, diet modification, and relaxation exercises gradually brought about positive change in the patient's condition. Although his naturally anxious personality and his hesitation to eliminate red meat and eggs from his diet challenged the course of treatment, he managed to make the necessary changes. He went on to win a place on the team and successfully completed his studies.

Self-Help Strategies

—Calm the Liver by reducing anger, irritability, or perfectionist tendencies.
—Cool the Stomach.
—Harmonize the Spleen.

3) Inexplicable weight gain and fluid retention are due to Spleen dysfunction.

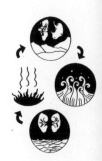

Another syndrome due to a Deficient Spleen occurs when the Spleen does not process food properly, resulting in fluid retention and weight gain. An excess of food and fluid are not converted into usable energy; the fluid accumulates, and weight fluctuations can be dramatic. Accompanying symptoms could include cold hands and feet, fatigue, a loose stool, a feeling of heaviness—especially in the hands and feet—fatigue in the limbs, and thirst that results in fullness or bloatedness after drinking.

Self-Help Strategies

—Regulate eating habits.
—Try to worry less, stop obsessive thoughts.
—Reduce or completely cut out raw, cold foods.

4) Deficient Kidney Fire results in a Weak Spleen that cannot process fluid and forms weight-increasing edema.

The Spleen and Kidney meridians are intimately related to each other and the endocrine system. Women are most often affected by disharmonies in these systems, which influences their weight. Eating quantities of raw and cold foods; drinking alcohol; keeping late hours; overworking or overstudying; physical or emotional stress; or excessive sexual activity can combine to produce a general feeling of cold, heaviness, fatigue or a lack of energy, hair loss; lower back pain with a chilled feeling; cold and aching knees; a loose stool; urinary blockage with edema, particularly in the lower body.

Peter treated a woman in her mid-30s who complained of puffiness and overweight. Her skin was very white and soft and she said she had been suffering from chronic diarrhea for a year. She tried over-the-counter drugs for the loose stool, but they did not help much. Her tongue was slightly swollen with teeth marks around the edges and was covered with a greasy margarine-like coat. She said she felt cold easily and was often thirsty, but whenever she drank she immediately felt full. Her appetite was minimal.

This woman ate a typical "fashion magazine diet," consisting of raw fruits and vegetables, a little meat and fish, and bread. She was diagnosed as having Dampness congestion (edema, bloating) due to Spleen Deficient Qi (no energy to convert food to energy). The Spleen is the source of juices of the body that circulate in the blood, saliva, and lymph. Dampness refers to edema or swelling, a surplus of fluid spilling over into the tissue. After the tissue becomes saturated, fluid runs into the joints, sinuses, abdomen, lungs, and the space between skin and muscle. Moxibustion was used to clear Damp congestion (edema), and she was put on a diet of cooked foods—consisting of steamed and cooked vegetables, broths, stews, and whole grains—to strengthen the digestive system. Herbs were later prescribed to further balance the energy. Her diarrhea stopped in two sessions, her appetite improved, and her mood changed. She became more positive and full of energy, and she shed the excess weight without strain.

Self-Help Strategies

—Stop aggravating the Spleen.
—Clear the fluid.
—Cut down on work and stress to tone the Kidney.

5) Eating at the wrong time of day

Normal weight depends, in part, on eating meals at the proper times. A 40-year-old man of medium height, who had been in Japan for eight years, came to see Peter for treatment. In the time he had been in Japan, his weight had increased from 75 kg to 108 kg. A Western medical check-up found his blood pressure to be within the normal range and his heart normal. He had no other major health problems.

Upon further questioning, Peter learned that the patient ate only one meal a day, a large dinner at 8 p.m. He never ate breakfast and had only a small snack for lunch. He drank large quantities of liquid—mostly water—never exercised, and sat reading in the evenings after dinner. He went to sleep around 10:30 to 11:00 p.m. and said he slept restlessly.

Basically, the man's weight problems were caused by imbalanced eating: consuming a large meal too late in the evening while starving during the day. In Oriental medicine, it is believed that each organ reaches a peak of activity for two hours a day. The peak time for the two main digestive organs, the Stomach and Spleen, are between 7 and 9 A.M. and between 9 and 11 A.M., consecutively. The morning hours are, therefore, considered the best time of day to consume a large meal.

In the patient's case, his meal came at the opposite end of the day, when the activity of the Stomach naturally slows down. Consequently, the food he ate was not being adequately broken down and transformed into usable energy. Furthermore, starving himself during the day had sent his system into survival mode, which slowed down his metabolism and resulted in his body retaining fat in anticipation of famine.

Treatment consisted of acupuncture, utilizing points such as ST. 36 and L.I. 11 to stimulate metabolism. The man's diet was modified so that he ate several small meals a day (although he had difficulty training himself to eat breakfast for the first several weeks), a smaller dinner at 7 P.M., and he was encouraged to take a walk after his evening meal. He gradually incorporated regular exercise into his routine. As a result, he lost 10 kg in eight weeks, had much more energy, and slept better. The last time Peter heard from him, he reported that he had become an avid fan of oatmeal with raisins for breakfast.

Self-Help Strategies

—Eat 2 to 3 times, or eat several small meals during the day.
—Eat well in the morning or early in the day.
—Keep evening meals light but nutritious.

Other problems with weight are understood as imbalances involving the thyroid gland, which is related to the Heart, Liver, and Spleen systems in Oriental medicine. Unexplained weight gain or loss should be treated by a professional.

Internal Applications

• Foods that injure the Stomach/Spleen should be reduced or eliminated altogether: iced drinks, cold or chilled foods, caffeinated beverages, dairy products, refined sugar, and heavy red meats.

• Avoid consuming large quantities of liquid if edema is a problem.

• Avoid liquid diets and extreme purges like the plague. They can damage the Spleen and make it extremely difficult for the body to ever regulate weight naturally.

• A Stomach/Spleen-nurturing diet of fresh vegetables—leafy greens and roots—eaten cooked and warm, fish and chicken, cooked tofu, whole grains and cereals, and legumes may make a startling difference.

• Spice foods lightly. Do not cover your fresh and lightly steamed vegetables with heavy, creamy, cheesy sauces.

• Dried tangerine peel, dioscorea, fresh ginger and garlic, Chinese red dates and lycium berries, can be added regularly to soups, stews, and simmered dishes to stimulate the Qi and strengthen the Stomach.

• Azuki and kidney beans help control edema. Sword beans and soybeans are considered essential forms of protein for people who also have a problem of overweight. Eat them regularly. Drink a cup of warm bean broth twice a day (see Appendix for directions on making).

Azuki bean sprouts are excellent. Eat the beans or sprouts with brown rice, and top with black sesame seeds. Chew everything well.

• Eat fish. Fish is full of Omega-3 oils, essential fatty acids that yield an enzyme necessary to the synthesis of prostaglandins, which are controlling factors in circulation, reproduction, metabolism, and growth. Scallops are said to help prevent fatty build-up and rid the body of fatigue. They are contraindicated in cases of edema.

• Kombu, a thick, wide seaweed used to make dashi (broth) in Japanese cooking, is recommended for its high mineral and low caloric content, and its ability to help lower blood pressure and inhibit the process of hardening of the arteries. It also helps prevent fat accumulation in the body.

• Drink genmai tea (sometimes sold under the misnomer "popcorn tea"), decoctions of Foetid Cassia seeds (habu-cha), and dandelion tea in place of coffee and black tea. Gentian tea is very bitter and can be drunk occasionally, after overeating or for bloating. Infuse 3 g in $1^1/_2$ cups water, separate into four portions, and drink throughout the day after meals.

External Applications

• Take a sitz bath as often as possible. This aids circulation, relieves fatigue, energizes and makes the body feel lighter.

• Exercise. You may have decided you "hate" it, but you can decide to change your mind and "like" it. Or you can decide you love yourself too much not to do it.

Acupressure for regulating appetite

(See BodyMap for exact location of points and explantions for the meaning of abbreviations.)

> ST. 36—Stimulates the metabolism and the digestive function. Moxa here is fine.
> C.V. 12—Warms and strengthens the digestive system.

Massage and apply pressure to the back area from just below the scapula bones to just above the hip bones, about 2 fingerwidths to either side of the spine on the muscle ridge.

Daily abdominal Qi massage

A daily Qi massage is excellent for relieving gas and constipation. Practice every morning and evening in sets of 9, starting with the left hand over the right on top of the belly button, then swinging down the left to just above the pubic bone and up the right side. Keep the motion smooth and fluid; do not stop the action. Breathe very deeply, expanding the lower abdomen with the inhalation. Imagine a white ball of light under the palms that energizes and moves the Qi with the hand movement.

BodyMap Points

English/Chinese/Japanese
(Chinese transliteration is in Pin Yin style.)

Lung 肺經
LU. 6, *Kongzui, Kōsai* 孔最—radial side of the inner surface of the forearm about 4 fingerwidths from the elbow crease. For cough and asthma.

LU. 7, *Lieque, Rekketsu* 列缺—in a groove at the bony wrist prominence about 2 fingerwidths from the inner wrist crease, radial side of the forearm. For cough, asthma, sore throat.

LU.11, *Shaoshang, Shoshō* 小商—radial side of the thumb at the corner of the foot of the nail. Counters cough, sore throat, asthma.

Large Intestine 大腸經
L.I. 4, *Hegu, Gokoku* 合谷—in a depression in front of the junction of the thumb and the forefinger. Activates Qi in whole body; used for headache, red and swollen eyes, nosebleeds, sore throat, arm pain, cardiac pain.

L.I. 10, *Shousanli, Tesanri* 手千里—bend the arm 90 degrees with the palm facing the waist. From the center of the elbow crease, measure down 3 fingerwidths. Press to find the tender spot. For abdominal pain, vomiting, diarrhea, shoulder and upper arm aches.

L.I. 11, *Quchi, Kyokuchi* 曲池—bend the arm 45 degrees with the palm facing the waist. Press the middle of the elbow crease. For Heat diseases: red painful eyes, sore throat, pain in upper back, shoulders, neck, dry skin.

L.I. 20, *Yinsiang, Geikō* 迎香—in a groove at the side of and level with the nostrils. Clears nasal congestion, nosebleeds, facial swelling.

Spleen 脾經
SP. 6, *Sanyinjiao, Saninkō* 三陰交—4 fingerwidths above the inner ankle bone, posterior to the tibia. Balances Kidney and Liver energies, tones the lower Yin channels, calms the mind, invigorates the circulation of Qi and Blood.

SP. 9, *Yinlingquan, Inryōsen* 陰陵泉—in a depression at the lower border of the medial condyle of the tibia. Removes Damp in the Middle and Lower Burners; clears fluid stagnation.

Stomach 胃經
ST. 6, *Jiache, Kyōsha* 頰車—clench teeth and feel for hard muscle in front of angle of jaw. Relax the mouth and a hollow will form; press there. For toothache, painful neck.

ST. 7, *Xiaguan, Gekan* 下關—place index and second fingers in front of the ear lobe; the second finger should fit into a groove below the cheekbone. For ear and tooth pain.

ST. 25, *Tianshu, Tensu* 天樞—about 3 fingerwidths horizontally (bilaterally) away from the bellybutton. For abdominal pain and distention, diarrhea, edema, menstrual irregularities.

ST. 36, *Zusanli, Ashisanri* 足三里—4 fingerwidths below the outer knee eye, on the lateral edge of the shinbone, in fleshy part at the point where it divides under pressure, 2 centimeters lateral to the crest of the tibia.

Readjusts Stomach/Spleen function, tonifies whole body, regulates heartbeat and rhythm. Also for stomach ache, distention, indigestion, vomiting, aching knee and tibia, swollen feet, diaphragm or throat blockage.

Heart 心經
HT. 7, *Shenmen, Shinmon* 神門—on the ulnar side of the inner wrist crease where a pulse can be felt. Regulates flow of Blood and Qi, calms the Shen.

Small Intestine 小腸經
S.I. 3, *Houxi, Gokei* 後溪—on the ulnar side of the hand at the end of the crease, behind the joint, when a loose fist is formed. Calms afternoon fever, night sweats, relieves edema.
S.I. 19, *Tinggong, Shikyū* 聽宮—between the tragus of the ear and the mandible joint where a depression forms when the mouth is wide open. Relieves pain, indicated for tinnitus, deafness, and madness.

Kidney 腎經
KI. 3, *Taixi, Taikei* 太溪—in a depression behind the inner ankle bone, in front of the Achilles tendon. Supplements Kidney Yin and invigorates Kidney Yang. Used for sore throat, deafness, asthma, irregular menses, insomnia, impotence, urinary frequency, lumbar pain.

Bladder 膀胱經
BL. 2, *Zanzhu, Sanchiku* 攢竹—in a notch at the inner corner of the eyebrow. For headache, visual dizziness, blurred vision, red and painful eyes, twitching eyelids.
BL. 10, *Tianzhu, Tenchū* 天柱—at the top of the trapezius muscle where it meets the base of the skull. Relieves neck and shoulder pain and Tai Yang headache.
BL. 12, *Fengmen, Fūmon* 風門—two fingerwidths lateral to 2nd thoracic vertebra; for cough, fever, headache, stiff neck, back and lumbar pain.
BL. 17, *Geshu, Kakuyu* 膈兪—on an imaginary line from the lower tip of the scapula bone to the space below the 7th thoracic vertebra. 2 fingerwidths bilateral to the spine. Main point for moving Stagnant Blood.
BL. 18, *Ganshu, Kanyu* 肝兪—about 2 fingerwidths bilateral to the lower border of the 9th thoracic vertebra. For hypochondriacal pain, blurred vision, red eyes, and mental confusion.
BL. 23, *Shenshu, Jinyu* 腎兪—on an imaginary line from the tip of the 12 rib to the space below the second lumbar vertebra point, about 2 fingerwidths bilateral to the spine. Promotes Blood production via Jing.
BL. 30, *Baihuanshu, Hakkannyu* 白環兪—about 2 fingerwidths from the midline of the back, level with the fourth sacral foramen. For irregular menses, seminal emission, and pain in the lower back and ribs.
BL. 40, *Weizhong, Ichū* 委中—midpoint of the crease at the back of the knee. For knee and lumbar pain. Do not use moxibustion.
BL. 60, *Kunlun, Konron* 崑崙—in the depression behind the outer ankle bone, in front of the Achilles tendon. For headache, stiff neck, shoulder and lumbar pain.

Liver 肝經
LIV. 3, *Taichong, Taishō* 太衝—in the hollow in front of the junction of the big and second toes. Calms and soothes the Liver, treats headache at the vertex, fullness in abdomen.
LIV. 14, *Qimen, Kimon* 期門—in the 6th intercostal space, 2 ribs below the nipple. For chest pain and pain under the ribs.

Gallbladder 膽經

G.B. 2, *Tinghui, Chōe* 聽會—in the depression in the front of the ear, where pulsation can be felt. Opens the ears, moves Qi, dispels Wind.

G.B. 3, *Shangguan, Jōkan* 上關—above the bone in front of the ear, where a hollow appears when the mouth is wide open. Frees the channels, boosts hearing; for headache, deafness, tinnitus, toothache.

G.B. 20, *Fengchi, Fūchi* 風池—in the hollow at the base of skull between the trapezius and the sternocleidomastoid muscles. Lateral to BL.10. Clears Wind and Cold from head, clears nasal congestion, dispels pain in head.

Pericardium 心包經

P.C. 6, *Neiguan, Naikan* 內關—about 3 finger-widths above the inner wrist crease between the two thick tendons on the inner forearm. Lies opposite T.H. 5, Waiguan. For tinnitus, shoulder and upper back pain and stiffness, and vomiting.

Conception Vessel 任脈

C.V. 3, *Zhongji, Chūkyoku* 中極—about a thumb's width above the top of the pubic bone on the midline of the abdomen. Regulates urination and the Bladder.

C.V. 4, *Guanyuan, Kangen* 關元—about 4 finger-widths below the navel on the midline of the abdomen. Use moxibustion to tone the Primary (Yuan) Qi, reinforce yang, and tone the qi in general.

C.V. 9, *Shuifen, Suibun* 水分—about 1 thumb's width above the navel on the midline of the abdomen. Promotes the Spleen function, clears fluid stagnation, acts as a diuretic, warms the Middle Burner.

C.V. 12, *Zhongwan, Chūkan* 中脘—on the center line directly in the center of an imaginary line drawn from the navel to where the ribs join below the sternum. Warms and strengthens the digestive system, corrects the Central Qi, warms the center, tonifies the whole body.

C.V. 17, *Shanzhong, Danchū* 膻中—in the center of the sternum between the nipples, level with the fourth intercostal space. Clears the Lung, transforms Phlegm, clears mucus, frees up the diaphragm.

C.V. 22, *Tiantu, Tentotsu* 天突—on the center line in the hollow above the sternum below the Adam's apple. Clears Phlegm, and blockages in the throat, eases asthma, and calms cough.

Governor 督脈

GV. 1, *Changqiang, Chōkyō* 長強—for moxibustion use at the tip of the tailbone. Aids intestinal Qi, stops diarrhea, disperses swelling, relieves pain.

GV. 4, *Mingmen, Meimon* 命門—on the spine in the space below the second lumbar vertebra. Used to clear headache, tinnitus, spinal column and lumbar pain, vaginal discharge, intestinal pain, rectal prolapse, and various forms of internal bleeding.

GV. 14, *Dazhui, Taishō* 大椎—in the depression in the spinal column below the 7th cervical (the large one) vertebra. Frees the Yang Qi of the whole body, clears the Heart, calms the Shen, regulates Qi. For common cold, cough, stiffness in the neck and spine.

GV. 20, *Baihui, Hyakue* 百會—at the crown of the head at the crossing of two imaginary lines: the first drawn from the crown apex down to the tops of the ears, and the second along the center line of the skull. Clears Wind/Heat in head, nasal obstruction, raises fallen Yang Qi, "pulls up the center" for prolapse and hemorrhoids.

Triple Heater 三焦經

T.H. 4, *Yangchi, Yōchi* 陽池—in a depression on the back of the wrist, from the base of the joint of the fingers, move straight back to the center of the wrist. For wrist, arm, shoulder, and throat pain, tinnitus, eye and neck swelling.

T.H. 5, *Waiguan, Gaikan* 外關—about 3 fingerwidths above the outer wrist crease, in a space between the ulnar and the radius bones of the forearm.

T.H. 17, *Yifeng, Efū* 翳風—behind lobule of ear, in a depression between the mandible and the mastoid process. When pressed causes pain in the ear. For tinnitus, deafness, clenched jaw, cheek swellings.

T. H. 21, *Ermen, Jimon* 耳門—in a depression by the protuberance of the flesh in front of the ear at the notch at the top of the tragus. For tinnitus, discharges from ear, toothache.

Extra Point, *Yintang, Indō* 印堂—above the bridge of the nose between the eyebrows. For frontal headache, rhinorrhea, and blurred vision.

Extra Point, *Uranaitei* 裏內庭—press the second toe down to the sole of the foot. Located at the point where it touches. For indigestion, stomach problems, rash. Use moxibustion.

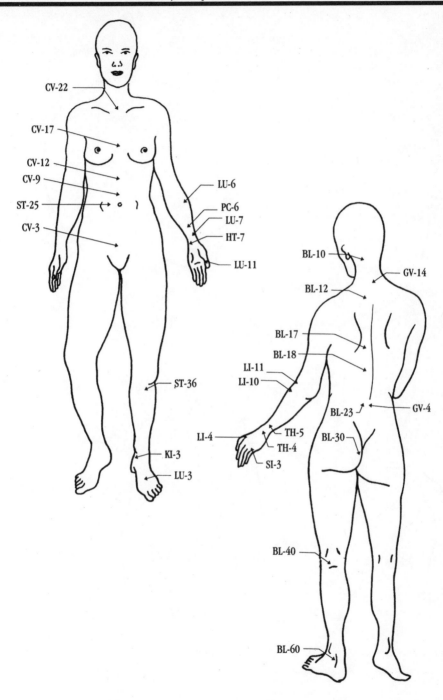

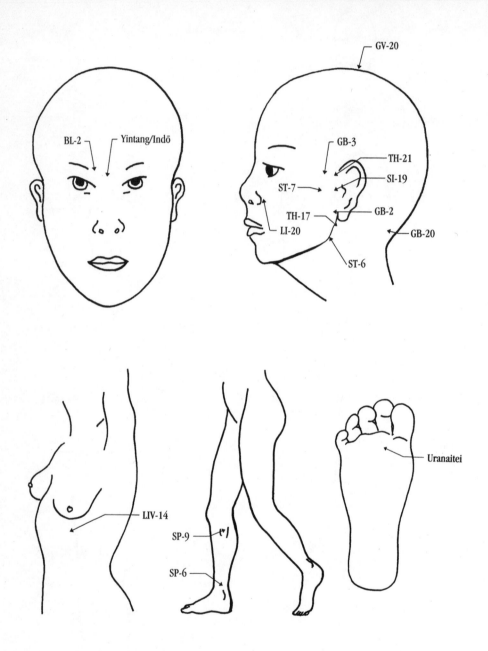

Appendices

I. Emergency Self-Help Kit

Of all the recommendations we have made, keeping an emergency self-help kit is probably going to be the one that will have the greatest effect on your life. Preparing a box of equipment and some medicines to have on hand for emergencies will make using natural remedies so much easier you will wonder why you haven't done it sooner. You may want to keep a list of remedies for common illnesses in the box. You could also order and keep some herbs there for conditions you and your family suffer from frequently. We recommend labeling herbs with their medicinal properties, making it easier to find and employ a remedy even in the middle of the night. You may want to label commercially prepared Chinese medicine the same way.

Equipment for the Self-Help Kit

- ace bandages
- adhesive tape
- bamboo strainer
- ceramic teapot
- cotton balls
- earthenware, fireproof pot
- essential oils: eucalyptus, lavender
- fabric bag or pouch to hold herbs in bath
- foot-soaking bucket
- gauze
- grater for roots and vegetables
- hair-dryer
- heating pad
- herb cooker
- hot-water bottle
- large plastic tub for sitz baths
- massage lotion with camphor
- muslin, cotton cloth, cheesecloth, old cut-up towels
- moxibustion sticks
- plastic wrap
- scissors
- Tiger Balm
- White Flower Oil or Kwan Loong Oil

Commercially Prepared Herbal Chinese Medicines*

• Cold, sore throat, fever, congestion (take at first sign of cold)	Yin Chiao Chieh Tu Pien 6 tabs every 3 hours
• Cold, sore muscles, chills, headache	Zhong Gan Ling 6 tabs every 3 hours
• Dry cough	Lo Han Cough Juice
• Cough with yellow phlegm that is difficult to expectorate, or with clear, abundant mucus	Pinella Expectorant
• Respiratory allergy and hay fever	Bi Yan Pian symptoms 6 tablets 4 times a day Prolonged use: 10 tabs twice daily
• PMS symptoms: bloating, cramps,	Wu Chi Pai Feng mood swings, irregular cycle, 10 pills twice a day fatigue Acute: 10 pills 4 times a day

* These medicines can be purchased from several companies listed in the Shopping section.

- Insomnia
- Migraine headache
- Hangover, nausea,
  indigestion, diarrhea

Healthy Brain Pills
Corydalis Yan Hu Suo Analgesic
Pill Curing
2 vials every 4 hours

Basic Food Ingredients to Keep around the House

barley
black and white fungus (dried)
cayenne pepper
Chinese cinnamon
Chinese licorice
Chinese red dates
garlic
ginger
honey
hot Japanese yellow mustard
Job's tears

kombu seaweed
lemons
lotus seeds
lycium berries
miso paste

onions, scallions, leeks
rice, brown and sweet
rice vinegar
salt
sesame oil
sesame seeds, black and white
shiitake mushrooms (dried)
soy sauce
sunflower seeds
teas: oolong, chrysanthemum, black, green, dandelion, jasmine,
    roasted Job's tears tea (hatomugi-cha)
umeboshi pickled plums
walnuts
wasabi
whole wheat flour

II. Preparing Organ Meats

You will find that organ meats are often indicated to balance many conditions listed in the Self-healing sections of the book. We are aware of the fact that many readers of this book probably eat very little meat, and for personal and health reasons believe it is better not to. Ultimately, you will eat how you like, but for those people who want to try incorporating more organ meats into their diets, we recommend purchasing meat of animals that have been free-range and organically fed and using the following methods for detoxifying the liver, kidney, lung (the filtering and elimination organs of the animal), and heart before eating them.

Salting Method

Purchase liver, kidney, lung, or heart as fresh as possible from your local butcher. Clean the meat, slice the liver, lung or heart; cut the kidney in half and remove the white tendons. Sprinkle sea salt liberally over the meat, cover, and leave overnight in the refrigerator, allowing it to sweat out any toxins. Thoroughly rinse before cooking.

Steaming Method

Slash the surface of the liver, lung, and heart meat a few times or cut it into bite-size pieces; clean out the center of the kidney as described above. Place the meat into a steamer, and steam for 30 to 45 minutes. Rinse well before adding to slow-cooking soups, stews, and simmered dishes.

III. Conditions Treatable by Acupuncture

As we mention in the Introduction, Oriental medicine can be used to cure or aid the healing of almost every imbalance and illness. According to Dr. Felix Mann, an early researcher in the efficacy of Oriental medicine, diseases and conditions that may be treated with acupuncture include:

Head: neuralgia, headaches, migraine, fainting, tics, spasms, cerebral arteriosclerosis causing senility (early stages)

Limbs and musculature: fibrositis, muscular rheumatism, sciatica, lumbago, swelling, discoloration, cramps, cold hands and feet, edema, writer's cramp, weakness, some types of trembling, neuralgia of the shoulders and arms, tennis elbow, rheumatoid or osteoarthritis, weakness or feeling of excess heaviness in the limbs, frozen shoulder

Digestion: duodenal and stomach ulcer, hyperacidity, gastritis, dyspepsia, inability to eat ordinary foods, no appetite, undigested stools, pale stools, eructations, gas, abdominal distension, bad breath, dry mouth, bad taste in the mouth, heartburn, pyloric spasms, nausea, vomiting, atony, perianal pain or itch, hematemesis (the vomiting of blood), underfunction of the liver, tender liver, hepatitis, chronic cholecystitis, ulcerative colitis, pancreatitis, morning sickness, cold abdomen

Respiratory system: asthma, bronchitis, tracheitis, shortness of breath, pulmonary congestion, pulmonary edema, recurrent colds, coughs, and mild pulmonary infections

Cardiovascular system: angina pectoris, pseudo angina pectoris, pain or heaviness over the cardiac area, palpitations, tachycardia, bradycardia, arrhythmia, cardiac insufficiency, valvular defects, high or low blood pressure, arterial spasms, phlebitis, hemorrhoids, lymphangitis, adenitis, pallor, pins and needles, poor circulation, fainting, chronic feeling of cold in the four limbs or all over the body

Urinary system: renal insufficiency, pyelitis, cystitis, some types of renal colic, lumbago, bladder irritation and spasm, bed-wetting, lack of control of bladder, early prostatic hypertrophy.

Reproductive system: pelvic pain, painful periods, irregular periods, excessive flow, vaginal discharge, vaginal pain, itching, menopausal trouble, hot flashes, ovarian pain, impotence, frigidity, sterility, lack of sexual desire, nymphomania, mastitis, menopausal hair loss*

Sight: weak eyesight, tired, strained eyes, black spots, zig-zags in front of eyes, pain behind or around eye, conjunctivitis, blepharitis, iritis*, glaucoma*

Ear, nose, and throat: hay fever, rhinitis, nosebleeds, sneezing, loss of smell*, sinusitis, catarrh, gingivitis, tonsillitis, laryngitis, loss of voice, tinnitus, pharyngitis

Skin: acne, itching, eczema, urticaria, abscesses, herpes, neurodermatitis

Nervous system, psychiatric factors: nervousness, depression, anxiety, fears, obsessions, timidity, stage fright, neurasthenia, wish to die, agitation, outbursts of temper, excessive loquacity, insomnia, nocturnal terror, facial palsy, neuralgia after shingles*, trembling

General: anemia, fatigue, lassitude, excessive perspiration, excessive sleep, excess yawning, sensitivity to changes in temperature, motion sickness, postoperative weakness, weakness after severe illness.

To this list we would add the broad category of immuno-deficiency, which plays a major role in increasing the body's susceptibility to mold-like bacteria (for example, yeast infection, or *Candida albicans*), fungi, parasites, viruses (such as Epstein-Barr and *Herpes simplex*), allergies, and cancer.

---

* Acupuncture is effective treatment in some instances where this symptom manifests, but not all. Discuss the problem with a practitioner for a better idea of its efficacy in your case.

IV. Warnings

Ma huang. In November, 1994, the Food and Drug Administration issued a consumer warning against a product containing *ma huang* (*Ephedra sinica* Stapf.) and kola nut, Nature's Nutrition Formula One, sold by Alliance U.S.A. of Richardson, Texas. After receiving more than 100 reports of injuries and adverse reactions in connection with this product, the FDA ordered the company to remove the kola nut, a source of caffeine, from the product. After "inadequate response" from Alliance, the FDA recalled the product. After the company again failed to comply to the FDA's demands, the agency issued a warning against Nature's Nutrition Formula One. Alliance has since reformulated its product. While the problem with the product seems to be the mixing of two stimulating herbs in unsafe proportions, the FDA, meanwhile, is evaluating the safety of ephedrine-containing products. (Source: *FDA Consumer Information* report, February 28, 1995.) *Ma huang* is an old and valuable herb in Oriental medicine, but it *is* stimulating and drying. Consult with a practitioner before taking it.

Comfrey. Since 1985, reports the Food and Drug Administration, at least seven cases of liver disease, one resulting in death, have been associated with the oral use of comfrey. Comfrey contains pyrrolizidine alkaloids, which, if taken for a prolonged period of time, expose the liver to the possibility of developing cirrhosis of the liver. Comfrey is "a safety concern," says the agency.

On the other side, herbalists point out that the woman who died of liver damage related to comfrey had been taking 6 comfrey/pepsin digestive capsules with a quart of comfrey tea every day for 6 months, without the supervision of a professional herbalist. This information was not included in the FDA bulletin that we received regarding comfrey.

To the best of our knowledge, there has never been a report of liver damage or cancer related to the use of comfrey when it has been taken in small doses over a short period of time. An appropriate, standard dose is 1 tsp. dried leaf or 2 tsp. bruised fresh leaves (not the root) in 8 ounces of hot water. Steep for 15 minutes and strain. Drink 1 cup per day for not more than 10 days to help break up bronchial congestion, discharge mucus in the lungs, and soothe ulcers. Talk to a professional herbalist before you take it, and don't take it if you have a liver condition.

Chinese licorice. This herb is the most commonly used of all Chinese herbs. It is considered tonic to Qi, is used as an expectorant and demulcent, to strengthen digestion, treat gastric-duodenal ulcers and abdominal pain, and to improve dryness of the Lungs, coughs, and colds. It is also used as a detoxifier and is known as a "guiding herb," or one that harmonizes well with other herbs in a formula and guides the herbs to the correct location in the body.

Anyone with a heart condition, particularly edema with a heart condition, should not take licorice. Do not take it regularly for a prolonged period of time, since it can be quite drying.

Shou Wu Chih. The Health Protection Branch of Health Canada has advised the public not to consume this commercially prepared herbal tonic manufactured by The United Pharmaceutical Manufactory of Kwangchow in the People's Republic of China. The product is a dark brown liquid, sold in light green, 500 ml bottles, in bright orange boxes. It is said to contain unspecified amounts of digitalis-like compounds that can cause heart palpitations and other serious adverse reactions. As of April, 1995, the HPB had received three reports of heart palpitations from consumers using the product. The Food and Drug Administration in the United States had received no complaints concerning the product as of June, 1995.

V. Recipes (listed alphabetically)

Azuki Bean Broth

When cooking azuki beans add about 1 liter extra water while cooking, cook the beans until soft, and reserve the extra water. Let cool slightly before drinking. The liquid can be refrigerated and warmed before ingesting, once, twice, or three times a day, depending on your condition. Strengthens the Kidneys, has diuretic properties, and regulates body fluids.

Brown Rice Cream

This is indicated for weak digestion, stomachache, loss of appetite, nausea, and for after vomiting.

1 c brown rice
7 c water

1. Toast the brown rice in a frying pan with no oil until it browns.
2. Cook in proportion of 1:7 with water on low heat.
3. Once it is very soft (you will have to taste test it), strain through a cheesecloth to remove the fiber and lumps.

Brown Rice Porridge

Warming and toning, porridge is recommended for almost any condition; additional ingredients specific to individual conditions are listed in the Self-care sections of Part II.

1. Cook rinsed or presoaked rice in water in a proportion of 1:8 or 9 in a heavy-lidded pot or in a rice cooker at the lowest heat possible.
2. Add herbs, meat, dried shrimp, or scallops from the beginning of cooking.
3. Presteam or salt organ meats before adding to the rice.
4. Before serving, add chopped trefoil, scallions, daikon radish sprouts, watercress, and/or slivered ginger. Season with a pinch of salt or soy sauce.

Change of Season Tea[1]

2–3 g astragalus	2–3 g dioscorea
2–3 g codonopsis	2–3 g lycium berries

Add the herbs to $1\frac{1}{2}$ cups water and simmer until reduced by a third. Drink whenever you are under heavy stress, are feeling run-down, or when the season is changing to boost the immune system.

Dang Gui Broth

Make a soup with this by adding fresh root vegetables, tofu or tempeh, meat if you like, and whatever spices you prefer. Cooking with the herbs is an effective way to derive their medicinal benefits, and the foods probably taste better than drinking the decoctions. Add a few slices of dang gui to chicken—a naturally delicious pair; cooked with garlic, onion, ginger, Hokkaido pumpkin, winter squash, rutabaga, turnips, or carrots, they make a fortifying soup or stew for body and Blood.

2–3 g dang gui	2–3 g Chinese red dates
2–3 g codonopsis	2–3 g peony root (optional)
2–3 g dioscorea	

Add 2 to 3 grams of each herb to a 2-quart or 2-liter pot (preferably a large earthenware one) of water. Bring to a boil and then turn down the heat to simmer for 10–15 minutes. Strain.

Dashi Broth

This is a classic recipe for arguably the most frequently used ingredient in Japanese cooking. Dashi is the base for nearly all simmered dishes, hot noodles, many dressings, and salad-like dishes. Its taste is light and adds that ineffable Japanese quality to whatever it has been added. The ingredients can be combined, although they are separate in the recipes below. The broth can be made ahead of time and stored in the refrigerator for up to a week.

> 1 cup water
> 3–4 inch-long strips of kombu, or
> 2 dried shiitake mushrooms, or
> 3 g (one small pack) bonito flakes, or
> 5–10 g fish shavings (for a heavier broth) per cup water per person

1. If using shiitake mushrooms, first soak them in a saucepan. After the mushrooms have softened somewhat, cook on medium heat and bring to a boil. Turn down the heat and cook for 5–7 more minutes. Strain out the mushrooms, cut off the stems, and use mushrooms in another dish.
2. If using kombu, add to the water in a saucepan, cook on medium heat, and bring to a boil. Turn off and strain.
3. If using pre-packaged bonito flakes, bring water to a boil, add the flakes, then turn off the heat and let the flakes steep for 5–10 minutes. Strain through a cheesecloth.
4. If using thicker fish flakes, add to water in a saucepan, bring to a boil, turn down heat to simmer, and cook for 8–10 minutes. Strain through a cheesecloth. This heavier broth is best for soba and udon. Use one cup water per person.

Di Huang Wine

Good for cleansing and increasing Blood and strengthening the Heart and Kidneys.

> 100 g di huang   30 g granulated sugar or honey
> 1 liter vodka or another 45° alcohol   optional: ¹/₂ cup port wine

Add the ingredients to a wide-mouth bottle and let age for a month until they turn a dark, rich brown color. Drink 20 ml, or one *sake* cupful once or twice a day with meals.

The Essential Egg

This oil is extremely bitter. Dilute with 5 drops to 15 drops of water and take daily for anemia, Kidney and Liver trouble, a weak constitution, low blood pressure, hemorrhoids, and vaginal problems.

1. Egg yolk essence can be made by using 10 to 20 egg yolks. First, make sure you have a bowl handy to put the egg oil into. Then another bowl, separate the eggs and set the whites aside.
2. Place the yolks in a pan over low heat. Mix well and scramble, stirring constantly with a wooden spoon. Allow the mixture to darken. As it gets darker turn up the flame, keep stirring, and the mixture will take on a sawdust consistency.
3. Continue cooking until the eggs give off an oil. Quickly press this with a spoon and drain off into the bowl you have set out in advance. Twenty eggs will yield about half a cup of liquid. It's very important to stir the mixture constantly and to have a container at hand so the liquid can be poured off as soon as it forms, or it

will evaporate. Requires about half an hour to make.

Four Things Vegetable Soup

(Serves 4)

10 g cooked di huang	2 quarts or liters clear chicken broth
10 g dang gui	3–4 dried shiitake mushrooms
10 g ligusticum	150 g taro or *sato imo* potato
10 g peony root	1 bunch bok choy
2 tsp. salt (or to taste)	3 tbsp. *sake*

1. Add the herbs to 5 cups of broth and simmer over low heat until the liquid is reduced by half.
2. Add two more cups broth and the dried mushroom. Peel the taro or *sato imo*, chop it into easy-to-eat pieces, and boil separately until it gives off large amounts of starchy, viscous liquid. Drain into a colander, then add to the soup.
3. Slice the bok choy, add to lightly salted boiling water for a minute until soft. Quickly drain and cool under cold running water. Squeeze the water out of the leaves.
4. Add salt and *sake* to the soup broth. Shortly before the end of cooking, remove the mushrooms, cut off stems, slice, and add them back to the soup. When ready to eat, add greens to each portion.

Garlic Liquor

Good for strengthening sexual energy, Stomach, and Intestines, this also warms the hands and feet, fights colds, and its antiseptic properties help fight infection.

800 g garlic	3–4 bay leaves
1 cup honey	1 liter 45° alcohol

Peel and roughly chop the garlic, add to honey, bay leaves, and alcohol in a wide-mouth jar. The liquor is effective after 3 months, but after a year the antibiotic properties of the garlic fully permeate the alcohol. Dose: 20 ml, one *sake* cupful, after meals. No more than that. Avoid drinking on an empty stomach. Drinking too much of this could reverse its effects, weakening the Blood and drying out the skin.

Kabocha Pumpkin and Azuki Bean Stew

The colors, textures, and taste of the Hokkaido pumpkin and the azuki are so complementary that traditionally they were called "first cousins" when simmered together in this dish.

(Serves 5–6)

360 g azuki beans	1 tbsp. soy sauce
1 small winter squash: Hokkaido pumpkin,	4 tbsp. honey
or buttercup, butternut, or acorn squash	$^1/_2$ tsp. salt
6 c dashi broth	

1. Cook the azuki beans first by soaking overnight and boiling until soft.
2. Peel and cut pumpkin. Place in large pot with the dashi, and cook on medium heat until soft.
3. Add azuki beans, soy sauce, honey, and salt. Turn down heat, and simmer until liquid is reduced by half.
4. Feel free to add a couple of slices (grams) of Warming and toning herbs such as dang gui, codonopsis, astragalus, peony root, Chinese red dates, and/or cinnamon. These lend the stew an exotic Chinese herbal tang you've probably never tasted before, and it's fabulous.

Liver-Toning and Restoring Tea

3 g lycium berries   3 g peony root
3 g dang gui   3 g dioscorea

Add together in 1¹/₂ c water, simmer until reduced by one-third in an earthenware pot or a Chinese herb cooker. Divide into two portions and drink warm twice daily. Makes a healthful, tonifying tea for women's reproductive organs. The tea can be refrigerated for a day and reheated as needed; the herbs can be saved and boiled again the next day. This combination of herbs can also be boiled in 2 liters of water to make broth. Bring to a boil, then simmer until the dioscorea is completely cooked through, strain the herbs out, and use as a base for soups and stews.

Mood Swing Wine

This remedy is also good for a heavy head when you've got a hangover, high blood pressure, tired eyes, or headache, and is a general restorative.

100 g dried chrysanthemum leaves
¹/₂ cup honey
1 liter 45° alcohol

Mix ingredients together in a wide-mouth bottle and let sit for 2 to 3 months. Drink 20 ml after meals once a day. This is quite bitter, so you may want to increase the amount of honey or add a tad more when you drink it.

Red Date Wine

Red dates are a traditional tonic nutrient and guiding herb. Energetically Sweet and Neutral, they are said to "clear the Nine Openings" of the body, and improve circulation; they are slightly sedative and relax the smooth muscles.

1 cup red dates, pitted or unpitted
750 ml 45° clear alcohol
¹/₂ cup honey

Add the ingredients to a wide-mouth jar and store for one month in a cool, dry place. Shake regularly. Drink 20 ml, or a *sake* cupful, once a day in the afternoon after a meal for insomnia, headache, anxiety, neurosis, restlessness, depression, and general nervousness. Contraindicated if headache is accompanied by constipation. Do not drink if you have any problem with gallstones.

Saffron Wine

Recommended in cases of anemia, weak or Cool/Cold body constitutions, menstrual irregularities, and other Blood Deficient imbalances.

1 tsp. saffron
1 liter of 45° alcohol
optional: ¹/₂ cup honey or granulated sugar

Let this sit for a week before drinking. Dose: 20 ml, or a *sake* cupful, nightly after meals.

Endnote

[*1] The above formula is frequently prescribed in the Far East and appears in many books on herbal medicine, but this particular recipe comes from Ron Teegarten's *Chinese Tonic Herbs* (New York: Japan Publications, Inc., 1984), p.105.

Glossary (Italicized words are in the order of Japanese, Chinese, and Latin.)

agar. Translucent strips or white powder that swell in cold water and dissolve in hot water, made of extracts of a type of red algae. Contain bulk that alleviates constipation, and stabilizing agents that gel foods. Also called Chinese gelatin, Japanese gelatin or *kanten*; agar-agar is a Malaysian word.

amazake. A sweet white beverage made from water and *koji*, the mold-innoculated rice used to make miso. Warming and Sweet, it assists Yang energy, regulates, tonifies, and benefits Qi, tones and activates the Blood, removes Blood Stagnation, expels Cold, and produces fluids. Available at natural foods stores.

anma. The oldest form of massage known in Japan, introduced to Japan from China. See *tui na*.

astragalus. *Ōgi, Huang Ch'i, Astragalus membranaceous.* A Warming, tonic root used to tone and energize the entire body; facilitates the movement of energy out of the body, strengthens the arms and legs, protects the immune function, tones the Lung and Blood, regulates fluid metabolism, and prevents edema. Is used in combination with ginseng to improve respiratory endurance and with dang gui to improve circulation.

azuki beans. Sweet/Sour, small red beans, similar in shape and taste to kidney beans, second in importance only to soybeans in Japan. Often used in desserts, pastries, soups; the seeds can be sprouted and eaten in salads and soups.

bancha. A generic term for Japanese unfermented green tea.

bok choy. Also *pak choi* in Chinese; *chingensai; Brassica rapa* var. *chinensis.* A crisp, leafy green with green or white stems, it comes in long bunches with "soup spoon"-shaped stem bottoms, or in flat bunches in deep, rich green, called Rosette bok choy. Can be stir-fried, added to soups at the end of cooking, and to meat and noodle dishes.

bonito flakes. *Katsuobushi*, in Japanese. Shavings from the dried, salty bonito fish that are sold prepackaged, or sections of the dried fish can be purchased and shaved as needed with a special shaver.

bupleuri. *Saikō, Chai Hu, Radix Bupleuri.* Used to release Stagnant Liver Qi with symptoms of dizziness, vertigo, chest and side pain, emotional instability, or menstrual problems. Also for disharmony between the Liver and Spleen: epigastric and side pain, constriction in the chest, abdominal bloating, nausea and indigestion. Also for hemorrhoids, and anal or uterine prolapse and diarrhea due to collapse of Spleen Qi. Combines with many herbs; use should be overseen by a practitioner.

butterbur. *Fuki, Petasites japonicus*, Japanese butterbur. A thick-stemmed, wide-leaved perennial that grows in the wild and is cultivated in Japan; is also cultivated in Great Britain. The flowers are used in tempura and added to soup, while the stems are simmered in soy sauce, mirin, and *sake*, or parboiled then used in other dishes.

codonopsis. *Tōsan, Tang Shen, Radix Codonopsis.* A Chinese tonic herb to reinvigorate and warm the body, is often used as a substitute for ginseng in formulas where the action of the ginseng would be too strong. Tones the digestive and respiratory systems, aiding digestion and the absorption of nutrients, stimulates Blood production, clears lungs of mucus and detoxifies the blood. Is used to clear the skin, and is given to nursing mothers.

dandelion coffee. *Tampopo kōhi.* This can be ordered from Japanese grocery stores and is well worth the effort. It is an excellent coffee substitute as well as a Liver tonic. As of yet the authors have not found it stocked on market shelves in the West.

dang gui. Also *dong quai* in Chinese, *Tōki* in Japanese, *Radix Angelicae sinensis.* Known as the Chinese women's herb, both men and women can take this Blood-tonifying herb. It improves Blood circulation, clears skin, hastens the healing of external wounds and is slightly sedative, soothing irritation and "nerves." Contributes to healthy Blood composed of the proper proportion of elements.

dashi. A broth made from boiling water with bonito flakes, kombu, and/or shiitake mushrooms. The broth is strained and used as a base for numerous Japanese boiled or simmered dishes and soups.

di huang. *Jiō* in Japanese, *Rehmannia glutinosa*. The cooked root has Sweet, slightly Warm properties. Is used to treat anemia, dizziness, pale complexion, uterine hemorrhage, insomnia. Nourishes Kidney Yin. Used dried or fresh, clears Deficient Yin Heat: inflammatory conditions such as tuberculosis and other consumptive diseases. Since it is oily, people with delicate digestive systems may want to stay clear of it.

dioscorea. *Sanyaku* in Japanese, *Shan Yao* in Chinese, *Radix Dioscorea oppositae*. Also translated as dried wild mountain yam, and Chinese yam root; is frequently sold in dried form as jinenjo in natural food stores. Is a secondary tonic, Cooling, and used to tone the Yin, strengthen the spirit, build up body weight, increase intellect and longevity. Tones the Stomach/Spleen and Lungs, supplements Kidney Qi. The raw vegetable is common in Japan, called yamaimo, Japanese mountain yam, Chinese yam. From the yam family, is a climbing trailing plant that produces strangely shaped tubers. Is edible raw (yamaimo); it has a slippery sticky consistency. When peeled and grated, can be added to hot noodle soups or mixed with raw egg and soy sauce and eaten over hot rice. Sliced lengthwise, cover with an Oriental-style salad dressing containing lemon and sesame oil, add shredded perilla leaf.

Dit Dat Jao. Also called kung fu lotion. An herbal lotion that is applied externally to promote circulation of Qi and Blood, the quick healing of bruises, pulled muscles, and sprains.

dokudami. Also *Gyōseisō* in Japanese, *Yù Xing Cao*, *Houttuynia cordata Thunb*. An acrid, Cool herb used to clear Heat and detoxify the system, has diuretic properties and is also used to reduce edema, swelling, and abscesses. Is used to treat Lung Abscess or Lung Heat cough with thick yellow-green phlegm. Also has antimicrobial and antiviral effects, inhibits *Streptococcus pneumoniae*, *Staphylococcus aureus*, and a number of other viruses. Has also been used effectively in many small, uncontrolled studies against bacterial pneumonia, pulmonary abscesses, chronic lung disease, and skin problems, including herpes simplex.

ginkgo nuts. *Ginkgo biloba*. A hard-shelled, pale nut of the ginkgo tree that contains a light green, soft inside, which can be boiled or roasted. They can be purchased fresh or canned.

goldenseal. *Hydrastic canadensis*; *Ranunculaceae*. A bitter, drying herb from the West, has antibacterial properties, cleanses and dries mucus membranes, prevents excessive flow of mucus, alleviates swelling and inflammation, helps regulate menses, inhibits excessive bleeding, cleanses the Blood, aids digestion, is also used in treatment of liver diseases, hemorrhoids, vaginal yeast infection, and dysentery. Is a common cold and flu palliative.

habu-cha. Also *ketsumeishi*, *Jue Ming Tzu*, *Foetid Cassia* seeds; *Cassia tora L.* The seeds are decocted with dang gui to relieve constipation due to Dry intestines. In other formulas it clears Liver Fire, benefits red eyes, helps relieve sore neck and shoulders, headache, and patterns of Ascending Liver Yang. Also clears excessive Wind Heat with symptoms of itchy, red, and painful eyes and sensitivity to light. Lowers blood pressure, has an antibiotic effect, and increases metabolism of fats.

hatomugi. Literally, "pigeon barley." Common name for Job's tears (*Coix lacryma-jobi*; *Coicis lachryma-jobi*) in Japan. Can be cooked and eaten with brown rice or other whole grains. Roasted, it is drunk as a tea with Cooling properties. Is commonly drunk in summer and is used to cleanse the Blood and clear the skin. Can also be used as a mild, external treatment for skin problems. It is not refined barley that has been polished into small, white, pearl-shaped grains.

hijiki. A type of long brown algae, is full of essential minerals and iron. Combined with vegetables, tofu, soybeans, soy sauce, and mirin, it is simmered and chilled to make a salad-like dish. Also added to soups.

Japanese gentian. (See semburi.)

Job's tears. *Yokuinin*, *Yi Yi Ren*. Also called pearl barley, *Coix lacryma-jobi*. Has Cool, Sweet energy, helps drain Damp and clears Heat, strengthens the Spleen and tones the Lungs. This is not the refined barley (*Hordeum vulgare*) that is grounded into round pellets, "pearled barley," and is purchasable at the regular supermarket. The two are unrelated.

ketsumeishi. (See habu-cha.)

komatsuna. *Brassica rapa* var. *komatsuna*, mustard spinach. A hardy green leaf of the *Brassica* family, is actually neither a spinach nor a mustard; the leaves are a full, rich green with a mild flavor. It can be cooked much like spinach: steamed, added to the end of stir-fries and soups, or parboiled and squeezed to wring out the excess water, then dressed with soy sauce, sesame oil and lemon.

konnyaku. Also mistakenly called arrowroot jelly, it is a gelatinous food made of starch from the devil's tongue root. It is usually sold in blocks, round balls, or noodles, can be added to simmered vegetable dishes and soups. Is almost always found in winter soups, called *nabemono*. Lubricates the intestines, and its sandy gelatinous quality alleviates constipation. Can be found in Japanese and Oriental grocery stores and some natural foods stores in the United States.

kuzu, kudzu root. *Puerariae lobata et thunbergiana*; *Leguminosae*. A root that is powdered to make a starch used in traditional Japanese and macrobiotic cooking. Prepared with bancha tea, ginger root, and umeboshi pickled plum, is used traditionally in Japan as a remedy for colds, flu, fever, and digestive problems.

ligusticum. *Kōhon*, *Gao Ben*, *Rhizoma et Radix Ligustici sinensis*. An Acrid (Pungent), Warming Chinese herb, contains essential oils and resin that slightly irritate the mucous membranes and increase the flow of blood; warms the interior organs and stimulates metabolism. Used to alleviate headache, stiff neck, toothache, and acute lower back pain (patterns of Wind/Cold).

litchi. *Raichi*, *reishikaku* in Japanese, *Li Zhi He*. This sweet, warming fruit alleviates pain and activates Qi. It is used for hernia-like pain, abdominal pain caused by Stagnant Liver Qi, and stomach and epigastral pain caused by Stomach/Spleen Stagnation. Also treats hiccough, thirst, stomachache, scrofula, toothache. Contraindicated: Yin Deficiency and Internal Heat.

longan. Dried litchi fruit, commonly sold in Chinese food shops and pharmacies, has Warm, Sweet energy, is a Blood and Qi tonic, has mild sedative properties, and is used to treat weakness, anemia, insomnia, amnesia, forgetfulness, dizziness, convulsions, and anxiety associated with imbalance in the Heart meridian. Contraindications: Phlegm or Damp conditions.

lotus root. *Renkon*, *Lian Ou*. The rhizome of the aquatic lotus plant is crunchy, crisp, slightly sweet, and Cooling. It is peeled, soaked, and cooked in stir-fries, mixed with meat, stuffed, deep-fried in tempura; was traditionally sugared and eaten as an accompaniment to tea.

lycium berries. *Kukōshi*, *Gou Qi Zi*, *Lycii chinensis Mill*. A well-known Liver and Blood tonic in China, the berries are believed to increase vitality, brighten the eyes, strengthen and invigorate the legs, aid the complexion, calm the Heart and the nervous system. Buy full, bright-red dried berries and add them to soups and simmered dishes; reconstitute in hot water or *sake* and add to salads. Can be decocted in tea with schizandra or rehmannia (di huang) as a tonic brew. Contraindications: Deficient Spleen with Damp, and Excess Heat patterns.

ma huang. *Maō* in Japanese, *Ephedrae sinensis*. A warm, drying herb, it clears the Lungs of mucus, has stimulant properties. Is used world-wide as an anti-asthma drug. It promotes alertness while calming the mind and relieving stress; for this reason it was used by Chinese monks to help them stay awake during all-night meditations. Should be used in very small doses to protect loss of Yin and should be balanced with Yin herbs. Excessive intake could result in respiratory hyperactivity and heavy expulsion of mucus. It is best to discuss ma huang with a practitioner before taking it. The FDA issued a Consumer Warning against a supplement formula, Nature's Nutrition Formula One, in February, 1995, which contained ma huang and gotu kola; the company has since pulled its product from the shelves and reformulated it.

mirin. A sweetened *sake* used in cooking.

matsutake mushroom. *Tricoloma matsutake*. Large brown mushrooms that signify the coming of autumn in Japan. They are considered a delicacy and are quite expensive. Are often added to sweet rice with sliced mountain vegetables, mirin, and a touch of *sake* and soy sauce to make a special warming meal in fall.

mochi. Blocks of pounded glutinous rice, sold hard and dried, they are cooked over coals or toasted in an oven and dipped in soy sauce; can be added to soups or stews much like dumplings. Is Sweet, Warming, tones Qi and Blood, and builds strength and flesh.

mugwort. *Yomogi, Ai Ye, Folium Artemisia*. A bitter, acrid herb, is the leaf used in Chinese moxibustion. Can also be drunk internally as an infusion. Is an important women's herb, is said to Warm the womb and pacify the fetus during vaginal bleeding that threatens pregnancy. Alleviates abdominal menstrual pain, is used to treat a Cold Uterus causing infertility. Use cautiously if there is Heat in the Blood and Deficient Yin.

myoga. *Zingiber mioga*. Japanese ginger appreciated for its young, incandescent leaves. Is harvested young before the cloves open; is a delicate pink color. It grows wild in damp areas in the mountains of Japan and is also cultivated. Myoga is eaten raw, whole or sliced, and added to salads, tofu, and as a condiment to fish. The whole clove can be simmered with soy sauce, mirin, and lemon, or slices can be added near the end of cooking to clear soups. Aids the digestion.

napa cabbage. Another member of the *Brassica* family, also called Chinese cabbage, is frequently added to Oriental soups and stir-fries.

nori. A flat, deep emerald or green-black seaweed, has Cold, Salty, and Sweet properties. Tones Qi, Blood, and Yin, clears Heat, transforms sputum, softens hardness, and is diuretic. Treats goiter, edema, dysuria, cough, and hypertension.

ōbako. *Shazenshi, Che Qian Zi*, plantago seeds, *Semen plantaginis*. Diuretic, clears Heat, used to clear edema, Heat-type urinary dysfunction, and Damp Heat diarrhea; clears the eyes, expels Phlegm, and stops cough with copious yellow-green mucus. Contraindications: use cautiously if the Yang Qi is exhausted. Do not take if pregnant.

ohitashi. The name of green vegetables that have been parboiled, squeezed of excess water, then dressed lightly with soy sauce and other seasonings.

okara. The remains of tofu, is full of fiber, white in color, bland in taste and has the consistency of mashed potatoes. Can be purchased at grocery stores in Japan or from health food stores in the United States. Is cooked with a small amount of soy sauce, mirin, and fresh vegetables and chilled, if desired, to make a salad-type dish.

perilla. *Shiso, ao shiso, aka shiso* in Japanese, *Zi Su Ye, Folium Perillae frutescentis*, also beefsteak leaves. Disperses Cold, used to dispel fever, chills, headache, nasal congestion, and cough. Circulates the Qi and harmonizes the digestive system. Used for Spleen disharmony: digestive disturbance, nausea, vomiting, poor appetite, fullness in the chest or abdomen. Alleviates morning sickness and seafood poisoning. An herb with a distinctive flavor, it is eaten with sushi to counteract stomach parasites in raw fish. It was one of the first plants to have its oil extracted and it has a long history of medical usage. It can be added at the end of cooking to soup, but is best eaten raw as an accompaniment to fish and tofu.

peony root. *Shaku yaku, Bai Shao, Radix Paeonia albiflora*. A Bitter/Sour, Cold root, peony in Oriental medicine is nearly as popular as a women's herb as dang gui. It tones Blood, regulates the menses and other menstrual irregularities, and treats menstrual cramps and nervous conditions.

plum extract. *Bainiku Ekisu.* The extract is made of fresh green plums that are crushed and pressed for their juice, which is then simmered down to a thick syrup. Macrobiotic teacher Michio Kushi says it is helpful for stomach problems, headache, and food poisoning.

plum vinegar. The salty, sour brine from pickling *Prunus mume* to make *umeboshi.* It is used in place of vinegar in macrobiotic cooking and is said to have medicinal effects similar to other ume (plum) products. Stimulates digestion and intestinal functions.

poria. *Bukuryō, FúuLing, Sclerotium Poriae Cocos.* An herb used in Oriental medicine to remove Dampness, reduces water retention, strengthens the Spleen, calms the Heart and Shen.

red dates. *Taisō, Da Zao, Ziziphus jujube.* Nourish Qi and Blood, have a calming effect, increase weight, build strength, increase longevity and harmonize herbal formulas, used as a Yin counterpart to Yang tonic herbs (such as ginseng). The steamed black dates are tonifying to the Spleen.

safflower. *Kōka, Hong Hua, Flos Carthami tinctorii.* An Acrid (Pungent), Warm herb, when infused and taken internally helps regulate the menses. Helps bring out eruptive diseases (such as measles) and fevers. Commonly used externally in lineament for burns, bruises, and injuries. Contraindicated during pregnancy. Use cautiously if there is Deficient Qi and Blood or excessive menstruation.

sanshō. Also *kashō,* Sichuan pepper, Japanese pepper, *Zanthoxylum pipertum,* Hercules' club. Is sometimes referred to as a type of prickly ash (*Zanthoxylum americanum; Rutaceae*). A species of the citrus *mikan* family, sanshō originally referred to the berry of the indigenous Japanese *Asakura zansho* in Japan. Today most of the sanshō used in Japan and around the world is grown in China, of the *Fuyuzanshō* (Winter sanshō) and *Inuzanshō* (Dog sanshō) varieties. Is used medicinally as a stomachic, diuretic, and for its antiseptic properties. Also stimulates the metabolism, treats stomach prolapse, stomach parasites, enlarged stomach, and Cold in the Stomach. It warms the body and increases circulation.

schizandra. *Gomishi, Wu Wei Zu, Fructus Schisandrae chinensis.* A Sour, Warm berry. Alleviates coughing and wheezing; strengthens Deficient Kidneys and treats diarrhea, nocturnal emission, spermatorrhea, leukorrhea, and frequent urination. Stops excessive sweating, calms the Shen, is used for insomnia and forgetfulness.

seitan. Wheat gluten. Cooling and sweet, has Descending energy, tones Qi and Blood, clears Heat, sedates Yang, harmonizes the digestive system, reduces fever, and quenches thirst. Can be used as a substitute for meat; is often used in vegetarian and macrobiotic cooking.

semburi. Also *tōyaku,* Japanese sweet gentian, *Swertia japonica.* An extremely bitter herb used to promote a healthy stomach, treats tuberculosis; infusions also used externally for massage purposes to stimulate capillary movement near the skin.

senna. *Banshayō, Fan Xie Ye, Cassia angustifolia Vahl.* Literally, "purgative leaf of the barbarians." Infusions are used to move the stool downward; is used for constipation from Heat accumulating in the intestines. The tea is also taken to prevent Summer Heat fatigue and lassitude. Contraindicated during pregnancy or menses, for weak constitutions, in lactating mothers, for patients with chronic constipation. Do not take regularly; overdoses can cause abdominal pain, nausea, and vomiting.

seri. *Shui qin, Oenanthe stolonifera.* Translated as Chinese celery. Originally from China, where it is still commonly found in soups and simmered dishes and accompanying many meat and fish dishes.

soba. Common buckwheat, is used in the soba noodle; the flour is also used to make soba *crêpes.* Low in calories, rich in bioflavonoids, soba also contains vitamin E. The noodles are excellent hot or cold, dipped in a soy-sauce-based dipping sauce. Be sure to eat 100% buckwheat flour soba, although be forewarned that it can take a long time to cook and gives off a lot of starch, depending on the type of noodle. Some 100% buckwheat noodles can take 5-7 minutes to cook, while others may require two or more boilings. Some experimentation is necessary, particularly for products purchased in bulk that may not come with cooking instructions.

sweet rice. Glutinous white rice, also called sticky rice. Is Sweet and Warming, has Descending energy. Used to make mochi. It is a very sticky, short-grain rice.

takuan. Daikon radish root pickled in a mixture of bran and salt for at least three months. Said to aid digestion and induce bowel movement.

taro. Also *sato imo*, *kyōimo*, *Colocasia esculenta*, also sold as *albi* in the West. There are about half a dozen types of taro tubers known in Asia. They are spherical or cylindrical in shape, covered with a thick, hairy brown skin, and the inside is starchy white. Peel and boil like potatoes, adding a bit of soy sauce to the water. Mix with soups and stews; often mixed with parboiled snow peas. Do not eat raw.

Tei Kuan Yin tea. *Tekkannon-cha*. Literally, "Iron Goddess of Mercy" tea. A partially fermented (around 40%) variation of oolong tea, but the flavor is richer than many other oolong teas popularly sold in the West. It has a slightly Warming energy. Can be drunk all-year-round, although one may want to drink more Chinese unfermented (green) teas during the hot summer months.

tōchū tea. *Du Zhong* in Chinese. An herbal tea made from Eucommia bark, it is Sweet, Acrid (Pungent), and slightly Warming, tones the Kidneys and the Liver, strengthens the sinews (tendons) and bones, used for weak or aching lower back and knees, fatigue, spermatorrhea, frequent urination. Aids the smooth flow of Qi and Blood, promotes circulation. Also used to prevent miscarriage when the "fetus is restless" and a woman has significant back pain. Contraindicated in Deficient Yin patterns with Heat signs: redness or red tinge in the face, hot body, red eyes, stiff neck and shoulders, easily irritated, flaring temper.

trefoil. *Mitsuba*, *Cryptotaenia japonica*; also called Japanese wild chervil, Japanese wild parsley. Literally, "three leaves," is indigenous to Japan but is similar to *Cryptotaenia canadensis* (honewort), once gathered by native American Indians. Has flat green leaves with serrated edges forming three leaflets at the end of a long, succulent stalk. Its distinctive, fresh taste complements Japanese egg custard (*chawan-mushi*) and *sukiyaki*. Add at the end of cooking.

tui na. Traditional Chinese massage, includes up to 13 different branches of styles. Techniques include those similar to relaxing Swedish massage, to deep-tissue massage, acupressure, and to resetting bones.

umeboshi. A salty, sour type of apricot (*Prunus mume*) pickled with red shiso leaf. The flesh can be removed from the pit and mashed. This is used in cooking, often eaten over white rice, or added as a filling to rice balls. It should not be confused with plum extract—ume ekisu (see above). It is mixed with bancha tea in a number of folk remedies; is said to aid the digestion and that eating one a day helps prevent colds.

wakame. A type of seaweed commonly used in Japan. Long dark green strips that are sold fresh, salted, or dried; used in soups and salads. Energetically Cold and Salty, seaweed clears Heat, lubricates, tones the Yin, softens hardness, transforms sputum, and is commonly used in the treatment of edema, abdominal swelling and obstruction, and goiter.

wasabi. *Shan ou cai*, *Wasabia japonica*, also Japanese horseradish. Grows wild in the mountains and is cultivated for mass consumption; the green roots are used fresh, grated very finely, and served as a condiment with sushi, sashimi, and soup. Is also dried and made into a paste or can be bought commercially prepared. Has a pungent, hot flavor.

White Flower Oil. A camphorous oil sold in Hong Kong and Chinatowns; has strong dispersing properties, is commonly used to relieve headache, nasal congestion, and muscle pain. Kwan Loong Oil, a pain-relieving aromatic oil produced in Singapore and containing menthol and other herbs, is similar.

yamaimo. (See **dioscorea**.)

yuzu. A citrus with a distinctive fragrance and taste, it is added to miso, to winter simmered dishes called *nabe*, and to baths in winter.

Shopping

Of course there are many, many outlets for Oriental foods, herbs, and medicine in the United States and Canada. The retail shops listed here are simply my favorites. Many of the foods and herbs included in this book may be purchased at your local natural foods shop, and what you cannot find there, you can find through the mail-order companies that follow.

Retail outlets

Angelica's, 147 First Ave., New York, NY 10003. Tel: (212) 529-4335. Has a knowledgeable staff and a large supply of herbs. There's also an herbal library open for public perusal and one of the most extensive herbal book selections in Manhattan.

Kam Man Food Products, Inc., 200 Canal St., New York, NY. Tel: (212) 571-0171. Has one of the widest arrays of Chinese foods, spices, herbs, and commercially available medicines on the East coast, plus cooking utensils, teapots, and a great (inexpensive!) selection of teas. To place an order by mail, call and ask for Ming.

Great China Herb Company, 857 Washington St., San Francisco, CA 94108. Tel: (415) 982-2195. Its colossal bags stuffed with herbs fill all available store space, plus canisters storing loose herbs that run the full length of one wall. A serious shopper could get lost in here for hours.

Katagiri & Co., Inc., 224 East 59th St., New York, NY 10022. Tel: (212) 755-3566; Fax: (212) 752-4197. Los Angeles: 865 East Sandhill Ave., Carson, CA 90746. Tel: (310) 323-1817; Fax: (310) 1730. Vancouver: 1239 Odlum Drive, Vancouver, B.C. V5L 3L8. Tel: (604) 253-4336; Fax: (604) 729-4868. Carries a wide range of Japanese foods and teas at Japanese prices; it feels like Tokyo in here. They also accept special orders by mail.

Ten Ren Tea and Ginseng Co., Inc., 75 Mott St., New York, NY, 10013. Tel: (212) 349-2286; Fax: (212) 349-2180. Has branches in Flushing, New York; Toronto, Canada; and Yokohama, Japan. An elegant shop with tin tea canisters filled with a wide range of top-quality, loose Chinese teas. They also carry canned teas, teacups, and tea-making utensils. They are more than happy to let customers taste teas before buying. Ten Ren Tea also does a thriving mail-order business; call toll-free (1-800-292-2049) for a product and price list.

Also, for our readers in the U.K. and Australia:

U.K.

Number One Herb Company
36, Bankhurst Rd.
London SE6 4XN
Tel/ Fax: (0181) 690-4840
For granules and tablets.
Sells bulk herbs, raw herbs, tinctures, and teas.

East-West Herbs, Ltd.
Langston Priory Mews
Kingham, Oxfordshire OA4 6UP
Tel: (01608) 658-862
Fax: (01608) 658-816

Australia

China Herb Co. (Australia), Pty Ltd.
82-84, George St., Red Fern, NSW 2016
Tel: (02) 698-5555   Fax: (02) 698-5755
Granules, tablets, Chinese patent medicines.

By Mail

BLT Supplies, Inc., 3501 Queens Boulevard, Long Island City, NY 11101. Tel: (718) 392-5671, (800) 322-2860. For several varieties of Dit Dat Jow, also White Flower Oil, and Tiger Balm.

Chinese Herb Suppliers, San Francisco, CA 94108. Tel: (415) 982-2195. For loose herbs for cooking herbal decoctions and broths. Sells all of the tonic herbs in bulk form listed in this book.

East West Products, P.O. Box 1210, New York, NY 10025-1210. Tel: (212) 864-1342. For organically grown teas, meridian system-toning teas, Chinese herbs, herb "soup" blends, Dit Dat Jow, tree flower oil, herbal ointments, herbal bath blends, adaptogenic formulas including shiitake and reishi mushrooms, Siberian ginseng, and single herb extracts.

Eden Foods, 701 Tecumseh Rd., Clinton, MI 49236. Tel: (517) 456-7424; Fax: (517) 456-7025. For macrobiotic and Japanese foods such as soba, udon, sea vegetables, kuzu, wasabi, miso paste, and umeboshi. Contact them for a free booklet of recipes and serving suggestions for Japanese foods.

Four Seasons Health Products, 1801 Lincoln Boulevard, Suite 261, Venice, CA 90291. Tel: (310) 392-2559. Herbal and ginseng cookers with 3- and 6-cup capacity, all the Chinese tonic herbs included in this book, many superfood supplements, and a wide array of herbal formulas.

Frontier Herbs, 3021 78th St., P.O. 299, Norway, IA 52318. Tel: (800) 786-1388, (319) 227-7996; Fax: (800)717-4372. Herbs from all over the world, sold in dried, bulk, capsule, and tincture form. Also environmentally sound health and skin care products.

Granum, Inc., 2901 N.E. Blakeley St., Seattle, WA 98105. Tel: (206) 525-0051; Fax: (206) 523-9750. For macrobiotic and Japanese foods. Sells a wide range of organically grown teas, condiments, sesame oil, brown rice vinegar, kuzu, dried tofu, dried shiitake, mirin, dried sea vegetables, miso, ume extract, and organic umeboshi.

Lotus Fulfillment Services, P.O. Box 1008, 1100 Lotus Dr., Silver Lake, WI 53170. Tel: 414-889-8501; Fax: (414) 889-8591. For bulk herbs, herbal extracts, incense, Chinese and Ayurvedic products and books.

Okada Yakkyoku, 2-14-2 Taishido, Setagaya-ku, Tokyo 154; Tel: 3418-7010, Fax: same. A mail-order source for crude herb dokudami, also Sei Ro Gan pills. Orders should be in Japanese (general catalogue available).

Isukura Yakkyoku, 2-9-5 Nihonbashi, Chiyoda-ku, Tokyo 103; Tel: 3273-7331, Fax: 3273-7334. A mail-order source for Gangenkaryū, a Chinese herbal medicine good for blood circulation. Catalog in Japanese only.

Moxibustion

Oriental Medical Supplies, 1950 Washington St., Braintree, MA 02184. Tel: 1-800-323-1839; Fax: (617) 335-5779. For loose, stick, and stick-on moxibustion, incense, hot and cold packs, and *haramaki* belly supports (keeps abdomen and Kidneys warm).

Recommended Reading

Preventative Health, Immune Strength, Allergies

Dufty, William. *Sugar Blues*. New York: Warner Books, 1975. This is a classic on the effects of the white poison on the system. It's still an eye-opener despite the years that have passed since it first appeared.

Gagnon, Daniel and Amadea Morningstar. *Breathe Free: Nutritional and Herbal Care for Your Respiratory System*. Wilmot, Ws.: Lotus Press, 1991. An essential book for people with respiratory problems. Combines Eastern and Western holistic approaches. Very clearly written.

Muramoto, Naboru. *Healing Ourselves*. Swan House Publishing Company/Avon, 1973. A classic. The first book that provided young Oriental medicine students with accessible recipes for frequently used herbal formulas and teas. Not strictly Traditional Chinese Medicine (TCM)—has a heavy macrobiotic influence.

The Natural Medicine Collective, with Gary McLain. *The Natural Way of Healing: Asthma and Allergies*. New York: Dell Publishing, 1995. This, and anything else published by the collective, supplies clear explanations and is rigorously holistic in approach. Combines Western herbal tradition with some Oriental medicine.

Weil, Andrew. *Natural Health, Natural Medicine: A Comprehensive Manual for Wellness and Self-Care*. Boston: Houghton Mifflin Company, 1990. This is a wonderful introduction to the concept of self-responsibility for health.

ORIENTAL MEDICINE

Theory & Philosophy

Beinfield, Harriet and Efrem Korngold. *Between Heaven and Earth*. New York: Ballantine Books, 1991. Already a classic, this book demystifies the theory and practice of Oriental medicine, which is described in clear, yet poetic language.

Chuen, Lam Kam. *The Way of Energy: A Gaia Original*. New York: Fireside/Simon & Schuster, 1991.

Connelly, Dianne M. *Traditional Acupuncture: Law of the Five Elements*. Columbus, Md.: The Traditional Acupuncture Institute, 1994.

Flaws, Bob. *Endometriosis, Infertility and Traditional Chinese Medicine*. Boulder, Col.: Blue Poppy Press, 1989. Any woman with menstrual or reproductive system difficulties should read this.

Kaptchuck, Ted J. *The Web That Has No Weaver*. New York: Congdon & Weed, 1983. Another classic; Kaptchuck describes Oriental medicine principles with clarity and profound understanding.

Manaka, Yoshio and Ian A. Urquhart. *The Layman's Guide to Acupuncture*. New York: Weatherhill, 1972. A clear, thorough introduction to acupuncture.

Wolfe, Honora Lee. *The Breast Connection: A Laywoman's Guide to the Treatment of Breast Disease By Chinese Medicine*. Boulder, Col.: Blue Poppy Press, 1989. Traces the development of the disharmony that leads to breast cancer from early signs.

Wolfe, Honora. *Menopause: A Second Spring*. Boulder, Col.: Blue Poppy Press, 1992. A fresh look at alleviating the uncomfortable symptoms of menopause from an Oriental medicine approach.

Nutrition

Flaws, Bob and Honora Wolfe. *Prince Wen Hui's Cook*. Brookline, Mass.: Paradigm Publications, 1983. Oriented toward practitioners,this book provides in-depth analysis of the use of food to treat energetic imbalances.

Flaws, Bob. *Arisal of the Clear*. Boulder, Col.: Blue Poppy Press, 1991. This is a clear, concise introduction to the art of eating to balance and harmonize energy. Flaws wrote it after *Prince Wen Hui's Cook* when the latter proved too confusing for lay readers.

Larkcom,Joy. *Oriental Vegetables: The Complete Guide for the Gardening Cook*. New York: Kodansha International, 1991. How to identify, grow, and prepare vegetables native to Far East Asia.

Lu, Henry C. *Chinese System of Food Cures: Prevention & Remedies*. New York: Sterling Publishing Co., 1991.

Ni, Maoshing, with Cathy McNease. *The Tao of Nutrition*. Santa Monica, Ca.: Seven Star Communications, 1987.

Herbal Medicine

Reid, Daniel P. *Chinese Herbal Medicine*. Boston: Shambhala Publications, 1987. Everything you ever needed to know about the subject, appropriate for beginners. Great photographs.

Teegarden, Ron. *Chinese Tonic Herbs*. New York: Japan Publications, 1984. Makes the concept of using Chinese medicinal tonics less foreign and difficult. Full of valuable information.

Tierra, Lesley. *The Herbs of Life: Health and Healing Using Western and Chinese Techniques*. Freedom, Ca.: The Crossing Press, 1992. Tierra's combined approach is a joy to read and is easy to follow.

Tierra, Michael. *Planetary Herbology: An Integration of Western Herbs into the Traditional Chinese and Ayurvedic Systems*. Santa Fe, N.M.: Lotus Press, 1988.

Green, James. *The Male Herbal: Health Care for Men and Boys*. Freedom, Ca.: The Crossing Press, 1991. A thorough, well-written herbal for men.

Massage, Acupressure, and Reflexology

Dougans, Inge, with Susan Ellis. *The Art of Reflexology*. Rockport, Mass.: Element, 1992.

Hin, Kuan. *Chinese Massage and Acupressure*. New York: Bergh Publishing, Inc., 1994.

Serizawa, Katsusuke. *Tsubō: Vital Points for Oriental Therapy*. Briarcliff Manor, N.Y.: Japan Publications (U.S.A.), 1976.

Young, Jacqueline. *Self-massage: The complete 15-minutes a day massage system for health and self-awareness*. New York: Thorsons/HarperCollins, 1992.

Young, Jacqueline. *Acupressure for Health*. New York: Thorsons/HarperCollins, 1994.

Qigong, Tai'chi, and Yoga

Iyengar, B.K.S. *Light on Yoga*. New York: Schocken Books, 1979. A bible for hatha yoga practitioners.

Kilham, Christopher S. *The Five Tibetans*. Rochester, Vt.: Healing Arts Press, 1994. Simple yoga-style exercises.

Liao, Waysun. *Tai-chi Classics*. Boston: Shambhala Publications, 1990. Includes theory and philosophy of tai'chi.

Ming-Dao, Deng. *Scholar Warrior: An Introduction to the Tao in Everyday Life*. San Francisco: HarperCollins, 1990. Much more than a martial arts book, provides an in-depth, practical description of a warrior-scholar's lifestyle.

Yang, Jwing-Ming. *Qigong for Arthritis*. Jamaica Plain, Mass.: YMAA Publications Center (38 Hyde Park Ave., Jamaica Plain, MA 02130), 1991.

Body/Mind

Gawain, Shakti. *Creative Visualization*. New York: Bantam, 1988.

Hammer, Leon. *Dragon Rises Red Bird Flies: Psychology and Chinese Medicine*. Barrytown, N.Y.: Station Hill, 1980.

Moyers, Bill. *Healing and the Mind*. New York: Doubleday, 1993.

Requena,Yves. *Character and Health: The Relationship of Acupuncture and Psychology*. Brookline, Mass.: Paradigm Press, 1989.

Weil, Andrew. *Spontaneous Healing*. New York: Alfred A. Knopf, 1995.

Pain

Chaitow, Leon. *The Book of Natural Pain Relief*. New York: HarperCollins Paperback, 1993.

Chaitow, Leon. *The Acupuncture Treatment of Pain*, Rochester, Vermont: Healing Arts Press, 1990.

The Natural Medicine Collective, with Theresa Digeronimo. *The Natural Way of Healing: Chronic Pain*. New York: Dell Publishing, 1995.

Sex

Chang, Jolan. *The Tao of Love and Sex*. New York: Arkana, 1991.

Reid, Daniel P. *The Tao of Health, Sex & Longevity: A Modern Practical Guide to the Ancient Way*. New York: Fireside/Simon and Schuster, 1989. Much more than a book about sexual practice and hygiene; a rich compilation of research and experience.

Bibliography

Articles

"Acupuncture," *Consumer Reports*, January 1994, pp. 54–59.

"Blood Sugar Blues," *Nutrition News* 14, no.2 (1991).

"Brain Boosters," *Nutrition News* 16, no.9 (1992).

"Dance Down the Primrose Path," *Nutrition News* 17, no.12 (1993).

Eisenberg, David M., Ronald C. Kessler, Cindy Foster, Frances E. Norlock, David R. Calkins, and Thomas L. Delbanco. "Unconventional Medicine in the United States: Prevalence, Costs, and Patterns of Use." *New England Journal of Medicine*, 328, No.4 (January 28, 1993): pp. 246–252.

"The Facts on Fats and Oils," *Nutrition News* 9, no.6 (1986).

Food and Drug Administration. "FDA Warns Consumers Against Nature's Nutrition Formula One," *FDA Consumer Information*, U.S. Department of Health and Human Services, Brooklyn, New York, February 28, 1995.

Food and Drug Administration. "Legislative Summary of the 'Dietary Supplement Health and Education Act of 1994,'" *FDA Consumer Information*, U.S. Department of Health and Human Services, Brooklyn, New York, March 3, 1995.

Farley, Dixie. "Dietary Supplements." Reprinted from *FDA Consumer*, November 1993.

"Ginseng," *Nutrition News* 3, no.12 (1980).

"Grant Hospital offers alternative care," *Health Care Strategic Management* 13, no. 3 (March, 1995): p. 6.

Graves, Jacqueline M. "Growing Pains for Alternative Cures." *Fortune*, March 20, 1995, p. 16.

Hamlin, Suzanne. "Green Tea: More Than Just a Soothing Brew." *New York Times*, June 15, 1994.

"Immune Fitness," *Nutrition News* 11, no.1 (1988).

Jahnke, Roger. "Ancient Futures." *IHFN News*, Spring/Summer 1994, pp. 4–5.

"Menopause," *Nutrition News*, Special Edition, 1992.

"Omega-3 Oils," *Nutrition News* 8, no.9 (1985).

"Opening Your Heart," *Nutrition News* 8, no.2 (1993).

"Sleep Well,"*Nutrition News* 10, no.1 (1987).

"What to do about Colds & Flu," *Nutrition News* 12, no.2 (1989).

"Wild Siberian Ginseng," *Nutrition News* 11, no.2 (1988).

Books

Achterberg, Jeanne, Barbara Dossey, and Leslie Kolkmeier. *Rituals of Healing: Using Imagery for Health and Wellness*. New York: Bantam Books, 1994.

Balch, James F., and Phyllis A. Balch. *Prescriptions for Nutritional Healing*. New York: Avery Publishing Group, 1990.

Beinfield, Harriet, and Efrem Korngold. *Between Heaven and Earth: A Guide to Chinese Medicine*. New York: Ballantine Books, 1991.

Bensky, Dan, and Andrew Gamble, with Ted Kaptchuck. *Chinese Herbal Medicine: Materia Medica*. Seattle: Eastland Press, 1986.

Blofeld, John, ed. & trans. *I-Ching: The Book of Changes*. New York: Arkana/Viking Penguin, 1991.

Chaitow, Leon. *The Acupuncture Treatment of Pain*. Rochester, Vt: Healing Arts Press, 1990.

Chopra, Deepak. *Ageless Body, Timeless Mind*. New York: Harmony Books, 1993.

Chopra, Deepak. *Quantum Healing: Exploring the Frontiers of Body, Mind, Medicine*. New York: Bantam, 1990.

Connelly, Dianne M. *Traditional Acupuncture: Law of the Five Elements*. Columbus, Md: The Traditional Acupuncture Institute, 1994.

Ellis, Andrew, Nigel Weisman, and Ken Boss. *Fundamentals of Chinese Acupuncture*. Brookline, Mass.: Paradigm Publications, 1988.

Flaws, Bob. *Endometriosis, Infertility and Traditional Chinese Medicine*. Boulder, Col.: Blue Poppy Press, 1989.

Flaws, Bob, and Honora Wolfe. *Prince Wen Hui's Cook*. Brookline, Mass.: Paradigm Publications, 1983.

Frawley, David, and Vasant Lad. *The Yoga of Herbs: An Ayurvedic Guide to Herbal Medicine*. Santa Fe, N.M.: Lotus Press, 1986.

Gagnon, Daniel, and Amadea Morningstar. *Breathe Free: Nutritional and Herbal Care for Your Respiratory System*. Wilmot, Wis.: Lotus Press, 1971.

Gawain, Shakti. *Creative Visualization*. New York: Bantam, 1988.

Gladstar, Rosemary. *Herbal Healing for Women*. New York: Fireside/Simon & Schuster, 1993.

Green, James. *The Male Herbal: Health Care for Men and Boys*. Freedom, Ca.: The Crossing Press, 1991.

Hammer, Leon. *Dragon Rises Red Bird Flies: Psychology and Chinese Medicine*. Barrytown, N.Y.: Station Hill, 1980.

Hin, Kuan. *Chinese Massage and Acupressure*. New York: Bergh Publishing, 1994.

Iyengar, B.K.S. *Light on Yoga*. New York: Schocken Books, 1979.

Juhan, Deane. *Job's Body: A Handbook for Bodywork*. Barrytown, N.Y.: Station Hill Press, 1987.

Kaptchuck, Ted J. *The Web That Has No Weaver*. New York: Congdon & Weed, New York, 1983.

Kushi, Michio. Ed. Marc Van Cauwenberghe. *Macrobiotic Home Remedies*. New York: Japan Publications, 1985.

Lark, Susan. *PMS Self-Help Book*. Berkeley: Celestial Arts, 1984.

Lark, Susan. *The Menopause Self-Help Book*. Berkeley, Celestial Arts, 1992.

Larkcom, Joy. *The Complete Guide for the Gardening Cook*. New York: Kodansha International, 1991.

Lu, Henry C. *Chinese System of Food Cures: Prevention & Remedies*. New York: Sterling Publishing Co., 1986.

Manaka, Yoshio, and Ian A. Urquhart. *The Layman's Guide to Acupuncture*. New York: Weatherhill, 1972.

Ming-Dao, Deng. *Scholar Warrior: An Introduction to the Tao in Everyday Life*. San Francisco: HarperSF/HarperCollins, 1990.

Ming-Dao, Deng. *365 Tao Daily Meditations*. San Francisco: HarperSF/HarperCollins, 1992.

Mitchell, Stephen, trans. *Tao Te Ching*. New York: HarperCollins, 1989.

Muramota, Naboru. *Healing Ourselves*. New York: Swan House Publishing, 1973.

Murray, Michael, and Joseph Pizzorno. *Encyclopedia of Natural Healing*. Rocklin, Ca.: Prima Publishing, 1991.

Ni, Maoshing, with Cathy McNease. *The Tao of Nutrition*. Santa Monica, Ca.: Seven Star Communications, 1987.

Ni, Maoshing, trans. *The Yellow Emperor's Classic of Medicine*. Boston: Shambhala, 1995.

Porter, Bill. *Road to Heaven: Encounters with Chinese Hermits*. San Francisco: Mercury House, 1993.

O'Connor, John, and Dan Bensky, trans. and ed. *Acupuncture: A Comprehensive Text: Shanghai College of*

Traditional Medicine. Chicago: Eastland Press, 1981.

Reid, Daniel P. *Chinese Herbal Medicine*. Boston: Shambhala Publications, 1987.

Reid, Daniel P. *The Tao of Health, Sex & Longevity: A Modern Practical Guide to the Ancient Way*. New York: Fireside/Simon & Schuster, 1989.

Serizawa, Katsusuke. *Tsubō: Vital Points for Oriental Therapy*. Briarcliff Manor, N.Y.: Japan Publications, 1976.

Teegarden, Ron. *Chinese Tonic Herbs*. New York: Japan Publications, 1984.

Tierra, Lesley. *The Herbs of Life: Health and Healing Using Western and Chinese Techniques*. Freedom, Ca.: The Crossing Press, 1992.

Tierra, Michael. *Planetary Herbology: An Integration of Western Herbs into the Traditional Chinese and Ayurvedic Systems*. Santa Fe, N.M.: Lotus Press, 1988.

Unschuld, Paul, ed. *Introductory Readings in Classical Chinese Medicine*. Netherlands: Kluwer Academic Publishers, 1989.

Weil, Andrew. *Natural Health, Natural Medicine: A Comprehensive Manual for Wellness and Self-Care*. Boston: Houghton Mifflin Company, 1990.

Wolfe, Honora. *The Breast Connection: A Laywoman's Guide to the Treatment of Breast Disease by Chinese Medicine*. Boulder, Col.: Blue Poppy Press, 1989.

Wolfe, Honora. *Menopause: A Second Spring*. Boulder, Col.: Blue Poppy Press, 1992.

Japanese-language Books

Gakken, ed. *Kanpoh Jitsuyō Daijiten* (A Dictionary of Herbal Medicine for Actual Practice). Tokyo: Gakken. 1990.

Hyōdō, Masayoshi. *Itami no Hanashi* (Plain Talk on Pain). Tokyo: Kenyūkan, 1992.

Kenmoto, Yoshio. *Minkanyaku Hyakka* (A Hundred Types of Folk Medicine). Tokyo: Kenyūkan, 1990.

Marumoto, Yoshio. *Oishiku Naosō* (Curing Ourselves Tastefully). Tokyo: Bungei Shunchū, 1989.

Morishita, Kenichi, and Yasushi Satō, *Yasōcha de Utsukushiku Kenko ni naru Hō* (How to become Beautifully Healthy with Herbal Tea) Tokyo: Pegasus, 1983.

Nōbunkyō, ed. *Minkan Ryōbō* (Folk Medicine). Tokyo: Nōbunkyō, 1981.

Ōumi, Jun. *Yakutō: Shinkin na Yasō de Kenko furo* (Medicinal Baths: Healthy Baths with Local Herbs) Tokyo: Nōbunkyō, 1994.

Shigeno, Tekkan, and Shizuo Ōta. *Kampō wo Taberu* (Eating Herbal Medicine). Tokyo: San-Ichi Shobo, 1985.

Tanimoto, Yōzō. *Chūkokucha no Miryoku* (The Charm of Chinese Tea). Tokyo: Shibata Shoten, 1990.

Tōjō, Yuriko. *Kenko de Dekiru Shizen Ryōbō* (Do-able Natural Medicine with Health). Tokyo: Anata to Kenkosha, 1978.

Wenwei, Miao. Ishikawa Tsuyako, trans. *Chūkoku Yasō Monogatari* (Tales of Chinese Herbs). Tokyo: Toban Shoken, 1992.

Yamada, Terutane, and Shinichi Yamanouchi. *Kampō to Minkan Ryōbō* (Herbal Medicine and Folk Medicine). Tokyo: Nagaoka Shoten, 1992.

Index